Vitamin D: Physiology, Molecular Biology and Clinical Applications

Vitamin D: Physiology, Molecular Biology and Clinical Applications

Editor: Fiona Richard

AMERICAN
MEDICAL PUBLISHERS
www.americanmedicalpublishers.com

AMERICAN
MEDICAL PUBLISHERS
www.americanmedicalpublishers.com

Cataloging-in-Publication Data

Vitamin D : physiology, molecular biology and clinical applications / edited by Fiona Richard.
p. cm.
Includes bibliographical references and index.
ISBN 978-1-63927-564-9
1. Vitamin D. 2. Vitamin D--Physiological effect. 3. Vitamin D--Molecular aspects.
4. Vitamin D--Health aspects. 5. Vitamin D--Therapeutic use. 6. Vitamin D--Metabolism.
I. Richard, Fiona.
QP772.V53 V584 2023
612.399--dc23

American Medical Publishers,
41 Flatbush Avenue,
1st Floor, New York,
NY 11217, USA

ISBN 978-1-63927-564-9 (Hardback)

Contents

Preface

The purpose of the book is to provide a glimpse into the dynamics and to present opinions and studies of some of the scientists engaged in the development of new ideas in the field from very different standpoints. This book will prove useful to students and researchers owing to its high content quality.

Vitamin D is a vitamin which increases the absorption of phosphorus and calcium from the intestine and stimulates their deposition into bones. The two most important types of vitamin D are vitamin D3 and vitamin D2. Vitamin D3 is obtained by exposure to sunlight and dietary sources such as fish or other supplements. Whereas, few foods except mushrooms consist of vitamin D2, and primarily it is found in fortified foods and supplements. They both are varied by their side chain structure. The side chain of vitamin D3 consists of a broken ring; whereas vitamin D2 consists of a double bond among carbons 22 and 23 along with methyl group on carbon 24 in its broken ring. Vitamin D is essential for bone health of human beings. It is also helpful in decreasing the risk of chronic diseases such as cardiovascular diseases, autoimmune diseases and cancer. This book aims to understand the physiology, molecular biology and clinical applications of vitamin D. It is a valuable compilation of topics, ranging from the basic to the most complex studies on this topic. This book is appropriate for students seeking detailed information in this area of study as well as for experts.

At the end, I would like to appreciate all the efforts made by the authors in completing their chapters professionally. I express my deepest gratitude to all of them for contributing to this book by sharing their valuable works. A special thanks to my family and friends for their constant support in this journey.

Editor

1

Passive Commuting and Higher Sedentary Time is Associated with Vitamin D Deficiency in Adult and Older Women: Results from Chilean National Health Survey 2016–2017

Patricio Solis-Urra [1,2,*], Carlos Cristi-Montero [2], Javier Romero-Parra [3], Juan Pablo Zavala-Crichton [4], Maria Jose Saez-Lara [5,6] and Julio Plaza-Diaz [6,7,8]

1. PROFITH "PROmoting FITness and Health through Physical Activity" Research Group, Department of Physical Education and Sport, Faculty of Sport Sciences, University of Granada, 18071 Granada, Spain
2. IRyS Research Group, School of Physical Education, Pontificia Universidad Católica de Valparaíso, Valparaiso 2374631, Chile; carlos.cristi.montero@gmail.com
3. Departamento de Ciencias Farmacéuticas, Facultad de Ciencias, Universidad Católica del Norte, Avda. Angamos 0610, Antofagasta 1270709, Chile; javier.romero@ucn.cl
4. Faculty of Education and Social Sciences, Universidad Andrés Bello, Viña del Mar 2531015, Chile; jzavala@unab.cl
5. Department of Biochemistry and Molecular Biology I, School of Sciences, University of Granada, 18071 Granada, Spain; mjsaez@ugr.es
6. Institute of Nutrition and Food Technology "José Mataix", Center of Biomedical Research, University of Granada, Avda. del Conocimiento s/n. Armilla, 18016 Granada, Spain; jrplaza@ugr.es
7. Department of Biochemistry and Molecular Biology II, School of Pharmacy, University of Granada, 18071 Granada, Spain
8. Instituto de Investigación Biosanitaria IBS.GRANADA, Complejo Hospitalario Universitario de Granada, 18014 Granada, Spain

* Correspondence: patricio.solis.u@gmail.com

Abstract: The aim was to investigate the associations between different physical activity (PA) patterns and sedentary time (ST) with vitamin D deficiency (<12 ng/mL) in a large sample of Chilean women. In this cross-sectional study, the final sample included 1245 adult and 686 older women. The PA levels, mode of commuting, ST, and leisure-time PA were self-reported. Vitamin D deficiency was defined as <12 ng/mL and insufficiency as <20 ng/mL. A higher ST was associated with vitamin D deficiency (odds ratio (OR): 2.4, 95%: 1.6–4.3) in adults, and passive commuting was associated with vitamin D deficiency in older (OR: 1.7, 95%: 1.1–2.7). Additionally, we found a joint association in the high ST/passive commuting group in adults (OR: 2.8, 95%: 1.6–4.9) and older (OR: 2.8, 95%: 1.5–5.2) with vitamin D deficiency, in respect to low ST/active commuting. The PA levels and leisure-time PA were not associated with vitamin D deficiency. In conclusion, mode of commuting and ST seems important variables related to vitamin D deficiency. Promoting a healthy lifestyle appears important also for vitamin D levels in adult and older women. Further studies are needed to establish causality of this association and the effect of vitamin D deficiency in different diseases in this population.

Keywords: Vitamin D; females; exercise; sedentary lifestyle; nutrition; elderly

1. Introduction

Vitamin D was first characterized as a vitamin in the 20th century and nowadays it is recognized as a prohormone [1]. Vitamin D has two major forms, vitamin D_2 (ergocalciferol) and vitamin D_3 (cholecalciferol). The first is derived from plant sources, is not largely human-made, and added to foods, and the latter is synthesized in human skin and is consumed in diets via animal-based foods intake, mainly fish oils [1]. The active form of vitamin D generates a number of extraskeletal biological responses including inhibition of breast, colon, and prostate cancer cell progression; effects on the cardiovascular system; and protection against a number of autoimmune diseases including multiple sclerosis and inflammatory bowel disease [2].

Vitamin D is important in biological process related with women's health, such as fertility, pregnancy outcomes, and lactation at young age [3]. Some observational studies have revealed that a decrease in the vitamin D levels in women is related with reduced fertility [4], antenatal and postpartum depression [3]; as well high parathyroid hormone, the increasing risk of suffering sarcopenia and impaired glucose metabolism in the general population [5,6]. Moreover, supplementation with vitamin D probably might reduce the rate of falls but not risk of falling in older people [4,7]. Normal levels of vitamin D are associated to a low frequency of pathogenesis and neoplasm progressions, as well as hypertension, diabetes, immune disorders such as multiple sclerosis, musculoskeletal conditions [8,9], or bone mass status, especially in women [10]. Although vitamin D deficiency is rare in developed countries, subclinical forms occur, and they have public health relevance since low vitamin D concentrations are highly prevalent among population living in high latitudes, mainly indoors, and among those who are older or dark skinned [11]. Sunlight is the primary source of vitamin D [12], a very rough general estimation indicates that about 80% of vitamin D supply comes from skin ultraviolet-B-induced production, whereas only 20% comes from dietary intake; however, this varies considerably depending on different factors such as seasonal/sun exposure habits, latitude, nutrition/supplement intake or ethnicity [13].

In 2013, a review identified 243 studies related with vitamin D status in Caribbean and Latin American countries. The final analysis only included 28 studies with two major characteristics: small samples sizes and low national representativeness. Countries with available data have shown that vitamin D insufficiency was classified in the range of mild, moderate, or severe public health problem, and the only country with a nationally representative sample in this study was Mexico [14]. In Chile, a study conducted in 2007 with 555 post-menopausal women showed a vitamin D deficiency in 47.5% of the population, defined as less than 17 ng/mL [15]. Recommendations of normal levels of vitamin D in plasma are above of 30 ng/mL, and different cut-points have been used to classify insufficiency or deficiency, according the population [16,17]. For instance, recent data from the Chilean population showed that 80% of older subjects with a low-energy hip fracture have presented insufficient vitamin D levels (less than 20 ng/mL) [18]. Moreover, in healthy older populations, vitamin D values were very similar, 83% of women and 55.3% of men presented parameters below 20 ng/mL [19].

Regular physical activity (PA) and low sedentary time (ST) have significant benefits for health at all ages [20]. The principal recommendation is some PA is better than doing none [21]. The adult population (aged from 18–64 years) and older population (aged 65 years and above) should do 150 minutes of moderate-intensity PA throughout the week or at least 75 minutes of vigorous-intensity PA throughout the week, or an equivalent combination of moderate- and vigorous-intensity activity (e.g., walking, cycling, or doing sports) [20]. Globally, around 23% of adults aged from 18 and above, were not active enough in 2010 (men 20% and women 27%) [4,7,22–25]. Physical activity increase may be about general PA level, leisure PA, mode of commuting, organized sports, among others and independently reducing ST [20].

Previously, low serum vitamin D levels have been associated with lower PA level, gait speed, and balance. Vitamin D level below 30 ng/mL was not associated to an increased risk of fractures; however, a subgroup of women with serum vitamin D levels below 20 ng/mL showed an increased risk tendency of fractures, which may be associated to an inferior PA and postural stability [26]. Another report demonstrates that serum vitamin D concentrations below 20 ng/mL are associated to a poor physical performance, that is to say to a decreased physical performance in older men and women [27]. On the other hand, evidence shows that cycling is associated to high UV exposure, and thus, to high serum vitamin D levels compared to most other outdoors activities that are practiced, including walk [28,29]. It has been established that not all activities are equivalent regarding to sunlight exposure. Thus, whereas some patterns of PA have been associated with vitamin D levels, there is a lack of studies considering ST of mode of commuting. Interestingly, it is necessary to establish a relationship of the aforementioned according to the different population, since it has been shown that older people would be at risk [30]. Furthermore, a better understanding of the effects, according to the population, could help to provide valuable lifestyle recommendation.

Finally, data from general Chilean population regarding vitamin D levels are scarce, and associations with PA patterns and ST might be important factors in the status of vitamin D and maintenance of health [22]. Therefore, the aim of the present study was to investigate associations between self-reported PA patterns, ST, and different serum vitamin D levels in a large sample of Chilean adults and older women, adjusting for a number of potential confounders.

2. Material and Methods

2.1. Study Population

The 2016–2017 Chilean National Health Survey was a representative household survey with a stratified multistage probability sample of 6233 non-institutionalized participants over 14 years old from the 15 regions in Chile, both urban and rural. This survey represents the first, largest, and representative measurement of serum vitamin D levels in Chilean people. Sample size was calculated with a relative sampling error of less than 30%, and absolute sampling error of 2.6% to national level. The participation rate was 90.2%. Detailed information about the survey has been described elsewhere [31]. Vitamin D measurement was taken from a subsample of fertile age women (15 to 49 years) and older people. In this cross-sectional study were included those who have complete vitamin D measurement, valid response in PA questions and correct anthropometric parameters. Final sample was divided in adults ($\geq$18 to <65 years) and older ($\geq$65 years) groups, both for Chilean women. The ethics committee of the Pontificia Universidad Católica de Chile and the Chilean Ministry of Health approved the study protocol and ethical consent forms.

2.2. Survey and Sample

Standardized protocols were used and all investigators (nurses and research technicians) underwent joint training sessions prior to implementation of the survey. The fieldwork for this survey was conducted between August 2016 and March 2017; while blood samples and laboratory tests were made between September 2016 and February 2017.

2.3. Serum Vitamin D Levels

A nurse took venous blood samples in morning hours. Serum was extracted from 1 mL of total blood. Standardized liquid chromatography-tandem mass spectrometry (LC–MS/MS) method was used for measurement of 25(OH)-Vitamin D_3 for Chilean National Health Survey 2016–2017, which allows laboratories and surveys to compare 25(OH)-Vitamin D_3 measurements [32]. Vitamin D levels were categorized according two different criteria: (i) specific criteria for Chilean population according to the Health Ministry of Chile [33] of deficiency as <12 ng/mL [34], and (ii) internationally frequent cut-points used criteria corresponding to insufficiency of <20 ng/mL) [16,17]. This method has better analytical specificity and sensitivity compared to immunoassay methods, and fixed analytical goals for imprecision ($\leq$10%) and bias ($\leq$5%) [35].

2.4. Physical Activity

The Global PA Questionnaire (GPAQ) (version 2) to measure PA was used. The physical active categories were defined according to standard criteria of the questionnaire. Those who had less of 600 metabolic equivalent of task (METS) per week were considered inactive and those who had 600 or more METS per week were considered active [36].

2.5. Leisure-Time Physical Activity

A question was made in the visit, the question was (i) *In the last month, Did you practice sport or did any PA out of work time, during 30 minutes or more each time*? The response options were: (i) Yes, three times a week or more; (ii) Yes, one or two times a week; (iii) Yes, less of four times per month; (iv) I do not practice sport. The responses then were categorized in "Yes" for those who exercise three times a week or more, and "no" for those who did not practice sport at least three times a week.

2.6. Commute Mode

A question was made in order to inquire the commute mode of every surveyed, (i) which is the mode of commuting that you use (at least one time per week?) The response options were: (i) drive a light car; (ii) drive a heavy car; (iii) light car passenger; (iv) heavy car passenger; (v) bicycle; (vi) walk; (vii) and other. The responses were categorized in "active commuting" for those had mode of commuting bicycle or walk, and "passive commuting" for the rest.

2.7. Sedentary Time

A question of the GPAQ to estimate ST was asked to every participant of the study. The question was (i) *How much time do you usually spend sitting or reclining on a typical day*? The participant had to respond in minutes and hours per day. This question was categorized according to low ST (<4 hours per day); middle ST (≥4 and <8 hours per day); and high ST (>8 hours per day) [37].

2.8. Covariates

Socio-demographic data were collected for all participants, including age (years), menopausal status (yes/no), achieved education level (primary/secondary/beyond secondary), region (I to XV) and dairy consumption (three times a day or less, once each day, each two days, once a week, once a month or definitely never). Further, participants were asked according their sunlight exposure during the last week, (i) How much sunlight have you been exposed to in the last week? The responses were: (i) much; (ii) little.

2.9. Statistical Analysis

Data were presented as mean, standard deviation (SD), and percentages (%). Independent t-test and chi-square test were used to compare differences between adults and older women for continuous and categorical variables, respectively. Firstly, separated multivariable logistic regression model were employed to obtain odds ratio (OR) and confidence interval (CI 95%) in respect to different cut-points, adjusted by age (years), menopausal status (yes/no), achieved education level (primary/secondary/beyond secondary), region (I to XV), dairy consumption (three times a day or less, once each day, each two days, once a week, once a month or definitely never), and sunlight exposure (much/little). Finally, joint associations of ST and commute mode according to different criteria were tested. Here, ST was categorized as low ST (<4 hours per day) and high ST (≥4 hours per day) and it was combined with active and passive commuting. Thus, low ST/active commuting was used as reference group, high ST/active commuting, low ST/passive commuting, high ST/active commuting were second, third, and fourth groups, respectively. The performed model was adjusted by the same covariates mentioned previously plus PA level (active/inactive). For the interpretation of odds ratio, the effect size cut points of 1.68, 3.47, and 6.71 were used, according to small, medium, and large effect size [38]. Analyses were performed using SPSS-IBM (Software, v.21.0 SPSS Inc., Chicago, IL, USA), and a value of $p < 0.05$ was considered statistically significant. The Figure 1 was performed using the ggplot2 package in R and Supplementary Materials Figure S1 with leaflet package.

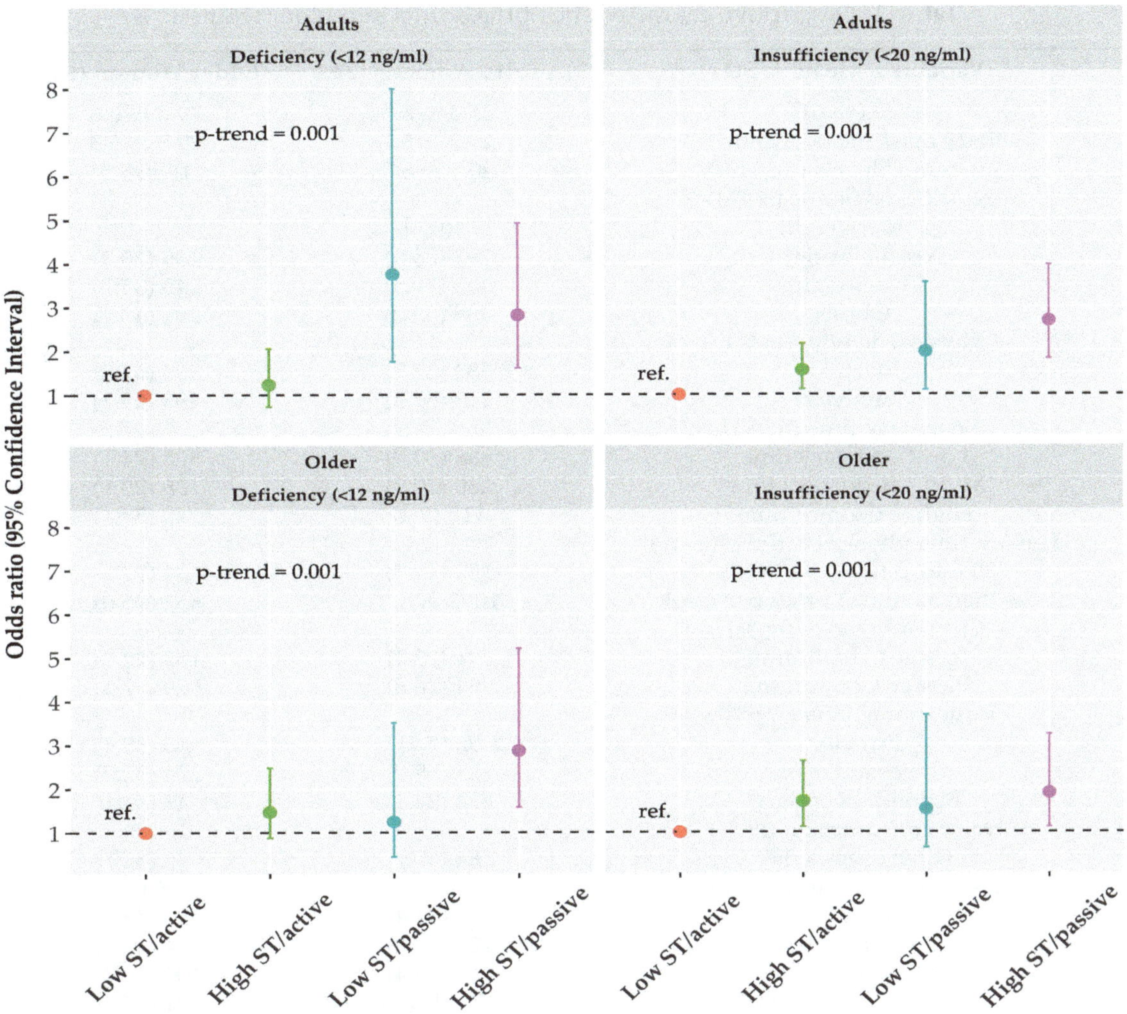

Figure 1. Odds ratio of the joint association between sedentary time (ST) and mode of commuting with different cut-points of vitamin D deficiency in adults and older women. The reference categories are groups with low ST (<4 hours/day) in combination with active commuting.

Figure 1 (bottom panels) shows joint OR for vitamin D deficiency for older women according the sedentary group and mode of commuting group. It can be appreciated from Figure 1 that for the cut-points of <12 ng/mL, compared to the reference group, the high ST/active group presents an OR of 1.476 (CI: 0.877–2.487, $p = 0.143$) the low ST/passive group presents an OR of 1.25 (CI: 0.444–3.514, $p = 0.673$) and high ST/passive group presents an OR of 2.875 (CI: 1.584–5.218, $p = 0.001$) for vitamin D deficiency. Furthermore, according to cut-points of <20 ng/mL, it can be appreciated in Figure 1 an OR of 1.712 9CI: 1.116–2.627, p: 0.014) for high ST/active, OR of 1.531 (CI: 0.638–3.676, $p = 0.34$) low ST/passive and OR of 1.905 (CI = 1.119–3.242, $p = 0.018$) high ST/active groups.

3. Results

The present study included only those who had a complete vitamin D measurement, valid responses in PA questions, and correct anthropometric measurements. The sample with serum vitamin D measurement was 2326. The final sample was divided into adults (≥18 years) and older (≥65 years) Chilean women groups. The final sample with complete data of physical activity patterns and covariates included was 1931 women. Table 1 shows descriptive characteristics of participants separated by group of age.

Table 1. Descriptive characteristic of the adults and older women.

Variables, Mean ± SD	Adults Women (1245)	Older Women (686)
Age (years)	35.4 ± 8.5	73.6 ± 6.6
Body mass index (kg/m^2)	29.2 ± 5.7	29.3 ± 5.3
Vitamin D levels (ng/mL)	20.2 ± 8.0	18 ± 8.5
Nutritional Status (*n*: %)		
Underweight	7 (0.6)	6 (0.9)
Normal weight	297 (23.9)	139 (20.3)
Overweight	455 (36.5)	245 (35.7)
Obese	486 (39.0)	296 (43.1)
Physical activity (*n*: %)		
Inactive	532 (42.7)	393 (57.3)
Active	713 (57.3)	293 (42.7)
Sedentary time (*n*: %)		
Low Sedentary time	868 (69.7)	508 (74.1)
Middle Sedentary time	260 (20.9)	138 (20.1)
High Sedentary time	117 (9.4)	40 (5.8)
Leisure-time physical activity (*n*: %)		
30 min, 3 times per week	153 (12.3)	34 (5.0)
Less than 30 min, 3 times per week	1092 (87.7)	652 (95.0)
Commute mode (*n*: %)		
Active Commuting	291 (23.4)	157 (22.9)
Passive Commuting	954 (76.6)	529 (77.1)
Educational Level (*n*: %)		
Primary	96 (7.7)	415 (60.4)
Secondary	725 (58.2)	224 (32.7)
Beyond secondary	424 (34.1)	47 (6.9)
Dairy consumption (*n*: %)		
Three times a day	84 (6.7)	46 (6.7)
Less than three times a day	79 (6.3)	55 (8)
Once a day	428 (34.4)	293 (42.7)
Every two days	223 (17.9)	124 (18.1)
At least once a week	242 (19.4)	104 (15.2)
At least once a month	73 (5.9)	22 (3.2)
Never	116 (9.3)	42 (6.1)
Menopausal status (*n*: %)		
Yes	48 (3.9)	693 (93.1)
No	1197 (96.1)	47 (6.9)
Vitamin D deficiency (<12 ng/mL) (*n*: %)		
<12 ng /mL	204 (16.4)	181 (26.4)
≥12 ng /mL	1041 (83.6)	505 (73.6)
Vitamin D insufficiency (<20 ng/mL) (*n*: %)		
<20 ng /mL	642 (51.6)	445 (64.9)
≥20 ng /mL	603 (48.4)	241 (35.1)
Sunlight exposure (*n*: %)		
Little	722 (58)	502 (73.2)
Much	523 (42)	184 (26.8)
Region (latitude *) (*n*: %)		
XV. Arica y Parinacota (−18.474)	94 (7.6)	30 (4.4)
I. Tarapacá (−20.213)	64 (5.1)	27 (3.9)
II. Antofagasta (−23.652)	57 (4.6)	23 (3.4)
III. Atacama (−27.366)	70 (5.6)	20 (2.9)
IV. Coquimbo (−29.953)	61 (4.9)	45 (6.6)
V. Valparaíso (−33.035)	125 (10)	85 (12.4)
XIII. Metropolitana (−33.456)	186 (14.9)	104 (15.2)
VI. L. Bdo. O'Higgins (−34.170)	74 (5.9)	33 (4.8)
VII. Maule (−35.426)	88 (7.1)	60 (8.7)
VIII. Bíobío (−36.826)	138 (11.1)	59 (8.6)
IX. La Araucanía (−38.739)	66 (5.3)	27 (3.9)
XIV. Los Ríos (−39.814)	56 (4.5)	48 (7)
X. Los Lagos (−41.469)	55 (4.4)	40 (5.8)
XI. Aysén (−45.575)	64 (5.1)	38 (5.5)
XII. Magallanes y Antártica (−53.154)	47 (3.8)	47 (6.9)

SD, standard deviation. * Coordinates have been calculated based on the world geodetic system (standard WGS84).

The anthropometric and nutritional values show similar results in both groups. The distribution of underweight, normal weight, overweight, and obese was the same for adult and older women. Vitamin D levels expressed as ng/mL were 20.2 for adult women and 18.0 for older women. Adult women exhibited higher vitamin D levels compared with older women, as well as higher PA patterns, leisure-time PA, educational level, and sunlight exposure. In contrast, ST, dairy consumption and menopausal status were lower in adult women compared to older population. Finally, the commute mode was similar in both groups. Table 2 shows the results of logistic regression analysis for each PA pattern according different cut-points and separated by adults and older women.

3.1. Adults

Table 2 (left side) shows the OR of vitamin D deficiency for adults. It can be seen that middle and high ST groups are associated with vitamin D deficiency (OR between 1.7 to 2.6, all $p < 0.001$) in both cut-points. Furthermore, Table 2 shows that passive commuting are also associated with vitamin D deficiency only for cut-points less than 20 ng/mL. PA level pattern and leisure-time PA pattern were not associated with vitamin D deficiency (all $p > 0.05$).

Figure 1 was constructed using two variables, ST and commute mode. These variables were categorized as low and high, and passive or active, respectively. The OR of the joint association between ST and mode of commuting was determined with different cut-points of vitamin D deficiency in adult women (Figure 1, upper panels) and older women (Figure 1, bottom panels). Reference categories were groups with low ST (<4 hours/day) in combination with active commuting. It can be appreciated from Figure 1 that for the cut-points of <12 ng/mL, compare to reference group, the high ST/active group presents OR of 1.231 (CI: 0.735–2.060, $p = 0.43$), the low ST/passive group presents OR of 3.754 (CI: 1.761–8.000, $p = 0.001$) and high ST/passive group presents OR of 2.821 (CI: 1.614–4.931, $p = <0.001$) for vitamin D deficiency. Furthermore, according to cut-points of <20 ng/mL, it can be appreciated an OR of 1.555 (CI: 1.120–2.158, $p = 0.008$), OR of 1.980 (CI: 1.102–3.558, $p = 0.022$) and OR of 2.689 (CI: 1.822–3.967, $p = <0.001$), for high ST/active, low ST/passive and high ST/active groups, respectively.

3.2. Older

Table 2 (right side) shows the OR of vitamin D deficiency for older women. Middle ST group shows a high vitamin D deficiency and high ST group showed a tendency association ($p = 0.004$ and 0,074, respectively) only in <12 ng/mL cut-points. Passive commuting is associated with vitamin D deficiency in both cut-points. PA level group and leisure-time PA group were not associated with vitamin D deficiency (all $p > 0.005$).

Table 2. Odds ratio for vitamin D deficiency according to different criteria for each physical activity pattern.

	Adults (1245)						**Older (686)**					
Outcome		(<12 ng/mL)			(<20 ng/mL)			(<12 ng/mL)			(<20 ng/mL)	
	OR	(95% CI)	*p*	OR	(95% CI)	*p*	OR	(95% CI)	*p*	OR	(95% CI)	*p*
Sedentary time												
Low sedentary time	1.0	Ref.		1.0	Ref.		1.0	Ref.		1.0	Ref.	
Middle sedentary time	2.4	1.6–3.6	**<0.001**	1.7	1.2–2.3	**0.001**	1.9	1.2–2.9	**0.004**	1.152	0.8–1.7	0.505
High sedentary time	2.6	1.6–4.3	**<0.001**	2.1	1.4–3.2	**0.001**	1.9	0.9–3.8	0.074	1.672	0.8–3.6	0.184
Physical activity level												
Active	1.0	Ref.		1.0	Ref.		1.0	Ref.		1.0	Ref.	
Inactive	0.9	0.7–1.3	0.6	1.0	0.8–1.3	0.795	1.2	0.8–1.7	0.393	1.2	0.9–1.7	0.207
Leisure-time physical activity												
30 min 3 times/week	1.0	Ref.		1.0	Ref.		1.0	Ref.		1.0	Ref.	
Less 30 min 3 times/week	1.0	0.8–1.3	0.795	1.1	0.7–1.5	0.717	1.2	0.5–2.9	0.644	1.3	0.6–2.6	0.502
Commuting												
Active commuting	1.0	Ref.		1.0	Ref.		1.0	Ref.		1.0	Ref.	
Passive commuting	1.1	0.7–1.6	0.755	1.5	1.2–2.0	**0.003**	1.7	1.1–2.7	**0.020**	1.7	1.1–2.4	**0.007**

OR: Odds ratio. CI: confidence interval. Results of binary regression logistic analysis adjust by age, region, dairy consumption, menopause, education level, and sunlight exposure. Significant values (<0.05) in bold.

4. Discussion

We examined the association between PA patterns and ST with vitamin D deficiency and insufficiency in a nationally representative sample of Chilean women. The results showed that passive commuting is associated with vitamin D deficiency and insufficiency in older women, whereas high ST is associated with vitamin D deficiency and insufficiency in adult women. Additionally, we identify a joint effect of high ST/passive commuting on vitamin D deficiency and insufficiency in both groups. The magnitude of the effect was between small to medium.

To our knowledge, this is the first study that analyzes how different patterns of PA and ST are related with vitamin D levels in Chilean population. Interestingly, active adult women and inactive older women shares the same value, as well as inactive adult women correspond to active older women, creating a mirror effect. The vitamin D levels expressed as ng/mL was 20.2 for adult women and 18.0 for older women. These results were similar to another study in a little sample of Chilean older people (n = 57 participants); the aforementioned study have reported that women presented lower levels than men 15.6 ± 5.8 and 19.2 ± 6.0 ng/mL, respectively.

In Europe, vitamin D insufficiency (<20 ng/mL) is present in 36.0% of younger and 24.4% of older participants [39], while there is a high variability between countries. Contrary, to our results, the prevalence of vitamin D insufficiency was higher in young people compared to older participants; an explanation given by the authors is that older population are healthier and quite more active than younger participants. These differences are connected, in some cases, to institutionalization factors, especially combined with concurrent health and mobility problems, such as reduced skin efficiency to produce endogenous vitamin D levels [40], poor dietary vitamin D intake as well poor general nutritional status [41]. Thus, the evidence is not conclusive regarding vitamin D levels according to age, since other risk factors have been identified as skin pigmentation, latitude, health status, vitamin D intake by fortified food or any behavior related to sunlight exposure such as the use of lighter-weight clothes, or indoor working [42–44].

Physical Activity has been proposed to be an important determinant of vitamin D status in Caucasian adults. Jerome et al. [45] showed that sedentary students possessed significantly lower vitamin D levels compared to trained athletes' students that live at high latitudes, even if these sedentary students had a higher vitamin D food intake. Furthermore, leisure-time PA has also been associated to vitamin D levels in cancer survivor patients; however, differences between outdoor and indoor PA were found [46]. In our sample, self-report PA levels, as well as leisure PA, were not associated to vitamin D deficiency or insufficiency. A previous study showed that people who practice mountain sports are associated to a lower risk of serum vitamin D deficiency, while this association was not observed for people who practice nautical sports [47]. Moreover, a previous study of US population reported similar results, although the association was strongest to PA measure by accelerometers than by self-report [48]. Therefore, this could be a reason of non-association in our data. Our data were self-reported and does not discriminate between outdoor or indoor physical activities, therefore the method of measure of PA, outdoor/indoor factor and the different population (cancer patients versus healthy women) could explain these findings.

Hibler was one of the first in to associate ST with serum vitamin D levels. Their results support that PA is positively associated to high vitamin D levels, nonetheless they do not show associations between ST and vitamin D levels [49]. Furthermore, it was not found in association with between ST and vitamin D levels in a Brazilian sample. These contradictory findings could be due to the differences between analyzed populations, since the Brazilian study considered adolescents and participants suffering colorectal adenoma [22,49]. On the other hand, no previous studies that correlate the commute mode with vitamin D deficiency or insufficiency were found, only some activities that increase the UV-light exposition. In this sense, our results provide valuable information that shows the beneficial effect of active commuting on vitamin D levels, since the commute mode has been related positively with better health [50], low type 2 diabetes risk [51], cancer, cardiovascular disease, and all-mortality causes [52].

The joint association between commute mode, ST, and serum vitamin D levels has not been studied. Physical Activity time and ST were jointly evaluated in the previous Chilean national health survey, in order to estimate cardiovascular risk. The active/low sedentary behavior group presented lower cardiovascular risk factors such as hypertension, obesity, and type 2 diabetes [53]. Collectively, active commuting changes were associated to better PA patterns [54]. Therefore, both active commuting as low ST could be an important strategy to increase serum vitamin D levels and avoid the deficiency, considering the arguments exposed above where PA pattern has been estimated as a determinant variable, specifically in postmenopausal women [55].

Vitamin D deficiency is related to musculoskeletal diseases such as rickets and osteomalacia, or several infectious and metabolic processes [56]. Thus, it has been recommended the increase of vitamin D intake [57]. Indeed, in a Chilean population it has been demonstrated the combined beneficial effect of vitamin D supplementation plus exercise on vitamin D serum levels, bone density and functional capacity [58]. Despite this, two recent systematic-reviews, shows that vitamin D supplementation do not have a significant effect on fracture incidence [59] and musculoskeletal health [60]. On the other hand, aging is associated to a progressive bone mass decrease, thus remain physically active is one of the main strategies to combat this continuous loss [13,61]. An alternative to PA is the active commuting, most prevalent behavior associated to active commuting in older population is walking; especially in this population, the benefits of active commuting represents the possibility of independence and autonomy [62,63]. That allows increased sunlight exposure, and therefore, a greater possibility of vitamin D absorption. These results could have important public health implications, since several health problems are associated to low vitamin D levels. In this sense, decrease ST and increase active commuting could be useful strategies against these problems.

The mechanism implicated in this relationship remains unclear, physical activity has been related to sun exposure and vitamin D levels. Nevertheless, this report, as well as other works, has found this same association regardless of sun exposure [47,64]. Another hypothesis is related to physical activity effect and bone metabolism, suggesting an interaction between calcium and vitamin D absorption [65]. Additionally, it has been proposed a close link between sedentary time and increase adiposity, since adiposity is related to decline vitamin D levels [66,67]. Hence, in light to support these hypotheses, more researches are needed.

Important strengths in this study include the population-based sampling method and the wide consideration of potential confounders. However, this study has some limitations. The principal limitation is that cross-sectional study design does not allow to draw causal relationships as was addressed above. Thus, it is not possible to establish whether PA can lead to a vitamin D deficiency or participants with vitamin D deficiency have less PA. Another limitation is about sunlight exposure; despite having considered a question about sunlight exposure, self-report nature and dichotomy response do not grant accurate information about the real amount exposure. On the other hand, the specific vitamin D intake estimation could not be obtained from the used questionnaire and PA questionnaires utilized in our paper often fail to provide sufficient detail on activity type, frequency, duration, and intensity, especially in older adults. Finally, another limitation was the lack of calorie measures of total energy, fat and sugar intake, which could not be obtained from the questionnaire used.

5. Conclusions

We found that high ST is associated with vitamin D deficiency in adult women as well as, passive commuting is associated with vitamin D deficiency. Moreover, there is a joint association of high ST/passive commuting on vitamin D deficiency and insufficiency in both groups. These novel results may add key information for public policy in Chile related to health system approach. In this sense, lifestyle recommendations are needed in order to establish specific recommendations, since the patterns of PA and ST could affect differentially vitamin D status according to age. Further research directions should establish the causal effect of PA and ST patterns, as well as establish the vitamin D deficiency implications in different pathologies in the studied Chilean population.

Supplementary Materials: Figure S1: Vitamin D levels of all survey participants along Chilean territory. Population from North of Chile exhibit higher serum vitamin D levels compared to the population from the south territory, being rather deficient for the latter. It is noteworthy, that no region's present population hold the recommended serum vitamin D levels, which is higher than 30 ng/mL.

Author Contributions: P.S.-U. and J.P.-D. conceived the hypothesis and conducted the statistical analyses; P.S.-U. and J.P.-D. drafted the manuscript; C.C.-M., J.R.-P, J.P.Z.-C., M.J.S.-L. critically revised the drafted manuscript. All authors took part in the interpretation of data, the drafting of the manuscript, and the critical revision of the manuscript.

Acknowledgments: We thank all participants for their cooperation and the Chilean Health Ministry and Department of Public Health, The Pontificia Universidad Católica de Chile for designing and conducting the third National Health Survey 2016–2017.

References

1. Gil, Á.; Plaza-Díaz, J.; Mesa, M.D. Vitamin D: Classic and Novel Actions. *Ann. Nutr. Metab.* **2018**, *72*, 87–95. [CrossRef] [PubMed]
2. Holick, M.F. Vitamin D Deficiency. *N. Engl. J. Med.* **2007**, *357*, 266–281. [CrossRef] [PubMed]
3. Aghajafari, F.; Letourneau, N.; Mahinpey, N.; Cosic, N.; Giesbrecht, G. Vitamin D Deficiency and Antenatal and Postpartum Depression: A Systematic Review. *Nutrients* **2018**, *10*, 10. [CrossRef] [PubMed]
4. Pilz, S.; Zittermann, A.; Obeid, R.; Hahn, A.; Pludowski, P.; Trummer, C.; Lerchbaum, E.; Pérez-López, F.R.; Karras, S.N.; März, W. The Role of Vitamin D in Fertility and during Pregnancy and Lactation: A Review of Clinical Data. *Int. J. Environ. Res. Public Health* **2018**, *15*, 2241. [CrossRef] [PubMed]
5. Visser, M.; Deeg, D.J.H.; Lips, P. Low Vitamin D and High Parathyroid Hormone Levels as Determinants of Loss of Muscle Strength and Muscle Mass (Sarcopenia): The Longitudinal Aging Study Amsterdam. *J. Clin. Endocrinol. Metab.* **2003**, *88*, 5766–5772. [CrossRef] [PubMed]
6. Mathieu, S.-V.; Fischer, K.; Dawson-Hughes, B.; Freystaetter, G.; Beuschlein, F.; Schietzel, S.; Egli, A.; Bischoff-Ferrari, H.A. Association between 25-Hydroxyvitamin D Status and Components of Body Composition and Glucose Metabolism in Older Men and Women. *Nutrients* **2018**, *10*, 1826. [CrossRef] [PubMed]
7. Cameron, I.D.; Dyer, S.M.; Panagoda, C.E.; Murray, G.R.; Hill, K.D.; Cumming, R.G.; Kerse, N. Interventions for preventing falls in older people in care facilities and hospitals. *Cochrane Database Syst. Rev.* **2018**, *9*, CD005465. [CrossRef]
8. Zhang, R.; Naughton, D.P. Vitamin D in health and disease: Current perspectives. *Nutr. J.* **2010**, *9*, 65. [CrossRef]
9. Agostini, D.; Zeppa, S.D.; Lucertini, F.; Annibalini, G.; Gervasi, M.; Marini, C.F.; Piccoli, G.; Stocchi, V.; Barbieri, E.; Sestili, P. Muscle and Bone Health in Postmenopausal Women: Role of Protein and Vitamin D Supplementation Combined with Exercise Training. *Nutrients* **2018**, *10*, 1103. [CrossRef]
10. Mouratidou, T.; Vicente-Rodríguez, G.; Gracia-Marco, L.; Huybrechts, I.; Sioen, I.; Widhalm, K.; Valtueña, J.; González-Gross, M.; Moreno, L.A.; HELENA Study Group. Associations of Dietary Calcium, Vitamin D, Milk Intakes, and 25-Hydroxyvitamin D With Bone Mass in Spanish Adolescents: The HELENA Study. *J. Clin. Densitom.* **2013**, *16*, 110–117. [CrossRef]
11. Zgaga, L.; Theodoratou, E.; Farrington, S.M.; Agakov, F.; Tenesa, A.; Walker, M.; Knox, S.; Wallace, A.M.; Cetnarskyj, R.; McNeill, G.; et al. Diet, Environmental Factors, and Lifestyle Underlie the High Prevalence of Vitamin D Deficiency in Healthy Adults in Scotland, and Supplementation Reduces the Proportion That Are Severely Deficient. *J. Nutr.* **2011**, *141*, 1535–1542. [CrossRef] [PubMed]
12. Scragg, R.; Rahman, J.; Thornley, S. Association of sun and UV exposure with blood pressure and cardiovascular disease: A systematic review. *J. Steroid Biochem. Mole. Biol.* **2018**. [CrossRef] [PubMed]

13. Pilz, S.; März, W.; Cashman, K.D.; Kiely, M.E.; Whiting, S.J.; Holick, M.F.; Grant, W.B.; Pludowski, P.; Hiligsmann, M.; Trummer, C.; et al. Rationale and Plan for Vitamin D Food Fortification: A Review and Guidance Paper. *Front. Endocrinol.* **2018**, *9*, 373. [CrossRef] [PubMed]
14. Brito, A.; Cori, H.; Olivares, M.; Mujica, M.F.; Cediel, G.; De Romaña, D.L. Less than Adequate Vitamin D Status and Intake in Latin America and the Caribbean: A Problem of Unknown Magnitude. *Food Nutr. Bull.* **2013**, *34*, 52–64. [CrossRef] [PubMed]
15. Rodríguez, P.J.A.; Valdivia, C.G.; Trincado, M.P. Vertebral fractures, osteoporosis and vitamin D levels in Chilean postmenopausal women. *Rev. Méd. Chile* **2007**, *135*, 31–36.
16. Holick, M.F.; Binkley, N.C.; Bischoff-Ferrari, H.A.; Gordon, C.M.; Hanley, D.A.; Heaney, R.P.; Murad, M.H.; Weaver, C.M. Evaluation, Treatment, and Prevention of Vitamin D Deficiency: An Endocrine Society Clinical Practice Guideline. *J. Clin. Endocrinol. Metab.* **2011**, *96*, 1911–1930. [CrossRef]
17. Ross, A.C.; Taylor, C.L.; Yaktine, A.L.; Del Valle, H.B. (Eds.) *Dietary Reference Intakes for Calcium and Vitamin D*; National Academies Press: Washington, DC, USA, 2011.
18. Schweitzer, D.; Amenabar, P.P.; Botello, E.; Lopez, M.; Saavedra, Y.; Klaber, I. Vitamin d levels among chilean older subjects with low energy hip fracture. *Rev. Med. Chile* **2016**, *144*, 175–180. [CrossRef]
19. Carrasco, G.M.; De Dominguez, L.A.; Martinez, F.G.; Ihle, S.S.; Rojas, A.V.; Foradori, C.A.; Marin, L.P. Vitamin d levels in older healthy chilean adults and their association with functional performance. *Rev. Med. Chile* **2014**, *142*, 1385–1391.
20. Piercy, K.L.; Troiano, R.P.; Ballard, R.M.; Carlson, S.A.; Fulton, J.E.; Galuska, D.A.; George, S.M.; Olson, R.D. The Physical Activity Guidelines for Americans. *JAMA* **2018**, *320*, 2020–2028. [CrossRef]
21. Foster, C.; Moore, J.B.; Singletary, C.R.; Skelton, J.A. Physical activity and family-based obesity treatment: A review of expert recommendations on physical activity in youth. *Clin. Obes.* **2017**, *8*, 68–79. [CrossRef]
22. Da Silva, A.C.M.; Cureau, F.V.; De Oliveira, C.L.; Giannini, D.T.; Bloch, K.V.; Kuschnir, M.C.C.; Dutra, E.S.; Schaan, B.D.; De Carvalho, K.M.B. Physical activity but not sedentary time is associated with vitamin D status in adolescents: Study of cardiovascular risk in adolescents (ERICA). *Eur. J. Clin. Nutr.* **2018**, 1. [CrossRef] [PubMed]
23. Hill, R.L.; Heesch, K.C. *The Problem of Physical Inactivity Worldwide Among Older People*; Springer: Berlin, Germany, 2018; pp. 25–41.
24. Mañas, A.; Del Pozo-Cruz, B.; Guadalupe-Grau, A.; Marín-Puyalto, J.; Alfaro-Acha, A.; Rodriguez-Mañas, L.; García-García, F.J.; Ara, I. Reallocating Accelerometer-Assessed Sedentary Time to Light or Moderate- to Vigorous-Intensity Physical Activity Reduces Frailty Levels in Older Adults: An Isotemporal Substitution Approach in the TSHA Study. *J. Am. Med. Dir. Assoc.* **2018**, *19*, 185.e1–185.e6.
25. Warburton, D.E.; Bredin, S.S. Lost in Translation: What Does the Physical Activity and Health Evidence Actually Tell Us? In *Lifestyle in Heart Health and Disease*; Elsevier: Amsterdam, The Netherland, 2018; pp. 175–186.
26. Gerdhem, P.; Ringsberg, K.A.M.; Obrant, K.J.; Åkesson, K. Association between 25-hydroxy vitamin D levels, physical activity, muscle strength and fractures in the prospective population-based OPRA Study of Elderly Women. *Osteoporos. Int.* **2005**, *16*, 1425–1431. [CrossRef] [PubMed]
27. Wicherts, I.S.; Van Schoor, N.M.; Boeke, A.J.P.; Visser, M.; Deeg, D.J.H.; Smit, J.; Knol, D.L.; Lips, P. Vitamin D Status Predicts Physical Performance and Its Decline in Older Persons. *J. Clin. Endocrinol. Metab.* **2007**, *92*, 2058–2065. [CrossRef]
28. Van den Heuvel, E.G.H.M.; Van Schoor, N.; De Jongh, R.T.; Visser, M.; Lips, P. Cross-sectional study on different characteristics of physical activity as determinants of vitamin D status; inadequate in half of the population. *Eur. J. Clin. Nutr.* **2013**, *67*, 360–365. [CrossRef] [PubMed]
29. De Rui, M.; Toffanello, E.D.; Veronese, N.; Zambon, S.; Bolzetta, F.; Sartori, L.; Musacchio, E.; Corti, M.C.; Baggio, G.; Crepaldi, G.; et al. Vitamin D Deficiency and Leisure Time Activities in the Elderly: Are All Pastimes the Same? *PLoS ONE* **2014**, *9*, e94805. [CrossRef] [PubMed]
30. Van Schoor, N.M.; Lips, P. Worldwide vitamin D status. *Best Pract. Res. Clin. Endocrinol. Metab.* **2011**, *25*, 671–680. [CrossRef] [PubMed]
31. Encuesta nacional de salud. *Encuesta Nacional de Salud (e.N.S) 2016-2017. Primeros Resultados*; Encuesta Nacional de Salud: Santiago, Chile, 2018.
32. Vogeser, M.; Parhofer, K. Liquid Chromatography Tandem-mass Spectrometry (LC-MS/MS) - Technique and Applications in Endocrinology. *Exp. Clin. Endocrinol. Diabetes* **2007**, *115*, 559–570. [CrossRef]

33. Ministerio de Salud. *Results Report of Vitamin D*; MINSAL: Santiago, Chile, 2018.
34. Gatti, D.; El Ghoch, M.; Viapiana, O.; Ruocco, A.; Chignola, E.; Rossini, M.; Giollo, A.; Idolazzi, L.; Adami, S.; Grave, R.D.; et al. Strong relationship between vitamin D status and bone mineral density in anorexia nervosa. *Bone* **2015**, *78*, 212–215. [CrossRef]
35. Orces, C.H. Association between leisure-time aerobic physical activity and vitamin D concentrations among US older adults: The NHANES 2007–2012. *Aging Clin. Exp. Res.* **2018**, 1–9. [CrossRef]
36. Armstrong, T.; Bull, F. Development of the World Health Organization Global Physical Activity Questionnaire (GPAQ). *J. Public Health* **2006**, *14*, 66–70. [CrossRef]
37. Díaz-Martínez, X.; Steell, L.; Martínez, M.A.; Leiva, A.M.; Salas-Bravo, C.; Labraña, A.M.; Durán, E.; Cristi-Montero, C.; Livingstone, K.M.; Garrido-Méndez, Á.; et al. Higher levels of self-reported sitting time is associated with higher risk of type 2 diabetes independent of physical activity in Chile. *J. Public Health* **2017**, *40*, 501–507. [CrossRef] [PubMed]
38. Chen, H.; Cohen, P.; Chen, S. How Big is a Big Odds Ratio? Interpreting the Magnitudes of Odds Ratios in Epidemiological Studies. *Commun. Stat. Simul. Comput.* **2010**, *39*, 860–864. [CrossRef]
39. Manios, Y.; Moschonis, G.; Lambrinou, C.P.; Mavrogianni, C.; Tsirigoti, L.; Hoeller, U.; Roos, F.F.; Bendik, I.; Eggersdorfer, M.; Celis-Morales, C.; et al. Associations of vitamin D status with dietary intakes and physical activity levels among adults from seven European countries: The Food4Me study. *Eur. J. Nutr.* **2017**, *57*, 1357–1368. [CrossRef]
40. MacLaughlin, J.; Holick, M. Aging decreases the capacity of human skin to produce vitamin D3. *J. Clin. Investig.* **1985**, *76*, 1536–1538. [CrossRef] [PubMed]
41. Lips, P.; Van Ginkel, F.C.; Jongen, M.J.; Rubertus, F.; Van Der Vijgh, W.J.; Netelenbos, J.C. Determinants of vitamin D status in patients with hip fracture and in elderly control subjects. *Am. J. Clin. Nutr.* **1987**, *46*, 1005–1010. [CrossRef] [PubMed]
42. Hilger, J.; Friedel, A.; Herr, R.; Rausch, T.; Roos, F.; Wahl, D.A.; Pierroz, D.D.; Weber, P.; Hoffmann, K. A systematic review of vitamin D status in populations worldwide. *Br. J. Nutr.* **2013**, *111*, 23–45. [CrossRef]
43. Cashman, K.D.; Dowling, K.G.; Škrabáková, Z.; González-Gross, M.; Valtueña, J.; De Henauw, S.; Moreno, L.; Damsgaard, C.T.; Michaelsen, K.F.; Mølgaard, C.; et al. Vitamin D deficiency in Europe: Pandemic? *Am. J. Clin. Nutr.* **2016**, *103*, 1033–1044. [CrossRef]
44. Casey, C.; Woodside, J.V.; McGinty, A.; Young, I.S.; McPeake, J.; Chakravarthy, U.; Rahu, M.; Seland, J.; Soubrane, G.; Tomazzoli, L.; et al. Factors associated with serum 25-hydroxyvitamin D concentrations in older people in Europe: The EUREYE study. *Eur. J. Clin. Nutr.* **2018**, *1*. [CrossRef]
45. Jerome, S.P.; Sticka, K.D.; Schnurr, T.M.; Mangum, S.J.; Reynolds, A.J.; Dunlap, K.L. 25(oh)d levels in trained versus sedentary university students at 64 degrees north. *Int. J. Circumpolar Health* **2017**, *76*, 1314414. [CrossRef]
46. Yang, L.; Toriola, A.T. Leisure-time physical activity and circulating 25-hydroxyvitamin D levels in cancer survivors: A cross-sectional analysis using data from the US National Health and Nutrition Examination Survey. *BMJ Open* **2017**, *7*, e016064. [CrossRef] [PubMed]
47. Touvier, M.; Deschasaux, M.; Montourcy, M.; Sutton, A.; Charnaux, N.; Kesse-Guyot, E.; Assmann, K.E.; Fezeu, L.; Latino-Martel, P.; Druesne-Pecollo, N.; et al. Determinants of Vitamin D Status in Caucasian Adults: Influence of Sun Exposure, Dietary Intake, Sociodemographic, Lifestyle, Anthropometric, and Genetic Factors. *J. Investig. Dermatol.* **2015**, *135*, 378–388. [CrossRef] [PubMed]
48. Wanner, M.; Richard, A.; Martin, B.; Linseisen, J.; Rohrmann, S. Associations between objective and self-reported physical activity and vitamin D serum levels in the US population. *Cancer Causes Control* **2015**, *26*, 881–891. [CrossRef] [PubMed]
49. Hibler, E.A.; Molmenti, C.L.S.; Dai, Q.; Kohler, L.N.; Anderson, S.W.; Jurutka, P.W.; Jacobs, E.T. Physical activity, sedentary behavior, and vitamin D metabolites. *Bone* **2016**, *83*, 248–255. [CrossRef] [PubMed]
50. Andersen, L.B. Active commuting is beneficial for health. *BMJ* **2017**, *357*, 1740. [CrossRef] [PubMed]
51. Rasmussen, M.G.; Grøntved, A.; Blond, K.; Overvad, K.; Tjønneland, A.; Jensen, M.K.; Østergaard, L. Associations between Recreational and Commuter Cycling, Changes in Cycling, and Type 2 Diabetes Risk: A Cohort Study of Danish Men and Women. *PLoS Med.* **2016**, *13*, e1002076. [CrossRef] [PubMed]
52. Celis-Morales, C.A.; Lyall, D.M.; Welsh, P.; Anderson, J.; Steell, L.; Guo, Y.; Maldonado, R.; Mackay, D.F.; Pell, J.P.; Sattar, N.; et al. Association between active commuting and incident cardiovascular disease, cancer, and mortality: Prospective cohort study. *BMJ* **2017**, *357*, j1456. [CrossRef]

53. Cristi-Montero, C.; Steell, L.; Petermann, F.; Garrido-Méndez, A.; Díaz-Martínez, X.; Salas-Bravo, C.; Ramirez-Campillo, R.; Alvarez, C.; Rodriguez, F.; Aguilar-Farias, N.; et al. Joint effect of physical activity and sedentary behaviour on cardiovascular risk factors in Chilean adults. *J. Public Health* **2017**, *40*, 485–492. [CrossRef]
54. Foley, L.; Panter, J.; Heinen, E.; Prins, R.; Ogilvie, D. Changes in active commuting and changes in physical activity in adults: A cohort study. *Int. J. Behav. Nutr. Phys. Act.* **2015**, *12*, 161. [CrossRef]
55. Millen, A.E.; Wactawski-Wende, J.; Pettinger, M.; Melamed, M.L.; Tylavsky, F.A.; Liu, S.; Robbins, J.; Lacroix, A.Z.; LeBoff, M.S.; Jackson, R.D.; et al. Predictors of serum 25-hydroxyvitamin D concentrations among postmenopausal women: The Women's Health Initiative Calcium plus Vitamin D Clinical Trial. *Am. J. Clin. Nutr.* **2010**, *91*, 1324–1335. [CrossRef]
56. Muscogiuri, G. Vitamin D: Past, present and future perspectives in the prevention of chronic diseases. *Eur. J. Clin. Nutr.* **2018**, *72*, 1221–1225. [CrossRef] [PubMed]
57. Mayor, S. Public Health England recommends vitamin D supplements in autumn and winter. *BMJ* **2016**, *354*, 4061. [CrossRef] [PubMed]
58. Bunout, D.; Barrera, G.; Leiva, L.; Gattás, V.; De La Maza, M.P.; Avendaño, M.; Hirsch, S. Effects of vitamin D supplementation and exercise training on physical performance in Chilean vitamin D deficient elderly subjects. *Exp. Gerontol.* **2006**, *41*, 746–752. [CrossRef] [PubMed]
59. Zhao, J.-G.; Zeng, X.-T.; Wang, J.; Liu, L. Association Between Calcium or Vitamin D Supplementation and Fracture Incidence in Community-Dwelling Older Adults: A Systematic Review and Meta-analysis. *JAMA* **2017**, *318*, 2466–2482. [CrossRef] [PubMed]
60. Bolland, M.J.; Grey, A.; Avenell, A. Effects of vitamin D supplementation on musculoskeletal health: A systematic review, meta-analysis, and trial sequential analysis. *Lancet Diabetes Endocrinol.* **2018**, *6*, 847–858. [CrossRef]
61. Rodríguez-Gómez, I.; Mañas, A.; Losa-Reyna, J.; Rodríguez-Mañas, L.; Chastin, S.F.M.; Alegre, L.M.; García-García, F.J.; Ara, I. Associations between sedentary time, physical activity and bone health among older people using compositional data analysis. *PLoS ONE* **2018**, *13*, e0206013. [CrossRef] [PubMed]
62. O'hern, S.; Oxley, J. Understanding travel patterns to support safe active transport for older adults. *J. Transp. Health* **2015**, *2*, 79–85. [CrossRef]
63. Musselwhite, C.; Holland, C.; Walker, I. The role of transport and mobility in the health of older people. *J. Transp. Health* **2015**, *2*, 1–4. [CrossRef]
64. Kluczynski, M.A.; LaMonte, M.J.; Mares, J.A.; Wactawski-Wende, J.; Smith, A.W.; Engelman, C.D.; Andrews, C.A.; Snetselaar, L.G.; Sarto, G.E.; Millen, A.E.; et al. Duration of Physical Activity and Serum 25-hydroxyvitamin D Status of Postmenopausal Women. *Ann. Epidemiol.* **2011**, *21*, 440–449. [CrossRef]
65. Al-Musharaf, S.; Krishnaswamy, S.; Yusuf, D.S.; Alkharfy, K.M.; Al-Saleh, Y.; Al-Attas, O.S.; Alokail, M.S.; Moharram, O.; Sabico, S.; Al-Othman, A.; et al. Effect of physical activity and sun exposure on vitamin D status of Saudi children and adolescents. *BMC Pediatr.* **2012**, *12*, 92.
66. Wortsman, J.; Matsuoka, L.Y.; Chen, T.C.; Lu, Z.; Holick, M.F. Decreased bioavailability of vitamin D in obesity. *Am. J. Clin. Nutr.* **2000**, *72*, 690–693. [CrossRef] [PubMed]
67. Scott, D.; Blizzard, L.; Fell, J.; Ding, C.; Winzenberg, T.; Jones, G. A prospective study of the associations between 25-hydroxy-vitamin D, sarcopenia progression and physical activity in older adults. *Clin. Endocrinol.* **2010**, *73*, 581–587. [CrossRef] [PubMed]

2

Long-Term Effects of Vitamin D Supplementation in Obese Children During Integrated Weight–Loss Programme—A Double Blind Randomized Placebo–Controlled Trial

Michał Brzeziński [1,2,*], Agnieszka Jankowska [1], Magdalena Słomińska-Frączek [3], Paulina Metelska [2,4], Piotr Wiśniewski [5], Piotr Socha [6] and Agnieszka Szlagatys-Sidorkiewicz [1]

1 Department of Paediatrics, Gastroenterology, Allergology and Paediatric Nutrition, Medical University of Gdańsk, 80–803 Gdańsk, Poland; ajankowska@gumed.edu.pl (A.J.); agnieszka.szlagatys-sidorkiewicz@gumed.edu.pl (A.S.-S.)
2 Department of Public Health and Social Medicine, Medical University of Gdansk, 80–210 Gdańsk, Poland; metelska.paulina@gumed.edu.pl
3 Department of Paediatrics, Copernicus Medical Center, 80-462 Gdańsk, Poland; madds@wp.pl
4 "6–10–14 for Health"–University Clinical Center, 80-952 Gdańsk, Poland
5 Department of Endocrinology and Internal Medicine, Medical University of Gdansk, 80–952 Gdańsk, Poland; piotr.wisniewski@gumed.edu.pl
6 Department of Gastroenterology, Hepatology and Feeding Disorders, The Children's Memorial Health Institute, 04–730 Warszawa, Poland; p.socha@ipczd.pl
* Correspondence: brzezinski@gumed.edu.pl

Abstract: Background: Vitamin D was studied in regards to its possible impact on body mass reduction and metabolic changes in adults and children with obesity yet there were no studies assessing the impact of vitamin D supplementation during a weight management program in children and adolescence. The aim of our study was to assess the influence of 26 weeks of vitamin D supplementation in overweight and obese children undergoing an integrated 12–months' long weight loss program on body mass reduction, body composition and bone mineral density. Methods: A double–blind randomized placebo–controlled trial. Vitamin D deficient patients (<30 ng/ml level of vitamin D) aged 6–14, participating in multidisciplinary weight management program were randomly allocated to receiving vitamin D (1200 IU) or placebo for the first 26 weeks of the intervention. Results: Out of the 152 qualified patients, 109 (72%) completed a full cycle of four visits scheduled in the program. There were no difference in the level of BMI (body mass index) change – both raw BMI and BMI centiles. Although the reduction of BMI centiles was greater in the vitamin D vs. placebo group (−4.28 ± 8.43 vs. −2.53 ± 6.10) the difference was not statistically significant ($p = 0.319$). Similarly the reduction in fat mass—assessed both using bioimpedance and DEXa was achieved, yet the differences between the groups were not statistically significant. Conclusions: Our study ads substantial results to support the thesis on no effect of vitamin D supplementation on body weight reduction in children and adolescents with vitamin D insufficiency undergoing a weight management program.

Keywords: vitamin D; obesity; weight–loss; body composition

1. Introduction

Worldwide prevalence of overweight and obesity is increasing both in adults and children [1,2]. It is observed on all continents, with the highest burden in those from lower socioeconomic and educational groups [1,3]. Obesity among others is associated with a wide range of metabolic disorders, such as insulin resistance, hyperinsulinemia, and impaired tolerance of glucose, abnormal fasting plasma glucose, symptomatic diabetes mellitus, lipid disorders and cardiovascular disorders, namely arterial hypertension [4–6]. Obesity alone is responsible for a significant increase in the risk of mortality in general population with [7]. In view of high risk of complications resulting from childhood obesity, early implementation of intervention programs seems to be vitally important, as in children and adolescents it is the first–choice intervention, although with limited effectiveness [8]. Several previous studies showed that integrated multidisciplinary weight–loss programs, which include the child's family as well, are the most effective [9–11]. Reduction of fat mass is associated with normalization of metabolic parameters, such as inflammatory markers, lipid profile, insulin resistance and arterial blood pressure [12–14]. Therefore, early and efficient intervention increases likelihood of staying healthy in the future. As pharmacological and surgical interventions in children are limited [15–17], trials looking for substances supporting lifestyle interventions were run, looking at several different dietary supplements, hers (green tea, yerba mate), DHA (docosahexaenoic acid) among others [18–22]. Vitamin D was also studied in regards to its possible impact on body mass reduction and metabolic changes in adults and children with obesity [23,24].

The role of vitamin D in energetic metabolism has been emphasized recently. Obese children frequently present with low blood concentrations of vitamin D [25–27]. This probably results from lower dietary intake of this vitamin by obese individuals on the one hand, and less outdoor physical activity on the other [28–30]. Moreover, a higher percentage of fat mass is associated with a lower blood concentration of vitamin D, which may, at least partially, result from its sequestration in adipose tissue [31]. Animal experiments with labelled vitamin D showed that this vitamin is accumulated in adipose tissue and slowly released to blood [32].

Consequently, a vitamin D deficiency in obese children seems to be associated with a significant increase of risk of many metabolic disorders associated with obesity, such as insulin resistance, hyperinsulinemia, impaired tolerance of glucose, abnormal fasting plasma glucose, symptomatic diabetes mellitus, lipid disorders and cardiovascular morbidity, namely arterial hypertension [5,6]. There is a number of observational studies which demonstrate the substantial role of vitamin D deficiency in developing metabolic syndrome and other complications of obesity [33–35]. However, we lack interventional studies to link these observations to demonstrate a causal relationship.

In this study we wanted to assess the influence of 26 weeks of vitamin D supplementation in overweight and obese children undergoing an integrated 12–months' long weight loss program on body mass reduction, body composition and bone mineral density [36].

2. Materials and Methods

Detailed information about the study protocol, participants and design of the interventional program has been previously published [36]. All study participants were recruited from "6–10–14 for Health" program run by University Clinical Center in Gdansk, Poland. The program is a multidisciplinary, interventional program dedicated to children aged 6–15 and their parents. All school children in Gdansk aged 6–15 are screened in a 3–4–year–interval by dedicated teams (pediatrician and or nurses). All children with BMI centile above 85th centile are invited to the "6–10–14 for Health" program. All participants of the "6–10–14 for Health" program and their family members (parents/caregivers) were offered 12–month integrated intervention, including individual medical (pediatric), dietetic, physical activity and psychological counselling, during one meeting (4 x 20–25min). This intervention was offered to all the participants in a 0–3–6–12 month scheme.

2.1. Trial Design

A double–blind placebo–controlled trial. Vitamin D deficient patients (<30 ng/ml level of vitamin D) participating in multidisciplinary weight program were randomized to two arms (1:1 ratio): receiving vitamin D (1200 IU) or placebo for the first 26 weeks of the intervention.

We hypothesized that the supplementation with vitamin D in obese children showing low serum 25(OH)D3 during weight–loss program could positively influence body mass index (BMI), muscle mass, bone mass and mineral density and biochemical markers of metabolic complications related to obesity compared to placebo.

The study was conducted at the Department of Paediatrics, Paediatric Gastroenterology, Allergology and Children Nutrition, the Medical University of Gdansk and within the framework of "6–10–14 for Health" Interventional Programme, University Clinical Centre in Gdansk.

2.2. Participants

Eligible participants were children aged 6, 9–11 and 14, according to the "6–10–14 for Health" program protocol:

Inclusion criteria: overweight (BMI ≥ 85th < 95th percentile) or obesity (BMI ≥ 95th percentile), identified on the basis of anthropometric parameters using Polish reference centile charts—OLAF project [37]; blood concentration of 25(OH)D3 < 30 ng/ml; written informed consent of legal caregivers.

Exclusion criteria: Chronic conditions (asthma or allergies, inflammatory diseases of connective tissue, gastrointestinal disorders, diseases of kidneys and liver, disorders of bone metabolism); contraindications to administration of vitamin D; administration of any preparation containing vitamin D, calcium, or steroid hormones during three months preceding the study.

2.3. Ethics Approval and Consent to Participate

The study is approved by Independent Bioethics Committee for Scientific Research at Medical University of Gdansk, Poland, [NKBBN/130–206/2015] dated 25.05.2015. The parents/caregivers gave their written consent before the start of any study procedure. The study protocol was peer reviewed by financial supporter (Fundacja Nutricia) independent commission, during the grant application process. Trial registration no: NCT 02828228; trial registration date: 8 June 2016 registered in: ClinicalTrials.gov.

2.4. Study Procedure

The study period covered four appointments within the "6–10–14 for Health" obesity management program at the 0, 3, 6 and 12 month mark. All visits included individual meetings with a pediatrician, dietician, physical activity specialist and psychologist. All child/parent dyads had individual meetings with all 4 specialists—one directly after other. Detailed information about the program can be found in previous publications [36]. During the first appointment, the caregivers of all children were asked to provide written consent to the child taking part in the trial. Refusal to participate in the trial did not influence participation in the interventional obesity management program. Children with low blood concentration of 25(OH)D3 (<30 ng/ml) were referred for DXA (dual–energy x–ray absorptiometry) within two weeks from the starting visit.

The enrolled subjects were randomly assigned to one of the two groups using computer generated randomization tables. Then participants were randomly assigned to one of the two trial groups:

- GROUP I (Vitamin D group): medical intervention, intervention of dietician, psychologist and physical education specialist, parental education + oral administration of vitamin D3 (1200 i.u. daily) for 26 weeks
- GROUP II (Placebo group): medical intervention, intervention of dietician, psychologist and physical education specialist, parental education + daily oral administration of placebo for 26 weeks.

Study time line chart is shown in Figure 1.

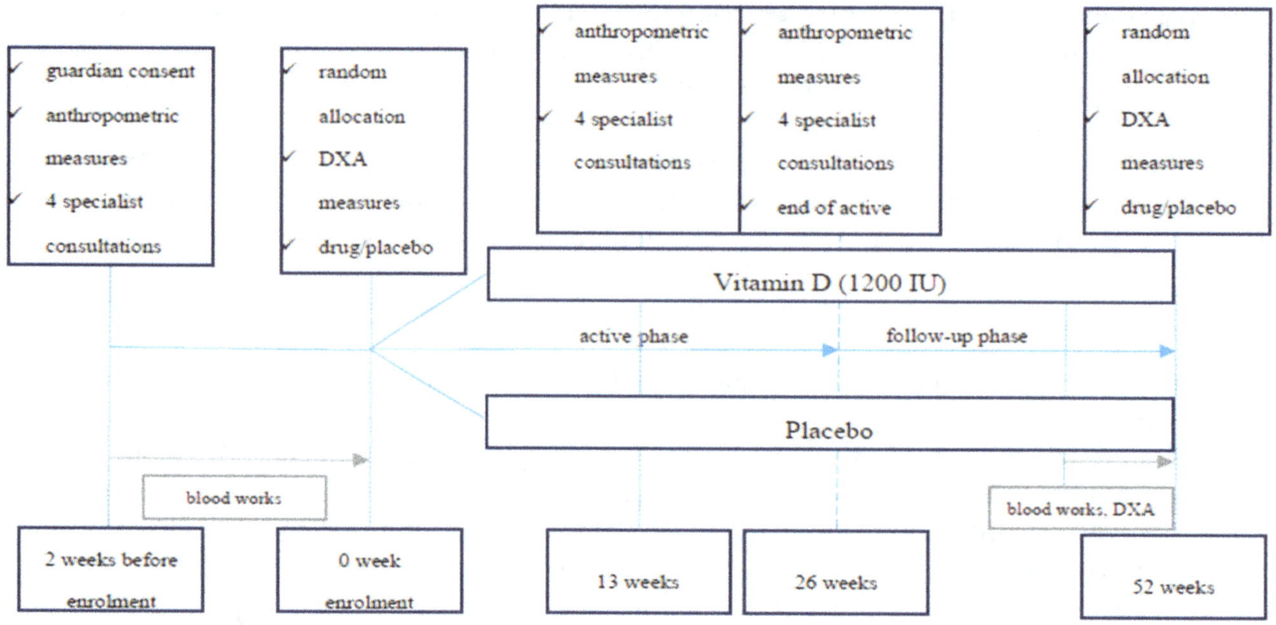

Figure 1. Patients' time line in the study.

2.5. *Randomization and Blinding*

The randomization list was generated by Office of Clinical and Scientific Research, University Clinical Centre (OCSR UCK), with no clinical involvement in the trial, via a computer program (StatsDirect) with an allocation ratio of 1:1 and with a block of 6. The allocation sequence was concealed from the researchers responsible for enrolling and assessing participants. Throughout the duration of the study, all investigators, participants, outcome assessors, and data analysts were blinded to the assigned treatment. Allocation to groups and drug/placebo distribution was performed by an independent researcher (M.S–F) not directly involved in the interventional program.

2.6. *Treatment Dispensing and Assessment of Compliance*

Both of the study treatments: vitamin D (1200 IU) and placebo were provided by the company (Sequoia) in identical capsules and packages (5 capsules in one blister, 6 blisters in a box). The sets of 7 boxes (6 months treatment) were prepared and blinded by Office of Clinical and Scientific Research, University Clinical Centre. Study treatment was dispensed by the investigator at the enrolment visit. At the final visit the sets of blisters and boxes were retrieved from the patient. The number of remaining capsules were documented to assess the compliance.

2.7. *Outcome Measures*

Primary endpoint: Change in BMI, BMI centile after 26 weeks of vitamin D supplementation. Secondary endpoints: change in body composition and bone mineral density and vitamin D level after 26 weeks of vitamin D supplementation. Additionally, we assessed changes in blood level of vitamin D.

2.8. *Sample Size*

Assuming probability of the event (at least 10% reduction in baseline BMI over the follow–up period) at 0.85 and 0.6 for the experimental and control group, respectively, minimum sample size providing 0.9 statistical power for alpha equal 0.05 or lower and beta equal 0.1 or lower was estimated at 130 (65 per group).

2.9. *Statistical Analysis*

Normal distribution of continuous variables was verified with the Shapiro–Wilk test. Descriptive statistics are presented as the mean or median and standard deviation from the mean. Between groups comparisons were carried out using the Mann–Whitney U test. Nonparametric tests were chosen because of the large number of significant Shapiro tests, which were used for normality assumption assessment. All statistical tests were two–tailed and performed at the 5% level of significance. All analyses were performed on the intention–to–treat basis, in which all of the participants in a trial are analyzed according to the intervention to which they were assigned, analyzing only participants who completed the whole weight management intervention program. Statistical analyses were performed with the Statistica 13 (TIBCO Software Inc., Tulsa, USA 2017).

3. Results

After obtaining and verifying the correctness of the recorded data (cross-checked with source data of 30% of patients), the data was decoded according to the protocol received from OCSR UCK in Gdansk.

After decoding, a full analysis of available anthropometric data and the results of densitometric examination was performed for patients divided into groups—receiving placebo and vitamin D.

A total of 170 patients were eligible for enrolment in the study during the enrolment period. A total of 152 patients were eventually included in the study (n = 8—no parental consent, n = 10—vitamin D intake during three months before the study). Subsequently the patients were randomly assigned to groups: 67 to the placebo group and 85 to the Vitamin D group. Out of the 152 qualified patients, 109 (72%) completed a full cycle of four visits scheduled in the program. In the placebo group, 64 patients completed the active phase of 26 weeks of supplementation, 53 completed the comprehensive treatment program (52 week duration).

The patient flow is shown in Figure 2.

Basic demographic and clinical data for both groups are presented in Table 1.

Table 1. Basic anthropometric and clinical data of studied groups (vitamin D and placebo) at visit 1.

	vitamin D (n = 85)		**placebo (n = 67)**		
	Mean ± SD	**(95% CI)**	**Mean ± SD**	**CI (–95%)**	p
age (years)	11.10 ± 2.84	10.49–11.72	10.70 ± 3.13	9.92–11.47	0.389
body mass (kg)	59.01 ± 21.04	54.47–63.55	56.89 ± 20.08	52.00–61.9	0.706
height (cm)	150.79 ± 16.69	147.19–154.39	149.31 ± 18.29	144.85–153.77	0.660
BMI	24.97 ± 4.12	24.08–25.86	24.53 ± 3.57	23.66–25.41	0.759
BMI centile	95.18 ± 3.24	94.49–95.88	95.23 ±3.43	94.41–96.06	0.812
no. of girls at visit 1	46		38		0.827
% of girls at visit 1	54.12%		56.72%		

$p < 0.05$ Mann–Whitney U test analysis.

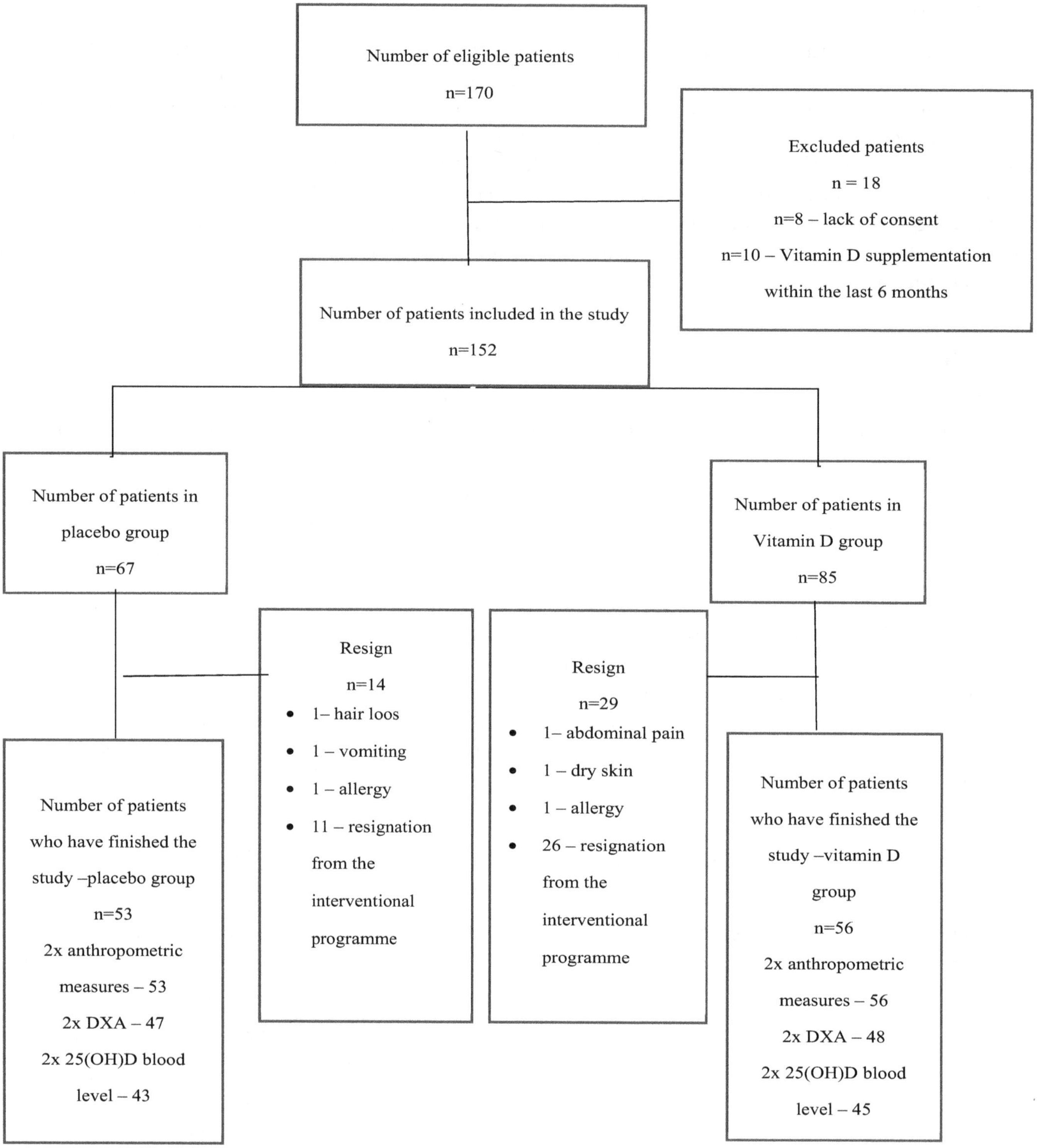

Figure 2. Patient flowchart in the study

There were no statistically significant differences between the vitamin D and placebo groups at the start of the study.

The differences between the groups in terms of main endpoints were subsequently assessed.

The results of basic anthropometric and 25(OH)D concentration tests are shown in Table 2.

Table 2. Results of basic anthropometric and 25(OH)D concentration tests in studied groups.

Variable	vitamin D			placebo			
	No	Mean ± SD	95% CI	No	Mean ±	95% CI	p
BMI visit 1	85	24.97 ± 4.12	24.08–25.86	67	24.53 ± 3.58	23.66–25.41	0.759
BMI visit 4	56	24.33 ± 3.97	23.27–25.39	53	24.68 ± 3.46	23.73–25.64	0.479
ΔBMI visit 4–1	56	–0.46 ± 1.80	−0.94–0.03	53	0.11 ±1.84	−0.40–0.61	0.203
BMI centile 1 visit	85	95.18 ± 3.22	94.49–95.88	67	95.23 ± 3.39	94.41–96.06	0.812
BMI centile 4 visit	56	90.91 ± 9.40	88.39–93.43	53	92.64 ± 7.53	90.56–94.71	0.303
Δ in BMI centiles visit 4–1	56	–4.28 ± 8.43	–6.54––2.03	53	−2.53 ± 6.10	−4.21––0.85	0.319
25 (OH) D level visit 1	85	19.35 ± 5.46	18.16–20.55	66	19.79 ± 5.15	18.52–21.06	0.622 *
25 (OH) D level visit 4	45	24.99 ± 5.54	23.33–26.66	43	18.3 ± 6.70	16.25–20.37	0.000 *
Δ 25 (OH) level visit 4–1	45	6.06 ± 5.80	4.32–7.81	43	−2.40 ± 5.97	−4.24––0.57	0.000 *

$p < 0.05$ Mann–Whitney U test, * t–student test for independent samples.

The results of bioelectric impedance measurements are shown in Table 3.

Table 3. Results of bioelectric impedance measurements in studied groups.

Variable	vitamin D			placebo			
	No	Mean	CI (–95%)	No	Mean	CI (–95%)	p
BI_FM (kg) visit 1	82	18.32 ± 8.01	16.56–20.08	64	17.80 ± 7.30	15.97–19.62	0.820
BI_FM (kg) visit 4	55	18.29 ± 8.07	16.11–20.47	53	18.13 ± 7.18	16.15–20.11	0.907
Δ BI_FM (kg) visit 4–1	54	−0.11 ± 4.09	−1.23–1.00	51	0.01 ± 4.01	−1.11–1.14	0.890
BI_FM (%) visit 1	54	31.15 ± 4.90	29.81–32.48	51	31.23 ± 5.91	29.57–32.89	0.741
BI_FM (%) visit 4	54	29.57 ± 6.03	27.92–31.21	51	29.39 ± 6.95	27.44–31.35	0.889*
Δ BI_FM (%) visit 4–1	54	−1.58 ± 4.04	−2.68–0.47	51	−1.83 ± 4.56	−3.12––0.55	0.951
BI_MM (kg) visit 1	82	38.46 ± 14.00	35.39–41.54	64	37.10 ± 13.65	33.69–40.51	0.586
BI_MM (kg) visit 4	56	40.12 ± 12.85	36.68–43.56	53	40.80 ± 12.92	37.24–44.36	0.886
Δ BI_MM (kg) visit 4–1	55	2.45 ±2.57	1.75–3.14	51	3.33 ± 2.75	2.56–4.10	0.091 *
BI_MM (%) visit 1	82	65.69 ±5.39	64.50–66.87	64	65.48 ± 5.03	64.22–66.73	0.350
BI_MM (%) visit 4	56	66.63 ±5.68	65.11–68.16	53	66.81 ± 6.52	65.01–68.61	0.896
Δ BI_MM (%) visit 4–1	55	1.42 ±4.02	0.33–2.51	51	1.48 ± 3.72	0.43–2.53	0.949

$p < 0.05$ Mann–Whitney U test, * t–student test for independent samples. BI—bioimpedance, FM—fat mass, Δ – delta–difference, MM—muscle mass.

The results of the dual X–ray absorptiometry (DXA) measurements are presented in Table 4.

Table 4. Results of dual X–ray absorptiometry (DXA) measurements in studied groups.

	Vitamin D			Placebo			
	No	Mean	CI (–95%)	No	Mean	CI (–95%)	p
Sp BMD visit 1	83	0.76 ± 0.18	0.72–0.80	67	0.74 ± 0.18	0.70–0.79	0.447
Sp BMD visit 4	47	0.82 ± 0.19	0.76–0.87	47	0.80 ± 0.19	0.75–0.86	0.623
Δ in Sp BMD visit 4–1	47	0.04 ± 0.04	0.03–0.06	47	0.06 ± 0.04	0.05–0.08	0.025 *
TBLH BMD visit 1	83	0.87 ± 0.14	0.84–0.90	67	0.86 ± 0.15	0.82–0.89	0.672
TBLH BMD visit 4	48	0.91 ± 0.14	0.87–0.95	47	0.90 ± 0.15	0.86–0.94	0.740
Δ in TBLH BMD visit 4–1	48	0.04± 0.03	0.04–0.05	47	0.04 ± 0.03	0.03–0.05	0.504*
TFM (kg) visit 1	83	25.18 ± 9.76	23.05–27.31	67	24.29 ± 9.08	22.08–26.51	0.652
TFM (kg) visit 4	48	25.17 ± 8.72	22.63–27.70	47	25.07 ± 8.96	22.44–27.70	0.959*
Δ in TFM visit 4–1	48	0.73 ±4.55	–0.59–2.05	47	0.68 ± 4.96	–0.77–2.14	0.734
TLM (kg) visit 1	83	32.52 ± 4.55	30.04–34.99	67	31.83 ± 10.94	29.16–34.50	0.823
TLM (kg) visit 4	48	34.41 ± 10.33	31.41–37.42	47	34.48 ± 12.19	30.90–38.06	0.976 *
TFM (%) visit 1	48	43.46 ± 3.82	42.35–44.57	47	43.30 ± 4.42	42.00–44.60	0.847
TFM (%) visit 4	48	41.89 ± 5.29	40.35–43.43	47	42.32 ± 5.50	40.71–43.94	0.695
Δ in TFM (%) visit 4–1	48	–1.57 ± 4.12	–2.77–0.38	47	–0.98 ± 3.97	–2.14–0.19	0.472 *
TLM (%) visit 1	48	56.54 ± 3.82	55.43–57.65	47	56.70 ± 4.42	55.40–58.00	0.847
TLM (%) visit 4	48	58.11 ± 5.29	56.57–59.65	47	57.68 ± 5.50	56.06–59.29	0.695
Δ in TLM (%) visit 4–1	48	1.57 ± 4.12	0.38–2.77	47	0.98 ± 3.97	–0.19–2.14	0.472

$p < 0.05$ Mann–Whitney U test, * t–student test for independent samples. Sp—spine, BMD—bone mineral density, Δ—delta–difference, TBLH—total body less head, TFM—total fat mass, TLM—total lean mass.

Both groups had a reduction in BMI centiles. Although the reduction was greater in the vitamin D vs. placebo group (–4.28 ± 8.43 vs. –2.53 ±6.10) the difference was not statistically significant ($p = 0.319$). Similarly the reduction in fat mass—assessed both using bioimpedance and DEXa was achieved, yet the differences between the groups were not statistically significant, as shown in Tables 3 and 4.

The analysis showed statistically significant differences between the groups only in 25(OH) D3 concentration in the measurements taken after the supplementation period (24.99 vs. 16.25; $p = 0.000$) and in the difference between second and first measurement of vitamin D levels (6.06 vs. –4.24; $p = 0.000$), and in the difference between second and first measurement of bone mineral density in the spine (Sp BMD) (0.04 vs. 0.06; $p < 0.0256$). The difference was higher in the placebo group.

There was no difference between the placebo group and the vitamin D group in BMI reduction, BMI centile, fat tissue in kg, % of fat tissue (assessed both by performing BIA and densitometry analysis).

Additionally, we have performed an analysis of correlations (Spearman rank correlation coefficient) between vitamin D levels at Visit 1 and 4 and changes of vitamin D level between the visits dependent on several anthropometric variables. Results are presented in Table 5.

Table 5. Correlation between vitamin D levels and anthropometric variables.

	25 (OH) D Level Visit 1	25 (OH) D Level Visit 4	Δ 25 (OH) Level Visit 4–1
BMI centile 1 visit	–0.088910	**–0.232998**	–0.066400
BMI centile 4 visit	–0.128452	**–0.297140**	–0.147392
Δ in BMI centiles visit 4–1	–0.059634	–0.141315	–0.138827
BI_FM (%) visit 1	**–0.248164**	**–0.238226**	–0.020100
BI_FM (%) visit 4	**–0.213330**	**–0.226632**	–0.019981
Δ BI_FM (%) visit 4–1	0.073786	–0.013645	–0.058235
BI_MM (%) visit 1	**0.214256**	0.202164	–0.005444
BI_MM (%) visit 4	**0.204376**	**0.233062**	0.045692
Δ BI_MM (%) visit 4–1	–0.077210	0.057706	0.107305
25 (OH) D level visit 1	1.000000	**0.322476**	**–0.426874**
25 (OH) D level visit 4	**0.322476**	1.000000	**0.692743**
Δ 25 (OH) level visit 4–1	**–0.426874**	**0.692743**	1.000000
TBLH BMD visit 1	**–0.357821**	–0.164349	0.102925
TBLH BMD visit 4	**–0.377036**	–0.222562	0.012532
Δ in TBLH BMD visit 4–1	0.079692	0.007924	–0.047583
TFM (%) visit 1	–0.177243	–0.206046	–0.111781
TFM (%) visit 4	–0.035164	–0.122583	–0.069020
Δ in TFM (%) visit 2–1	0.174996	–0.008749	–0.047612
TLM (%) visit 1	0.177243	0.206046	0.111781
TLM (%) visit 4	0.035164	0.122583	0.069020
Δ in TLM (%) visit 4–1	–0.174996	0.008749	0.047612

Spearman rank correlation coefficient; bolded when $p < 0.05$, BI—bioimpedance, FM—fat mass, Δ—delta–difference, MM—muscle mass, BMD—bone mineral density, TBLH—total body less head, TFM—total fat mass, TLM—total lean mass.

The results show that there were no important correlation between the initial BMI centile and vitamin D level at the first visit. Additionally the correlation did not show any significant influence of BMI changes on changes in vitamin D level after the supplementation period. There were significant negative correlations ($p < 0.05$) between fat mass % and levels of vitamin D during both visits—which can confirm the relation between the fat mass and blood level of vitamin D. Yet this was a rather weak correlation (–0.25 to –0.21). Further, it was not confirmed in DXA measurements.

4. Discussion

4.1. *Effect of Vitamin D Supplementation on Body Mass Reduction*

Presented study is the first randomized trial to assess potential effects of vitamin D supplementation in body mass reduction in overweight and obese children. Results of present study show that supplementation of vitamin D did not have a statistically significant, put potentially clinically important, influence on body mass (BMI, BMI centile) body composition or bone mineral density comparing to placebo groups during an organized obesity management program in children.

Biological role of vitamin D in etiopathogenesis of metabolic syndrome represents an interesting issue. Previous studies conducted among children revealed inverse relationship between blood concentration of vitamin D and waist circumference, systolic blood pressure, insulin resistance, fasting glucose, total cholesterol, triglycerides and LDL cholesterol, as well as positive association between the concentration of vitamin D and HDL cholesterol [25,38,39]. It seems that vitamin D can interfere with secretion of insulin both directly—binding to its receptors [VDR] on pancreatic β cells, and indirectly by modulating concentration of calcium in extracellular space [40].

Importantly, a positive association between the concentration of vitamin D and sensitivity to insulin was observed in obese children, along with an inverse relationship between the level of this vitamin and concentration of glycated hemoglobin (HbA1c) [41]. Supplementation with vitamin D in obese adolescents resulted in decrease of insulin resistance, while levels of inflammatory markers [CRP, TNF–α, IL–6] remained unchanged [42]. Till now, to the best of our knowledge, no studies were carried out in children or adolescents regarding the effects of vitamin D supplementation on body mass reduction during an organized lifestyle modification program. As we presented, adding a 1200 IU/day dose of vitamin D did not lead to higher changes in BMI (BMI centile) or fat mass as well as fat free mass changes in children aged 6–14. It needs to be stated that the results presented show that although there was a reduction in BMI in vitamin D group compared to placebo group (–0.46 ± 1.80 vs. 0.11 ±1.84) and BMI centiles also showed higher reduction in children supplemented with vitamin D (–4.28 ± 8.43 vs. –2.53 ±6.10) none of those results was statistically significant ($p = 0.203$ and $p = 0.319$ respectively). Similar results can be found in bioimpedance measurements, but not DXA assessment. Presented results would be presented as clinically valid. Although this 26-week long supplementation had an influence on blood concentration level of 25(OH) D in the active treatment group, only 6 out of all patients reached a level above 30 ng/ml in the final assessment (2 in the placebo group) 52 weeks after the start of the intervention. This shows that vitamin D can potentially have an impact on weight loss level but possibly due to resignation ratio or sample size we were not able to show that effect.

As previous studies in adolescents and adults showed, low (~1000 IU/daily) or high doses (up to 300,000 IU/month) of vitamin D supplementation have a very mixed results in influencing changes in fat mass, free fat mass or muscle mass [43–45]. Data regarding effect of vitamin D supplementation on body mass/body fat changes are limited to studies and meta–analyses/ reviews regarding adults with wide range of interventions (medical weight loss, bariatric surgery, low–caloric diet) were used together with vitamin D supplementation. Additionally those studies were focused on finding the optimal dose of supplementation to reach the optimal (>30 ng/l) level of vitamin D [44] or assessing the association of vitamin level and body fat. Meta-analysis of studies in obese adults showed that although there was an impact of vitamin D supplementation on body fat, the results were not statistically significant [43]. This study also acknowledges that the impact of vitamin D supplementation on body fat reduction has a linear effect up to 2000 IU/d, with no benefits in increasing the dose in adults. The only review regarding impact of vitamin D supplementation on bone mineral density was focused on general population—as no studies was directly focused on overweight/obese children. In addition, no sub–analysis was performed to show the effect depending on body mass. Winzenberg states that the impact of vitamin D supplementation can be higher in vitamin D deficient children, but the effect is small—in most studies standardized mean difference between groups was small (<0,3) [45]. Yet all of these measures are only proxy measures to changes in body weight as a primary outcome of supplementation of vitamin D in obese children/adolescents. As for now, no studies have demonstrated effectiveness of such a strategy for supporting body fat reduction throughout a long–term interventional process.

4.2. *Effect of Vitamin D Supplementation on Bone Mineral Density During Weight Loss*

Metabolic effects of obesity on growth and maturation of bones are still not fully understood. Moreover, the results of previous studies analyzing bone mass and density in obese individuals are highly inconclusive. While some authors claimed a decrease in bone mass relative to body weight [46], others did not document significant differences in bone mineral density [47] or showed an increase in body mass and bone size in obese children, adolescents and adults. Increased bone mass and density observed in obese individuals is postulated to be a response to greater mechanical load, direct influence of leptin or enhanced enzymatic activity of aromatase [48,49]. Nevertheless, obesity markedly increases the risk of bone fractures in children [50]. Vitamin D plays important biological role in the process of bone maturation and mineralization. Previous studies documented an inverse relationship between blood concentration of vitamin D and bone mineral density [51,52]. One meta–analysis revealed that supplementation of vitamin D can improve both bone mineral density and bone mass in individuals with low blood levels of this vitamin [45]. The effects of supplementation are particularly favorable in premenarcheal girls with normal body weight, in whom administration of vitamin D resulted in increases of both bone mass and fat–free mass [53]. An analysis of 58 morbidly obese teenagers showed that individuals with physiological blood concentration of PTH (parathyroid hormone) have normal bone mineral density, irrespectively of their vitamin D levels [54]. In contrast, a recently published study involving a small group of adolescents with obesity (n = 24) and normal body weight (n = 25) showed that obese people present with higher bone mineral density, irrespectively their blood concentration of vitamin D and despite lower level of physical activity than their normal-weight peers. Moreover, the differences in bone mineral density turned out to be independent from fat-free mass content. Furthermore, bone mineral density was associated with blood concentrations of leptin and insulin [55]. Our study shows clearly that we can observe an increase of bone mineral density both spinal and subtotal BMD with body mass reduction. Yet there is no impact of vitamin D supplementation on the level of bone density assessed using DXA. This shows that the body mass reduction itself impacts the bone mineralization the most.

Apart from many unquestioned favorable health effects of losing excessive weight, this process may also be associated with enhanced bone turnover and decrease in bone mineral density. In recently published systemic review, the decrease of bone mass was reported following calorie-restricting diet but not in exercise–induced weight-loss [56]. However, this evidence originates mostly from studies conducted among adults [57–59], and to the best of our knowledge, the issue in question was a subject of only one study of adolescents after bariatric surgeries [60]. The results from previous intervention studies suggest that a low-calorie albeit high-protein (ca. 30%) diet, containing high amounts of dairy products, can prevent the loss of bone mass and a decrease in bone mineralization [61]. Yet supplementation with high doses of vitamin D can have a negative effect on bone mineralization in adults—as a recent study by Burt et al. showed [62].

Study limitations:

This study has some limitations that need to be taken into account when assessing the usefulness of the results:

– Children aged 6–14 years old were included in the study—this is not a homogenic group when it comes to maturation/puberty status—and this has an impact on both the ability to decrease body mass and bone turnover and mineralization;

– We were giving one dose of vitamin D (1200 IU) to all participants independent the body mass and age, which could have result in less effective increase of 25(OH)D level, which in turn could have impacted the changes in body mass or bone mineral density;

– 26 weeks may be too short to establish the effects of vitamin D supplementation on the rate of skeletal mineralization

– There was an almost 30% drop–out, seen especially in the second part of the program—after finishing the active supplementation with vitamin D/placebo period. This was unlikely to be due to the treatment itself (as there were no important side effects registered). The level of lost to follow-up patients in the interventional program is similar to other such programs seen in Poland and other European countries [63,64].

– Finally, the sample sizes were smaller than anticipated and there is a possibility that with the estimated reduction of 10% of BMI reduction the study sample is underestimated. It is possible that the study was underpowered to detect smaller changes in BMI/BMI centiles as well as other parameters.

5. Conclusions

Available data on the efficacy of vitamin supplementation during weight loss are inconclusive and mostly limited to adults. Our study shows that there is a limited or no effect of vitamin D supplementation on body weight reduction in children and adolescents with vitamin D insufficiency. Being aware and understanding the potential limitation of our study—wide age group, one dose of vitamin D, small sample of the study we believe that further research in this field is needed.

Author Contributions: M.B. participated in the study design and coordination of the study, performed the statistical data analysis, drafted the paper and revised and approved the manuscript; A.J., M.S.-F., P.M., and P.W. participated in the study design, patient recruitment, data collection, revised and approved the manuscript; P.S. participated in the study design and revised and approved the manuscript; A.S.-S. participated in the study design and coordination of the study, data analysis, drafted, revised and approved the manuscript. All authors have read and agreed to the published version of the manuscript.

Acknowledgments: All authors would like to sincerely thank all participant, parents and members of the "6–10–14 for Health" team for their input into the study. Authors would also like to thank University Clinical Centre administration for help in performing the study.

References

1. Bentham, J.; Di Cesare, M.; Bilano, V.; Bixby, H.; Zhou, B.; Stevens, G.A.; Riley, L.M.; Taddei, C.; Hajifathalian, K.; Lu, Y.; et al. Worldwide trends in body-mass index, underweight, overweight, and obesity from 1975 to 2016: A pooled analysis of 2416 population-based measurement studies in 128·9 million children, adolescents, and adults. *Lancet* **2017**, *390*, 2627–2642.

2. Ng, M.; Fleming, T.; Robinson, M.; Thomson, B.; Graetz, N.; Margono, C.; Mullany, E.C.; Biryukov, S.; Abbafati, C.; Abera, S.F.; et al. Global, regional, and national prevalence of overweight and obesity in children and adults during 1980–2013: A systematic analysis for the Global Burden of Disease Study 2013. *Lancet* **2014**, *384*, 766–781. [CrossRef]

3. Bann, D.; Johnson, W.; Li, L.; Kuh, D.; Hardy, R. Socioeconomic inequalities in childhood and adolescent body-mass index, weight, and height from 1953 to 2015: An analysis of four longitudinal, observational, British birth cohort studies. *Lancet Public Health* **2018**, *3*, e194–e203. [CrossRef]

4. Kumar, S.; Kelly, A.S. Review of Childhood Obesity: From Epidemiology, Etiology, and Comorbidities to Clinical Assessment and Treatment. *Mayo Clin. Proc.* **2017**, *92*, 251–265. [CrossRef] [PubMed]

5. Kelly, A.S.; Barlow, S.E.; Rao, G.; Inge, T.H.; Hayman, L.L.; Steinberger, J.; Urbina, E.M.; Ewing, L.J.; Daniels, S.R. Severe obesity in children and adolescents: Identification, associated health risks, and treatment approaches: A scientific statement from the American Heart Association. *Circulation* **2013**, *128*, 1689–1712. [CrossRef] [PubMed]

6. Kinlen, D.; Cody, D.; O'Shea, D. Complications of obesity. *QJM An Int. J. Med.* **2018**, *111*, 437–443. [CrossRef]

7. Di Angelantonio, E.; Bhupathiraju, S.; Wormser, D.; Gao, P.; Kaptoge, S.; Berrington de Gonzalez, A.; Cairns, B.; Huxley, R.; Jackson, C.; et al.; Global BMI Mortality Collaboration Body-mass index and all-cause mortality: Individual-participant-data meta-analysis of 239 prospective studies in four continents. *Lancet* **2016**, *388*, 776–786. [CrossRef]

8. Brown, T.; Moore, T.H.; Hooper, L.; Gao, Y.; Zayegh, A.; Ijaz, S.; Elwenspoek, M.; Foxen, S.C.; Magee, L.; O'Malley, C.; et al. Interventions for preventing obesity in children. *Cochrane Database Syst. Rev.* **2019**, *2019*. [CrossRef]
9. Nemet, D.; Levi, L.; Pantanowitz, M.; Eliakim, A. A combined nutritional-behavioral-physical activity intervention for the treatment of childhood obesity—A 7-year summary. *J. Pediatr. Endocrinol. Metab.* **2014**, *27*, 445–451. [CrossRef]
10. Oude Luttikhuis, H.; Baur, L.; Jansen, H.; Shrewsbury, V.A.; O'Malley, C.; Stolk, R.P.; Summerbell, C.D. Interventions for treating obesity in children. *Cochrane Database Syst. Rev.* **2019**, *3*, CD001872. [CrossRef]
11. Masquio, D.C.L.; De Piano, A.; Campos, R.M.S.; Sanches, P.L.; Carnier, J.; Corgosinho, F.C.; Netto, B.D.M.; Carvalho-Ferreira, J.P.; Oyama, L.M.; Nascimento, C.M.O.; et al. The role of multicomponent therapy in the metabolic syndrome, inflammation and cardiovascular risk in obese adolescents. *Br. J. Nutr.* **2015**, *113*, 1920–1930. [CrossRef] [PubMed]
12. Ferreira, Y.A.M.; Kravchychyn, A.C.P.; Vicente, S.d.C.F.; Campos, R.M.d.S.; Tock, L.; Oyama, L.M.; Boldarine, V.T.; Masquio, D.C.L.; Thivel, D.; Shivappa, N.; et al. An interdisciplinary weight loss program improves body composition and metabolic profile in adolescents with obesity: Associations with the dietary inflammatory index. *Front. Nutr.* **2019**, *6*, 77. [CrossRef] [PubMed]
13. Reinehr, T. Calculating cardiac risk in obese adolescents before and after onset of lifestyle intervention. *Expert Rev. Cardiovasc. Ther.* **2013**, *11*, 297–306. [CrossRef] [PubMed]
14. Masquio, D.C.L.; De Piano, A.; Sanches, P.L.; Corgosinho, F.C.; Campos, R.M.S.; Carnier, J.; Da Silva, P.L.; Caranti, D.A.; Tock, L.; Oyama, L.M.; et al. The effect of weight loss magnitude on pro-/anti-inflammatory adipokines and carotid intima-media thickness in obese adolescents engaged in interdisciplinary weight loss therapy. *Clin. Endocrinol.* **2013**, *79*, 55–64. [CrossRef]
15. Cuda, S.E.; Censani, M. Pediatric Obesity Algorithm: A Practical Approach to Obesity Diagnosis and Management. *Front. Pediatr.* **2019**, *6*, 431. [CrossRef]
16. Boland, C.L.; Harris, J.B.; Harris, K.B. Pharmacological Management of Obesity in Pediatric Patients. *Ann. Pharmacother.* **2015**, *49*, 220–232. [CrossRef]
17. Domecq, J.P.; Prutsky, G.; Leppin, A.; Sonbol, M.B.; Altayar, O.; Undavalli, C.; Wang, Z.; Elraiyah, T.; Brito, J.P.; Mauck, K.F.; et al. Drugs commonly associated with weight change: A systematic review and meta-analysis. *J. Clin. Endocrinol. Metab.* **2015**, *100*, 363–370. [CrossRef]
18. Pooyandjoo, M.; Nouhi, M.; Shab-Bidar, S.; Djafarian, K.; Olyaeemanesh, A. The effect of (L-)carnitine on weight loss in adults: A systematic review and meta-analysis of randomized controlled trials. *Obes. Rev.* **2016**, *17*, 970–976. [CrossRef]
19. Huang, J.; Wang, Y.; Xie, Z.; Zhou, Y.; Zhang, Y.; Wan, X. The anti-obesity effects of green tea in human intervention and basic molecular studies. *Eur. J. Clin. Nutr.* **2014**, *68*, 1075–1087. [CrossRef]
20. Kim, S.Y.; Oh, M.R.; Kim, M.G.; Chae, H.J.; Chae, S.W. Anti-obesity effects of Yerba Mate (Ilex Paraguariensis): A randomized, double-blind, placebo-controlled clinical trial. *BMC Complement. Altern. Med.* **2015**, *15*, 338. [CrossRef]
21. Zalewski, B.M.; Szajewska, H. No Effect of Glucomannan on Body Weight Reduction in Children and Adolescents with Overweight and Obesity: A Randomized Controlled Trial. *J. Pediatr.* **2019**, *211*, 85–91. [CrossRef] [PubMed]
22. De Luis, D.; Domingo, J.C.; Izaola, O.; Casanueva, F.F.; Bellido, D.; Sajoux, I. Effect of DHA supplementation in a very low-calorie ketogenic diet in the treatment of obesity: A randomized clinical trial. *Endocrine* **2016**, *54*, 111–122. [CrossRef] [PubMed]
23. Lerchbaum, E.; Trummer, C.; Theiler-Schwetz, V.; Kollmann, M.; Wölfler, M.; Pilz, S.; Obermayer-Pietsch, B. Effects of vitamin D supplementation on body composition and metabolic risk factors in men: A randomized controlled trial. *Nutrients* **2019**, *11*, 1894. [CrossRef] [PubMed]
24. Al-Daghri, N.M.; Amer, O.E.; Khattak, M.N.K.; Sabico, S.; Ghouse Ahmed Ansari, M.; Al-Saleh, Y.; Aljohani, N.; Alfawaz, H.; Alokail, M.S. Effects of different vitamin D supplementation strategies in reversing metabolic syndrome and its component risk factors in adolescents. *J. Steroid Biochem. Mol. Biol.* **2019**, *191*, 105378. [CrossRef] [PubMed]
25. Aypak, C.; Türedi, Ö.; Yüce, A. The association of vitamin D status with cardiometabolic risk factors, obesity and puberty in children. *Eur. J. Pediatr.* **2014**, *173*, 367–373. [CrossRef]

26. Lee, D.Y.; Kwon, A.R.; Ahn, J.M.; Kim, Y.J.; Chae, H.W.; Kim, D.H.; Kim, H.-S. Relationship between serum 25-hydroxyvitamin D concentration and risks of metabolic syndrome in children and adolescents from Korean National Health and Nutrition Examination survey 2008–2010. *Ann. Pediatr. Endocrinol. Metab.* **2015**, *20*, 46. [CrossRef]
27. Voortman, T.; van den Hooven, E.H.; Heijboer, A.C.; Hofman, A.; Jaddoe, V.W.; Franco, O.H. Vitamin D Deficiency in School-Age Children Is Associated with Sociodemographic and Lifestyle Factors. *J. Nutr.* **2015**, *145*, 791–798. [CrossRef]
28. Kamycheva, E.; Joakimsen, R.M.; Jorde, R. Intakes of Calcium and Vitamin D Predict Body Mass Index in the Population of Northern Norway. *J. Nutr.* **2003**, *133*, 102–106. [CrossRef]
29. Pourshahidi, L.K. Vitamin D and obesity: Current perspectives and future directions. In Proceedings of the Nutrition Society; Cambridge University Press: Cambridge, UK, 2015; Volume 74, pp. 115–124.
30. Engberg, E.; Figueiredo, R.A.O.; Rounge, T.B.; Weiderpass, E.; Viljakainen, H. Heavy screen users are the heaviest among 10,000 children. *Sci. Rep.* **2019**, *9*, 11158. [CrossRef]
31. Pacifico, L.; Anania, C.; Osborn, J.F.; Ferraro, F.; Bonci, E.; Olivero, E.; Chiesa, C. Low 25(OH)D3 levels are associated with total adiposity, metabolic syndrome, and hypertension in Caucasian children and adolescents. *Eur. J. Endocrinol.* **2011**, *165*, 603–611. [CrossRef]
32. Rosenstreich, S.J.; Rich, C.; Volwiler, W. Deposition in and release of vitamin D3 from body fat: Evidence for a storage site in the rat. *J. Clin. Invest.* **1971**, *50*, 679–687. [CrossRef] [PubMed]
33. Fu, J.; Han, L.; Zhao, Y.; Li, G.; Zhu, Y.; Li, Y.; Li, M.; Gao, S.; Willi, S.M. Vitamin D levels are associated with metabolic syndrome in adolescents and young adults: The BCAMS study. *Clin. Nutr.* **2019**, *38*, 2161–2167. [CrossRef] [PubMed]
34. Denova-Gutiérrez, E.; Muñoz-Aguirre, P.; López, D.; Flores, M.; Medeiros, M.; Tamborrel, N.; Clark, P. Low serum vitamin D concentrations are associated with insulin resistance in Mexican children and adolescents. *Nutrients* **2019**, *11*, 2109. [CrossRef] [PubMed]
35. Mitri, J.; Nelson, J.; Ruthazer, R.; Garganta, C.; Nathan, D.M.; Hu, F.B.; Dawson-Hughes, B.; Pittas, A.G. Plasma 25-hydroxyvitamin D and risk of metabolic syndrome: An ancillary analysis in the Diabetes Prevention Program. *Eur. J. Clin. Nutr.* **2014**, *68*, 376–383. [CrossRef]
36. Szlagatys-Sidorkiewicz, A.; Brzeziński, M.; Jankowska, A.; Metelska, P.; Słomińska-Fraczek, M.; Socha, P. Long-term effects of vitamin D supplementation in vitamin D deficient obese children participating in an integrated weight-loss programme (a double-blind placebo-controlled study)—Rationale for the study design. *BMC Pediatr.* **2017**, *17*, 97. [CrossRef]
37. Kułaga, Z.; Litwin, M.; Tkaczyk, M.; Palczewska, I.; Zajączkowska, M.; Zwolińska, D.; Krynicki, T.; Wasilewska, A.; Moczulska, A.; Morawiec-Knysak, A.; et al. Polish 2010 growth references for school-aged children and adolescents. *Eur. J. Pediatr.* **2011**, *170*, 599–609. [CrossRef]
38. Reyman, M.; Verrijn Stuart, A.A.; Van Summeren, M.; Rakhshandehroo, M.; Nuboer, R.; De Boer, F.K.; Van Den Ham, H.J.; Kalkhoven, E.; Prakken, B.; Schipper, H.S. Vitamin D deficiency in childhood obesity is associated with high levels of circulating inflammatory mediators, and low insulin sensitivity. *Int. J. Obes.* **2014**, *38*, 46–52. [CrossRef]
39. Ganji, V.; Zhang, X.; Shaikh, N.; Tangpricha, V. Serum 25-hydroxyvitamin D concentrations are associated with prevalence of metabolic syndrome and various cardiometabolic risk factors in US children and adolescents based on assay-adjusted serum 25-hydroxyvitamin D data from NHANES 2001-2006. *Am. J. Clin. Nutr.* **2011**, *94*, 225–233. [CrossRef]
40. Song, Y.; Wang, L.; Pittas, A.G.; Del Gobbo, L.C.; Zhang, C.; Manson, J.E.; Hu, F.B. Blood 25-Hydroxy Vitamin D Levels and Incident Type 2 Diabetes. *Diabetes Care* **2013**, *36*, 1422–1428. [CrossRef]
41. Alemzadeh, R.; Kichler, J.; Babar, G.; Calhoun, M. Hypovitaminosis D in obese children and adolescents: Relationship with adiposity, insulin sensitivity, ethnicity, and season. *Metabolism* **2008**, *57*, 183–191. [CrossRef]
42. Belenchia, A.M.; Tosh, A.K.; Hillman, L.S.; Peterson, C.A. Correcting vitamin D insufficiency improves insulin sensitivity in obese adolescents: A randomized controlled trial. *Am. J. Clin. Nutr.* **2013**, *97*, 774–781. [CrossRef] [PubMed]
43. Golzarand, M.; Hollis, B.W.; Mirmiran, P.; Wagner, C.L.; Shab-Bidar, S. Vitamin D supplementation and body fat mass: A systematic review and meta-analysis. *Eur. J. Clin. Nutr.* **2018**, *72*, 1345–1357. [CrossRef]
44. Bassatne, A.; Chakhtoura, M.; Saad, R.; Fuleihan, G.E.H. Vitamin D supplementation in obesity and during weight loss: A review of randomized controlled trials. *Metabolism* **2019**, *92*, 193–205. [CrossRef] [PubMed]

45. Winzenberg, T.; Powell, S.; Shaw, K.A.; Jones, G. Effects of vitamin D supplementation on bone density in healthy children: Systematic review and meta-analysis. *BMJ* **2011**, *342*, 267. [CrossRef] [PubMed]

46. Goulding, A.; Taylor, R.W.; Jones, I.E.; McAuley, K.A.; Manning, P.J.; Williams, S.M. Overweight and obese children have low bone mass and area for their weight. *Int. J. Obes.* **2000**, *24*, 627–632. [CrossRef] [PubMed]

47. El Hage, R.; El Hage, Z.; Jacob, C.; Moussa, E.; Theunynck, D.; Baddoura, R. Bone Mineral Content and Density in Overweight and Control Adolescent Boys. *J. Clin. Densitom.* **2011'** *14*, 122–128. [CrossRef]

48. McVey, M.K.; Geraghty, A.A.; O'Brien, E.C.; McKenna, M.J.; Kilbane, M.T.; Crowley, R.K.; Twomey, P.J.; McAuliffe, F.M. The impact of diet, body composition, and physical activity on child bone mineral density at five years of age—Findings from the ROLO Kids Study. *Eur. J. Pediatr.* **2020**, *179*, 121–131. [CrossRef]

49. Rønne, M.S.; Heidemann, M.; Lylloff, L.; Schou, A.J.; Tarp, J.; Laursen, J.O.; Jørgensen, N.R.; Husby, S.; Wedderkopp, N.; Mølgaard, C. Bone Mass Development in Childhood and Its Association with Physical Activity and Vitamin D Levels. The CHAMPS-Study DK. *Calcif. Tissue Int.* **2019**, *104*, 1–13. [CrossRef]

50. Kessler, J.; Koebnick, C.; Smith, N.; Adams, A. Childhood obesity is associated with increased risk of most lower extremity fractures pediatrics. *Clin. Orthop. Relat. Res.* **2013**, *471*, 1199–1207. [CrossRef]

51. Cashman, K.D.; Hill, T.R.; Cotter, A.A.; Boreham, C.A.; Dubitzky, W.; Murray, L.; Strain, J.J.; Flynn, A.; Robson, P.J.; Wallace, J.M.; et al. Low vitamin D status adversely affects bone health parameters in adolescents 1-3. *Am. J. Clin. Nutr.* **2008**, *87*, 1039–1044. [CrossRef]

52. Pekkinen, M.; Viljakainen, H.; Saarnio, E.; Lamberg-Allardt, C.; Mäkitie, O. Vitamin D is a major determinant of bone mineral density at school age. *PLoS ONE* **2012**, *7*, e40090. [CrossRef] [PubMed]

53. Fuleihan, G.E.H.; Nabulsi, M.; Tamim, H.; Maalouf, J.; Salamoun, M.; Khalife, H.; Choucair, M.; Arabi, A.; Vieth, R. Effect of vitamin D replacement on musculoskeletal parameters in school children: A randomized controlled trial. *J. Clin. Endocrinol. Metab.* **2006**, *91*, 405–412. [CrossRef] [PubMed]

54. Lenders, C.M.; Feldman, H.A.; Von Scheven, E.; Merewood, A.; Sweeney, C.; Wilson, D.M.; Lee, P.D.K.; Abrams, S.H.; Gitelman, S.E.; Wertz, M.S.; et al. Relation of body fat indexes to vitamin D status and deficiency among obese adolescents. *Am. J. Clin. Nutr.* **2009** *90*, 459–467. [PubMed]

55. Maggio, A.B.R.; Belli, D.C.; Puigdefabregas, J.W.B.; Rizzoli, R.; Farpour-Lambert, N.J.; Beghetti, M.; McLin, V.A. High bone density in adolescents with obesity is related to fat mass and serum leptin concentrations. *J. Pediatr. Gastroenterol. Nutr.* **2014**, *58*, 723–728. [PubMed]

56. Soltani, S.; Hunter, G.R.; Kazemi, A.; Shab-Bidar, S. The effects of weight loss approaches on bone mineral density in adults: A systematic review and meta-analysis of randomized controlled trials. *Osteoporos. Int.* **2016**, *27*, 2655–2671. [CrossRef]

57. Rector, R.S.; Loethen, J.; Ruebel, M.; Thomas, T.R.; Hinton, P.S. Serum markers of bone turnover are increased by modest weight loss with or without weight-bearing exercise in overweight premenopausal women. *Appl. Physiol. Nutr. Metab.* **2009**, *34*, 933–941. [CrossRef]

58. Lindeman, K.G.; Greenblatt, L.B.; Rourke, C.; Bouxsein, M.L.; Finkelstein, J.S.; Yu, E.W. Longitudinal 5-year evaluation of bone density and microarchitecture after Roux-en-Y gastric bypass surgery. *J. Clin. Endocrinol. Metab.* **2018**, *103*, 4104–4112. [CrossRef]

59. Elaine, W.Y.; Bouxsein, M.L.; Putman, M.S.; Monis, E.L.; Roy, A.E.; Pratt, J.S.A.; Butsch, W.S.; Finkelstein, J.S. Two-year changes in bone density after Roux-en-Y gastric bypass surgery. *J. Clin. Endocrinol. Metab.* **2015**, *100*, 1452–1459.

60. Kaulfers, A.M.D.; Bean, J.A.; Inge, T.H.; Dolan, L.M.; Kalkwarf, H.J. Bone loss in adolescents after bariatric surgery. *Pediatrics* **2011**, *127*, e956–e961. [CrossRef]

61. Labouesse, M.A.; Gertz, E.R.; Piccolo, B.D.; Souza, E.C.; Schuster, G.U.; Witbracht, M.G.; Woodhouse, L.R.; Adams, S.H.; Keim, N.L.; Van Loan, M.D. Associations among endocrine, inflammatory, and bone markers, body composition and weight loss induced bone loss. *Bone* **2014**, *64*, 138–146. [CrossRef]

62. Burt, L.A.; Billington, E.O.; Rose, M.S.; Raymond, D.A.; Hanley, D.A.; Boyd, S.K. Effect of high-dose vitamin D supplementation on volumetric bone density and bone strength: A randomized clinical trial. *JAMA J. Am. Med. Assoc.* **2019**, *322*, 736–745. [CrossRef] [PubMed]

63. Inelmen, E.M.; Toffanello, E.D.; Enzi, G.; Gasparini, G.; Miotto, F.; Sergi, G.; Busetto, L. Predictors of drop-out in overweight and obese outpatients. *Int. J. Obes.* **2005**, *29*, 122–128. [CrossRef] [PubMed]
64. Ortner Hadžiabdić, M.; Mucalo, I.; Hrabač, P.; Matić, T.; Rahelić, D.; Božikov, V. Factors predictive of drop-out and weight loss success in weight management of obese patients. *J. Hum. Nutr. Diet.* **2015**, *28*, 24–32. [CrossRef] [PubMed]

3

Differential and Overlapping Effects of 20,23(OH)$_2$D3 and 1,25(OH)$_2$D3 on Gene Expression in Human Epidermal Keratinocytes: Identification of AhR as an Alternative Receptor for 20,23(OH)$_2$D3

Andrzej T. Slominski [1,2,3,*], Tae-Kang Kim [1], Zorica Janjetovic [1], Anna A. Brożyna [4,5], Michal A. Żmijewski [6], Hui Xu [1], Thomas R. Sutter [7], Robert C. Tuckey [8], Anton M. Jetten [9] and David K. Crossman [10]

1 Department of Dermatology, University of Alabama at Birmingham, Birmingham, AL 35294, USA; tkim@uabmc.edu (T.-K.K.); zjanjetovic@uabmc.edu (Z.J.); huixu@uabmc.edu (H.X.)

2 Comprehensive Cancer Center, Cancer Chemoprevention Program, University of Alabama at Birmingham, Birmingham, AL 35294, USA

3 Veteran Administration Medical Center, Birmingham, AL 35294, USA

4 Department of Medical Biology, Faculty of Biology and Environment Protection, Nicolaus Copernicus University, 87-100 Toruń, Poland; brozyna.anna@gmail.com

5 Department of Tumor Pathology and Pathomorphology, Oncology Centre-Prof. Franciszek Łukaszczyk Memorial Hospital, 85-796 Bydgoszcz, Poland

6 Department of Histology, Medical University of Gdańsk, 80-211 Gdańsk, Poland; mzmijewski@gumed.edu.pl

7 Feinstone Center for Genomic Research, University of Memphis, Memphis, TN 38152 USA; tsutter@memphis.edu

8 School of Molecular Sciences, The University of Western Australia, Perth, WA 6009, Australia; robert.tuckey@uwa.edu.au

9 Immunity, Inflammation, and Disease Laboratory/Cell Biology Group, National Institute of Environmental Health Sciences, NIH, Research Triangle Park, NC 27709, USA; jetten@niehs.nih.gov

10 Howell and Elizabeth Heflin Center for Human Genetics, Genomic Core Facility, University of Alabama at Birmingham, Birmingham, AL 35294, USA; dcrossman@uabmc.edu

* Correspondence: aslominski@uabmc.edu

Abstract: A novel pathway of vitamin D activation by CYP11A has previously been elucidated. To define the mechanism of action of its major dihydroxy-products, we tested the divergence and overlap between the gene expression profiles of human epidermal keratinocytes treated with either CYP11A1-derived 20,23(OH)$_2$D3 or classical 1,25(OH)$_2$D3. Both secosteroids have significant chemical similarity with the only differences being the positions of the hydroxyl groups. mRNA was isolated and examined by microarray analysis using Illumina's HumanWG-6 chip/arrays and subsequent bioinformatics analyses. Marked differences in the up- and downregulated genes were observed between 1,25(OH)$_2$D3- and 20,23(OH)$_2$D3-treated cells. Hierarchical clustering identified both distinct, opposite and common (overlapping) gene expression patterns. *CYP24A1* was a common gene strongly activated by both compounds, a finding confirmed by qPCR. Ingenuity pathway analysis identified VDR/RXR signaling as the top canonical pathway induced by 1,25(OH)$_2$D3. In contrast, the top canonical pathway induced by 20,23(OH)$_2$D3 was AhR, with VDR/RXR being the second nuclear receptor signaling pathway identified. QPCR analyses validated the former finding by revealing that 20,23(OH)$_2$D3 stimulated *CYP1A1* and *CYP1B1* gene expression, effects located downstream of AhR. Similar stimulation was observed with 20(OH)D3, the precursor to 20,23(OH)$_2$D3, as well as with its downstream metabolite, 17,20,23(OH)$_3$D3. Using a Human AhR Reporter Assay System we showed marked activation of AhR activity by 20,23(OH)$_2$D3, with weaker stimulation by 20(OH)D3. Finally, molecular modeling using an AhR LBD model predicted vitamin D3 hydroxyderivatives to be good ligands for this receptor. Thus, our microarray, qPCR, functional studies and molecular modeling indicate that AhR is the major receptor target for 20,23$(OH)_2$D3, opening an exciting area of investigation on the interaction of different vitamin D3-hydroxyderivatives with AhR and the subsequent downstream activation of signal transduction pathways in a cell-type-dependent manner.

Keywords: vitamin D; dihydroxyvitamin D; epidermal keratinocytes; nuclear receptor signaling; microarray

---

1. Introduction

Vitamin D3 (D3) is formed by ultraviolet B radiation (UVB)-mediated breaking of the B ring of 7-dehydrocholesterol (7DHC) followed by thermal isomerization of the resulting pre-vitamin D3 to D3 [1,2]. The vast majority of circulating D3 is generated in epidermal keratinocytes [3]. D3 is a prohormone that is activated by sequential hydroxylations at C25 (by CYP2R1 or CYP27A1) and C1α (by CYP27B1) to 1,25-dihydroxyvitamin D3 (1,25$(OH)_2$D3), the hormonally active form, referred to as the canonical pathway [4–7]. At the systemic level, C25 hydroxylation takes place in the liver with the resulting 25(OH)D3 being hydroxylated at C1α in kidneys [3–7]. The same pathway operates in peripheral tissues including epidermal keratinocytes, the major site of D3 formation [1].

In addition to the canonical pathway of vitamin D activation described above, novel CYP11A-mediated pathways have been discovered (reviewed in [8]). Specifically, CYP11A1, the first enzyme of steroidogenesis that hydroxylates and then cleaves the side chain of cholesterol to produce pregnenolone (reviewed in [9,10]), can also hydroxylate and cleave the side chain of 7DHC, and hydroxylate the side chain of D3 and D2 without cleavage [11–16]. The two major products of CYP11A1 action on D3, with defined stereochemistry, are 20*S*-hydroxyvitamin D3 (20(OH)D3) and 20*S*,23*S*-dihydroxyvitamin D3 (20,23$(OH)_2$D3) [17]. These pathways operate in cultured epidermal, human and pig keratinocytes, dermal fibroblasts, colon cancer cells, and have also been described ex vivo for placenta and adrenal glands [18–23]. Importantly, the major products of these pathways are detectable in vivo in human serum, epidermis and adrenal glands [24].

The classical, hormonally-active dihydroxy form of vitamin D3, 1,25$(OH)_2$D3, in addition to playing a fundamental role in body calcium and phosphorous homeostasis and in the proper functioning of the skeletomuscular system, has pleiotropic effects on different organs and cell functions (reviewed in [3,6,25–29]). These studies show that 1,25$(OH)_2$D3 has immunomodulatory properties, is involved in the regulation of reproduction, pregnancy, child development, neurodevelopment, regulation of global metabolic and endocrine homeostasis and functions of the cardiovascular system, and has anticancer activities (reviewed in [2,6,30–50]). At the cellular level, it regulates proliferation, differentiation, apoptosis, senescence, metabolism, migration, secretory activities, and protective and reparative mechanisms against oxidative stress and radiation. It is widely accepted that these functions are regulated by different signal transduction pathways initiated by 1,25$(OH)_2$D3 binding to the vitamin D receptor (VDR) at the genomic binding site, and to some degree at a nongenomic binding site, in a cell-type dependent manner (reviewed [6,45–47,51–54]). In the skin, 1,25$(OH)_2$D3 regulates the epidermal barrier and hair cycling and has radioprotective, anti-cancer and anti-inflammatory properties [1,3,52,53,55–59].

The novel secosteroids, produced by the non-canonical activation pathways initiated by CYP11A1, inhibit the proliferation of epidermal keratinocytes, melanocytes and dermal fibroblasts and promote the differentiation of keratinocytes. Furthermore, they inhibit fibrotic activities of fibroblasts and have immunomodulatory properties (reviewed in [19,49,60]). Importantly, 20(OH)D3 and 20,23$(OH)_2$D3 are non-calcemic at pharmacological doses [61–63] which is in contrast to the highly calcemic effects of 1,25$(OH)_2$D3 and 25(OH)D3. 20(OH)D3 and 20,23$(OH)_2$D3 also attenuate the symptoms of skin fibrosis, rheumatoid arthritis and have photoprotective properties [8,19,23,64,65]. The CYP11A1-derived secosteroids have pleiotropic phenotypic effects that are cell-type–dependent [19,23,60–62,65–75]. They can act as biased agonists of the VDR [19,60,76,77] and can act as inverse agonists on retinoic acid orphan receptors (ROR) α and γ [60,78].

To better define the signaling pathways and mechanisms underlying the similarities and differences between phenotypic activities of classical 1,25(OH)$_2$D3 and the major dihydroxy product of CYP11A1 action on vitamin D3, 20,23(OH)$_2$D3, we examined and compared the gene expression profiles of human keratinocytes exposed to these secosteroids. Bioinformatics analysis was performed and differences and similarities in the activities of these structurally similar but distinct dihydroxy-D3 species were compared.

2. Results and Discussion

The structures and sequences of the reactions producing 1,25(OH)$_2$D3 and 20,23(OH)$_2$D3 in the epidermis are shown in Figure 1.

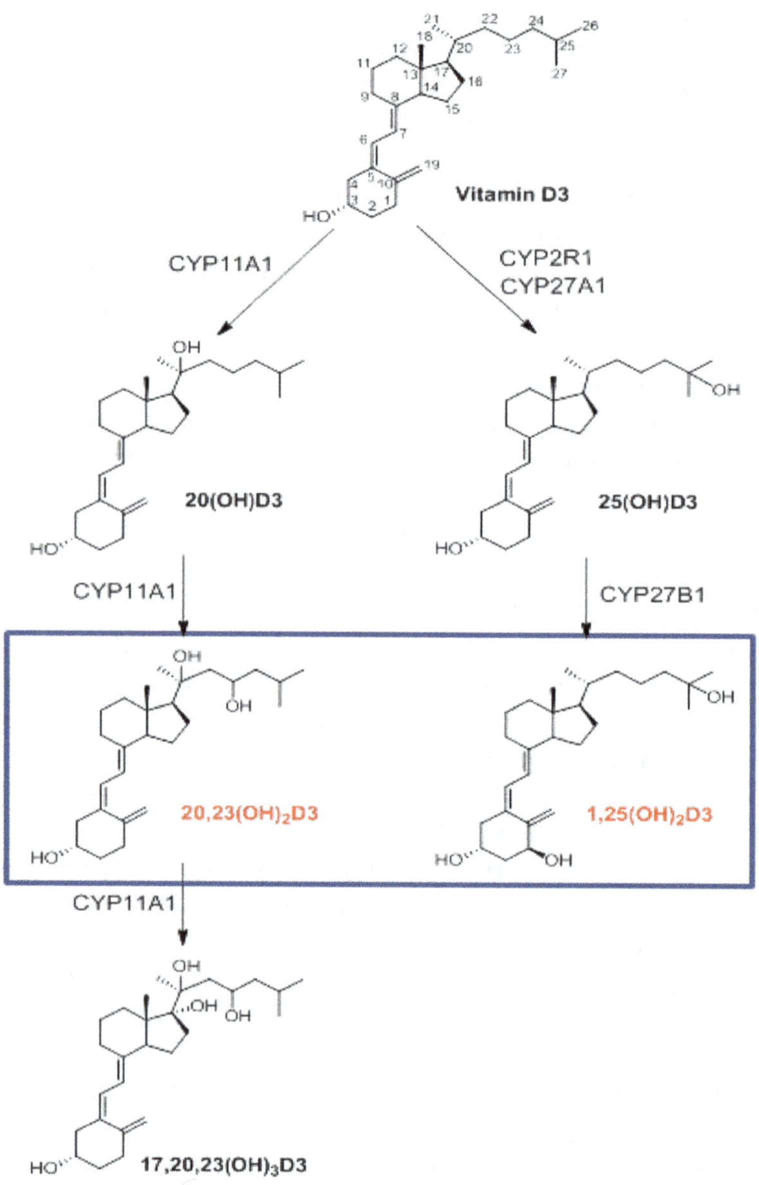

Figure 1. Epidermal pathways of vitamin D3 activation to produce 1,25(OH)$_2$D3 and 20,23(OH)$_2$D3 and the downstream metabolite 17,20,23(OH)$_3$D3. The rectangle marks the secosteroids used for microarray analyses.

The schematic outline of the experimental design is presented in Figure 2. Briefly, to test the divergence and overlap between the gene expression patterns, human neonatal epidermal keratinocytes combined from four African-American [79] donors were treated with 1,25$(OH)_2$D3 or 20,23$(OH)_2$D3 for 6 or 24 h. Microarray assays were performed using Illumina's HumanWG-6_V2 (Platform GPL13376) chip/array as described in Materials and Methods and the raw data has been deposited at the NCBI GEO (GSE117351).

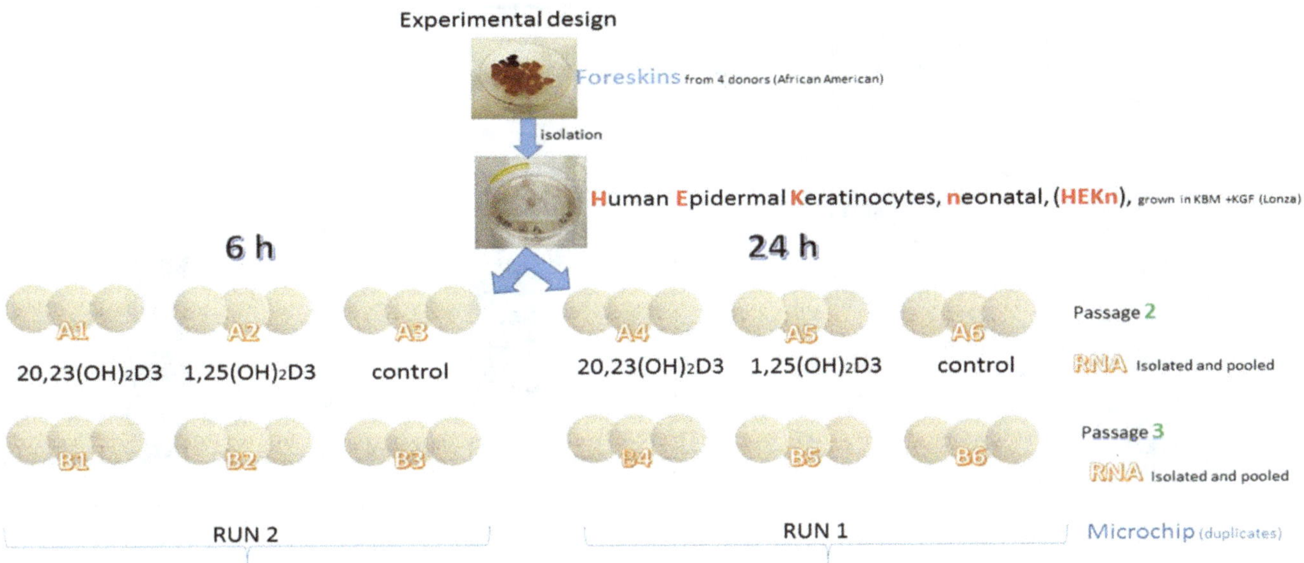

Figure 2. Outline of the experimental design.

The relative changes in gene expression (average of two independent experiments that used triplicate cell cultures), were normalized vs. vehicle control (0.1% ethanol). Table 1 shows marked differences in the number of genes up- or downregulated by either 1,25$(OH)_2$D3 or 20,23$(OH)_2$D3 using 1.5-, 2- and 4-fold cut-off values (FC). Average signal values for filtered gene clusters with FC $\geq \pm 1.5$ are shown in Supplemental excel file #1. Briefly, treatment with 1,25$(OH)_2$D3 for 6 h leads to changes in the expression of 148 vs. 37 genes for 20,23$(OH)_2$D3 when using 1.5-FC, and 38 vs. 21 and 3 vs. 0 when using 2- and 4-FC, respectively. After 24 h, this trend changed to 410 and 4079 genes regulated, respectively, by 1,25$(OH)_2$D3 and 20,23$(OH)_2$D3 with 1.5-FC value, and 119 and 1611 for 2-FC value and 12 and 199 genes for 4-FC value, respectively (Table 1).

Table 1. Number of genes up or downregulated in keratinocytes by 1,25$(OH)_2$D3 or 20,23$(OH)_2$D3 in comparison to vehicle control using 1.5-, 2- and 4-fold cut-off values.

Time	Genes	1,25$(OH)_2$D3			20,23$(OH)_2$D3		
		>1.5-Fold	>2-Fold	>4-Fold	>1.5-Fold	>2-Fold	>4-Fold
6 h	Upregulated	116	35	3	33	21	0
	Downregulated	32	3	0	4	0	0
24 h	Upregulated	266	98	12	2013	763	98
	Downregulated	144	21	0	2066	848	101

Hierarchical clustering identified patterns of genes responding to either 1,25$(OH)_2$D3 or 20,23$(OH)_2$D3, or to both. Selected gene clusters, representing the altered expression after 6 h of incubation as well as Venn diagrams are shown in Figure 3A. The heat maps corresponding to relative gene expression levels displayed both distinct or opposite, or common (overlapping) gene expression. For 2-FC there was only 1 common gene (CYP24A1) stimulated by both 1,25$(OH)_2$D3 (82 fold) and 20,23$(OH)_2$D3 (3.4 fold). This differential stimulation of CYP24A1 was further confirmed by qPCR

(Figure 3B) and is consistent with the literature on 1,25(OH)$_2$D3 [1,3,6,27,51] and 20,23(OH)$_2$D3 [69,80]. For 1.5-FC there were two common genes, CYP24A1 and the gene with a target id ILMN_131812 (identified as small ILF3/NF90-associated RNA A1 (SNAR-A1)), for which expression was stimulated.

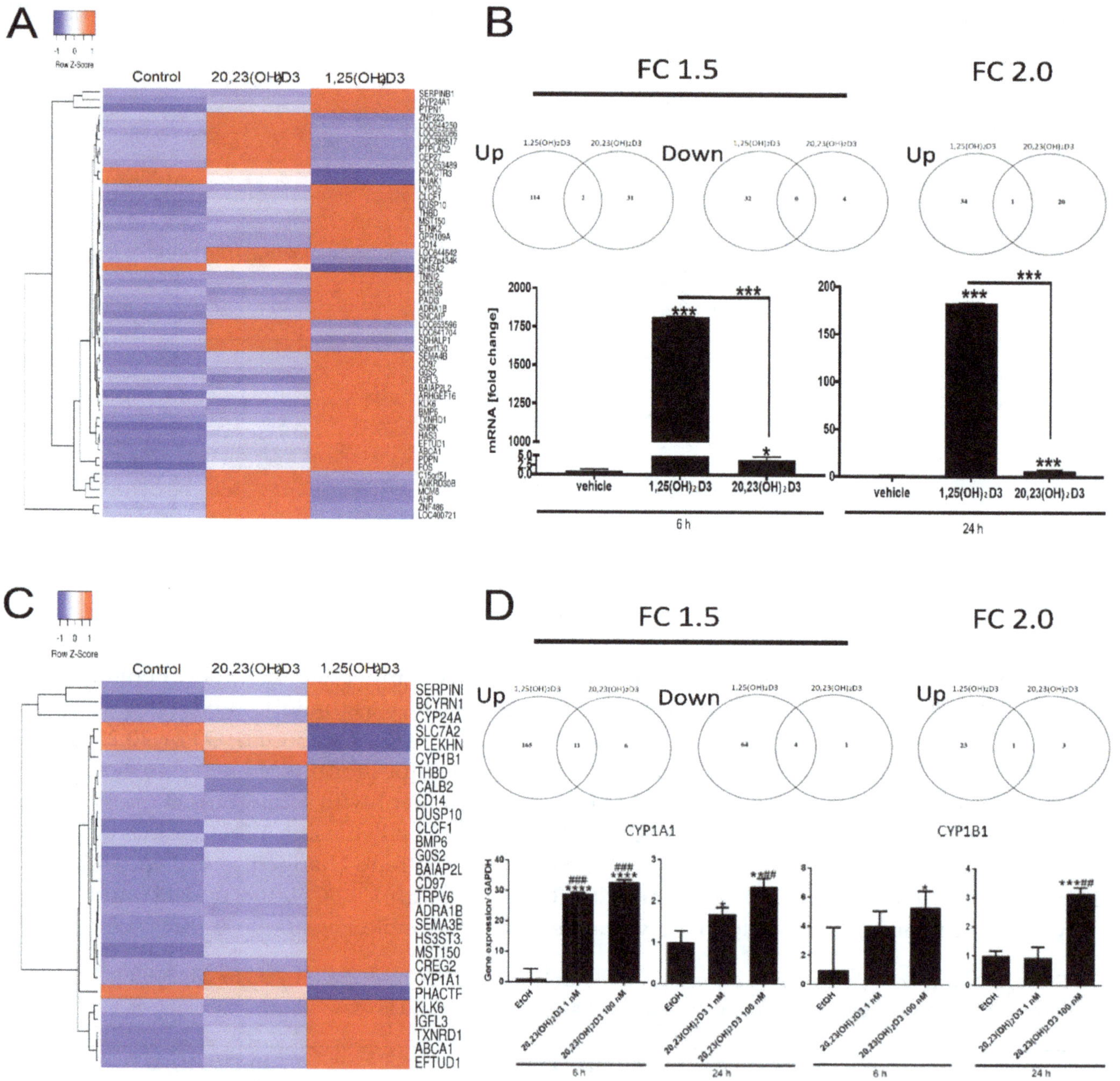

Figure 3. Changes in gene expression in human epidermal keratinocytes treated with 1,25(OH)$_2$D3 or 20,23(OH)$_2$D3 for 6 h. (**A**) Heat map of the gene expression pattern for experiment #1 with corresponding Venn diagrams for FC ≥ 2 and 1.5. (**B**) Effect of 10^{-7} M of 1,25(OH)$_2$D3 or 20,23(OH)$_2$D3 on *CYP24A1* expression in keratinocytes after 6 and 24 h treatment. (**C**) Heat map of the gene expression pattern for experiment #2 with corresponding Venn diagrams for FC-2 and 1.5. (**D**) Effect of 10^{-9} and 10^{-7} M of 20,23(OH)$_2$D3 on CYP1A1 and CYP1B1 expression in keratinocytes after 6 or 24 h treatment. Data represent means $\pm$ SD ($n = 3$) where * $p < 0.05$, ** $p < 0.01$, *** $p < 0.001$ and **** $p < 0.0001$ at student t-test; ## $p < 0.01$ and ### $p < 0.001$ at one-way ANOVA test.

Ingenuity pathway analysis using FC $\geq \pm 1.5$ was performed. The top canonical pathway induced by 1,25(OH)$_2$D3 was VDR/RXR signaling (Table 2) (Supplemental Figure S1A), which was expected [3,6,51,81,82]. This was followed by the roles of osteoblasts, osteoclasts and chondrocytes in rheumatoid arthritis; the role of macrophages, fibroblasts and endothelial cells in rheumatoid arthritis; and Toll-like receptor signaling (Table 2), which is consistent with previously reported functions of 1,25(OH)$_2$D3 [3,6,30,31,45,51,54]. Interestingly, the next top nuclear receptor signaling pathway activated by 1,25(OH)$_2$D3 was linked to the glucocorticoid receptor (GR) followed by the aryl hydrocarbon receptor [74], PPAR, PPARα/RXRα, LXR/RXR, and RAR (Table 2). The inclusion of these additional pathways could be secondary to the use of the same dimeric partner, RXR, and communication between receptors, or alternatively by activation by signaling pathways downstream of VDR. For example, it is already known that 1,25(OH)$_2$D3 can selectively activate local elements of hypothalamo-pituitary adrenal axis in keratinocytes [71]. The significance of additional nuclear receptor signaling is out of the scope of this paper and is a goal of our future research.

Table 2. Canonical pathways activated by 1,25(OH)$_2$D3 in human epidermal keratinocytes after 6 h of treatment. Nuclear receptors are marked in bold.

Ingenuity Canonical Pathways	*p*-Value	Overlap (%)	Downregulated	No Change	Upregulated	No Overlap with Dataset
VDR/RXR Activation	1.0×10^{-10}	12.8	34/78 (44%)	0/78 (0%)	43/78 (55%)	1/78 (1%)
Role of Osteoblasts, Osteoclasts and Chondrocytes in Rheumatoid Arthritis	2.2×10^{-7}	5.02	100/219 (46%)	0/219 (0%)	114/219 (52%)	5/219 (2%)
Role of Macrophages, Fibroblasts and Endothelial Cells in Rheumatoid Arthritis	4.4×10^{-6}	3.72	144/296 (49%)	0/296 (0%)	138/296 (47%)	14/296 (5%)
Toll-like Receptor Signaling	9.3×10^{-6}	8.11	39/74 (53%)	0/74 (0%)	33/74 (45%)	2/74 (3%)
Hepatic Cholestasis	1.2×10^{-5}	4.94	83/162 (51%)	0/162 (0%)	75/162 (46%)	4/162 (2%)
Glucocorticoid Receptor Signaling	1.5×10^{-5}	3.64	152/275 (55%)	0/275 (0%)	117/275 (43%)	6/275 (2%)
Role of Cytokines in Mediating Communication between Immune Cells	3.1×10^{-5}	9.09	32/55 (58%)	0/55 (0%)	20/55 (36%)	3/55 (5%)
IL-10 Signaling	8.5×10^{-5}	7.35	33/68 (49%)	0/68 (0%)	34/68 (50%)	1/68 (1%)
IL-6 Signaling	0.00012	5.17	57/116 (49%)	0/116 (0%)	59/116 (51%)	0/116 (0%)
p38 MAPK Signaling	0.000126	5.13	62/117 (53%)	0/117 (0%)	52/117 (44%)	3/117 (3%)
MIF Regulation of Innate Immunity	0.000151	9.76	19/41 (46%)	0/41 (0%)	21/41 (51%)	1/41 (2%)
Molecular Mechanisms of Cancer	0.000155	2.74	201/365 (55%)	0/365 (0%)	157/365 (43%)	7/365 (2%)
iNOS Signaling	0.0002	9.09	23/44 (52%)	0/44 (0%)	20/44 (45%)	1/44 (2%)
Aryl Hydrocarbon Receptor Signaling	0.000331	4.29	73/140 (52%)	0/140 (0%)	61/140 (44%)	6/140 (4%)
PPAR Signaling	0.000398	5.32	52/94 (55%)	0/94 (0%)	38/94 (40%)	4/94 (4%)
LPS/IL-1 Mediated Inhibition of RXR Function	0.000631	3.2	119/219 (54%)	0/219 (0%)	88/219 (40%)	12/219 (5%)
TNFR2 Signaling	0.000891	10.3	14/29 (48%)	0/29 (0%)	14/29 (48%)	1/29 (3%)
HMGB1 Signaling	0.001202	4.17	54/120 (45%)	0/120 (0%)	63/120 (53%)	3/120 (3%)
MIF-mediated Glucocorticoid Regulation	0.001318	9.09	16/33 (48%)	0/33 (0%)	16/33 (48%)	1/33 (3%)
ILK Signaling	0.001479	3.23	102/186 (55%)	0/186 (0%)	77/186 (41%)	7/186 (4%)
IL-17A Signaling in Fibroblasts	0.001549	8.57	20/35 (57%)	0/35 (0%)	15/35 (43%)	0/35 (0%)
Role of JAK2 in Hormone-like Cytokine Signaling	0.001549	8.57	18/35 (51%)	0/35 (0%)	14/35 (40%)	3/35 (9%)
PI3K Signaling in B Lymphocytes	0.001585	3.91	66/128 (52%)	0/128 (0%)	57/128 (45%)	5/128 (4%)

Table 2. *Cont.*

Ingenuity Canonical Pathways	*p*-Value	Overlap (%)	Downregulated	No Change	Upregulated	No Overlap with Dataset
Factors Promoting Cardiogenesis in Vertebrates	0.003236	4.35	52/92 (57%)	0/92 (0%)	37/92 (40%)	3/92 (3%)
TNFR1 Signaling	0.004169	6.12	27/49 (55%)	0/49 (0%)	20/49 (41%)	2/49 (4%)
Antioxidant Action of Vitamin C	0.004169	4.04	51/99 (52%)	0/99 (0%)	42/99 (42%)	6/99 (6%)
Acute Phase Response Signaling	0.005248	2.96	88/169 (52%)	0/169 (0%)	79/169 (47%)	2/169 (1%)
Differential Regulation of Cytokine Production in Macrophages and T Helper Cells by IL-17A and IL-17F	0.006166	11.1	7/18 (39%)	0/18 (0%)	11/18 (61%)	0/18 (0%)
PPARα/RXRα Activation	0.006607	2.79	98/179 (55%)	0/179 (0%)	67/179 (37%)	14/179 (8%)
Hepatic Fibrosis/Hepatic Stellate Cell Activation	0.007244	2.73	96/183 (52%)	0/183 (0%)	84/183 (46%)	3/183 (2%)
Type II Diabetes Mellitus Signaling	0.007586	3.42	50/117 (43%)	0/117 (0%)	64/117 (55%)	3/117 (3%)
Estrogen-Dependent Breast Cancer Signaling	0.008318	4.76	30/63 (48%)	0/63 (0%)	33/63 (52%)	0/63 (0%)
LXR/RXR Activation	0.008511	3.31	68/121 (56%)	0/121 (0%)	53/121 (44%)	0/121 (0%)
RAR Activation	0.008511	2.63	86/190 (45%)	0/190 (0%)	100/190 (53%)	4/190 (2%)

The top canonical nuclear receptor pathway induced by 20,23(OH)$_2$D3 was AhR signaling (Supplemental Figure S2A) with VDR/RXR being next (Supplemental Figure S3A) (Table 3). While the identification of the VDR/RXR as the target for 20,23(OH)$_2$D3 is consistent with previously reported functional data and molecular modeling [60,65,69,83], identification of the AhR as its primary target was unexpected and hence it was further analyzed in detail as described below. Table 4 shows that for 1,25(OH)$_2$D3 the nuclear signaling pathways VDR/RXR, followed by AhR, PPARα/RXRα, RAR and LXR/RXR, were among the top toxicity-related pathways identified. The top signaling pathways for 20,23(OH)$_2$D3 were linked to the activation of AhR and VDR/RXR (Table 5). Tables 6 and 7 show certain functional similarities between top diseases and bifunctions affected by both molecules. For example, cancer, and organismal injury and abnormalities, are the top two diseases affected by both molecules. These phenotypic similarities are consistent with previously reported studies comparing the biological effects of 1,25(OH)$_2$D3 and CYP11A1-derived D3-hydroxyderivatives, including 20,23(OH)$_2$D3, and indicate similarities between the effects on cell proliferation and differentiation, as well as similar anti-inflammatory, photoprotective and anti-cancer actions [23,60–62,64,72,80,84].

Table 3. Canonical pathways activated by 20,23(OH)$_2$D3 in human epidermal keratinocytes after 6 h of treatment. Nuclear receptors are marked in bold.

Ingenuity Canonical Pathways	*p*-Value	Overlap (%)	Downregulated	No Change	Upregulated	No Overlap with Dataset
2-ketoglutarate Dehydrogenase Complex	0.004898	25	2/4 (50%)	0/4 (0%)	2/4 (50%)	0/4 (0%)
Aryl Hydrocarbon Receptor Signaling	0.012589	1.43	64/140 (46%)	0/140 (0%)	70/140 (50%)	6/140 (4%)
Aldosterone Signaling in Epithelial Cells	0.014791	1.32	80/152 (53%)	0/152 (0%)	69/152 (45%)	3/152 (2%)
TCA Cycle II (Eukaryotic)	0.027542	4.35	14/23 (61%)	0/23 (0%)	9/23 (39%)	0/23 (0%)
Bupropion Degradation	0.0302	4	12/25 (48%)	0/25 (0%)	12/25 (48%)	1/25 (4%)
D-myo-inositol (1,4,5)-Trisphosphate Biosynthesis	0.032359	3.7	13/27 (48%)	0/27 (0%)	13/27 (48%)	1/27 (4%)

Table 3. *Cont.*

Ingenuity Canonical Pathways	*p*-Value	Overlap (%)	Downregulated	No Change	Upregulated	No Overlap with Dataset
Acetone Degradation I (to Methylglyoxal)	0.032359	3.7	13/27 (48%)	0/27 (0%)	13/27 (48%)	1/27 (4%)
Xenobiotic Metabolism Signaling	0.042658	0.738	133/271 (49%)	0/271 (0%)	122/271 (45%)	16/271 (6%)
Estrogen Biosynthesis	0.045709	2.63	17/38 (45%)	0/38 (0%)	20/38 (53%)	1/38 (3%)
Nicotine Degradation III	0.064565	1.85	23/54 (43%)	0/54 (0%)	22/54 (41%)	9/54 (17%)
Melatonin Degradation I	0.067608	1.75	25/57 (44%)	0/57 (0%)	24/57 (42%)	8/57 (14%)
Superpathway of Melatonin Degradation	0.072444	1.61	27/62 (44%)	0/62 (0%)	27/62 (44%)	8/62 (13%)
GM-CSF Signaling	0.072444	1.61	26/62 (42%)	0/62 (0%)	36/62 (58%)	0/62 (0%)
Nicotine Degradation II	0.074131	1.59	26/63 (41%)	0/63 (0%)	25/63 (40%)	12/63 (19%)
VDR/RXR Activation	0.091201	1.28	34/78 (44%)	0/78 (0%)	43/78 (55%)	1/78 (1%)
Acute Myeloid Leukemia Signaling	0.091201	1.27	39/79 (49%)	0/79 (0%)	38/79 (48%)	2/79 (3%)
TR/RXR Activation	0.097724	1.18	39/85 (46%)	0/85 (0%)	46/85 (54%)	0/85 (0%)
Regulation of Actin-based Motility by Rho	0.105196	1.1	45/91 (49%)	0/91 (0%)	39/91 (43%)	7/91 (8%)
Antioxidant Action of Vitamin C	0.114025	1.01	53/99 (54%)	0/99 (0%)	40/99 (40%)	6/99 (6%)
Rac Signaling	0.119399	0.962	47/104 (45%)	0/104 (0%)	55/104 (53%)	2/104 (2%)
Type I Diabetes Mellitus Signaling	0.125893	0.909	54/110 (49%)	1/110 (1%)	46/110 (42%)	9/110 (8%)
RhoA Signaling	0.138676	0.82	56/122 (46%)	0/122 (0%)	61/122 (50%)	5/122 (4%)
3-phosphoinositide Biosynthesis	0.175792	0.633	72/158 (46%)	0/158 (0%)	76/158 (48%)	10/158 (6%)
RhoGDI Signaling	0.190985	0.578	75/173 (43%)	0/173 (0%)	94/173 (54%)	4/173 (2%)
Superpathway of Inositol Phosphate Compounds	0.212814	0.513	87/195 (45%)	0/195 (0%)	96/195 (49%)	12/195 (6%)
Actin Cytoskeleton Signaling	0.233884	0.461	93/217 (43%)	0/217 (0%)	115/217 (53%)	9/217 (4%)
Signaling by Rho Family GTPases	0.249459	0.427	106/234 (45%)	0/234 (0%)	124/234 (53%)	4/234 (2%)
Protein Ubiquitination Pathway	0.268534	0.392	121/255 (47%)	0/255 (0%)	126/255 (49%)	8/255 (3%)

Table 4. Ingenuity toxicity list secondary to keratinocytes treatment with $1,25(OH)_2D3$ in humans for 6 h. Nuclear receptors are marked in bold.

Ingenuity Toxicity Lists	*p*-Value	Overlap (%)	Downregulated	No Change	Upregulated	No Overlap with Dataset
VDR/RXR Activation	1.0×10^{-10}	12.8	34/78 (44%)	0/78 (0%)	43/78 (55%)	1/78 (1%)
Hepatic Cholestasis	1.4×10^{-5}	4.85	85/165 (52%)	0/165 (0%)	76/165 (46%)	4/165 (2%)
Renal Necrosis/Cell Death	2.8×10^{-5}	2.59	241/501 (48%)	0/501 (0%)	242/501 (48%)	18/501 (4%)
Aryl Hydrocarbon Receptor Signaling	9.6×10^{-5}	4.35	79/161 (49%)	0/161 (0%)	67/161 (42%)	15/161 (9%)
Liver Necrosis/Cell Death	0.000525	2.87	131/279 (47%)	0/279 (0%)	136/279 (49%)	12/279 (4%)
Liver Proliferation	0.000776	3.08	110/227 (48%)	0/227 (0%)	106/227 (47%)	11/227 (5%)
Cardiac Hypertrophy	0.00138	2.24	207/401 (52%)	0/401 (0%)	171/401 (43%)	23/401 (6%)
LPS/IL-1 Mediated Inhibition of RXR Function	0.00138	2.79	124/251 (49%)	0/251 (0%)	93/251 (37%)	34/251 (14%)
Hepatic Stellate Cell Activation	0.001549	8.57	17/35 (49%)	0/35 (0%)	18/35 (51%)	0/35 (0%)
Increases Liver Steatosis	0.002188	4.82	43/83 (52%)	0/83 (0%)	37/83 (45%)	3/83 (4%)

Table 4. *Cont.*

Ingenuity Toxicity Lists	*p*-Value	Overlap (%)	Downregulated	No Change	Upregulated	No Overlap with Dataset
Mechanism of Gene Regulation by Peroxisome Proliferators via **PPARα**	0.003631	4.21	54/95 (57%)	0/95 (0%)	40/95 (42%)	1/95 (1%)
Hepatic Fibrosis	0.004169	4.04	42/99 (42%)	0/99 (0%)	54/99 (55%)	3/99 (3%)
Increases Liver Damage	0.005495	3.74	48/107 (45%)	0/107 (0%)	56/107 (52%)	3/107 (3%)
PPARα/RXRα Activation	0.007244	2.73	100/183 (55%)	0/183 (0%)	69/183 (38%)	14/183 (8%)
Acute Renal Failure Panel (Rat)	0.007943	4.84	31/62 (50%)	0/62 (0%)	24/62 (39%)	7/62 (11%)
RAR Activation	0.008511	2.63	86/190 (45%)	0/190 (0%)	100/190 (53%)	4/190 (2%)
Cardiac Necrosis/Cell Death	0.008913	2.23	141/269 (52%)	0/269 (0%)	114/269 (42%)	14/269 (5%)
Cardiac Fibrosis	0.008913	2.6	104/192 (54%)	0/192 (0%)	72/192 (38%)	16/192 (8%)
LXR/RXR Activation	0.008913	3.25	69/123 (56%)	0/123 (0%)	54/123 (44%)	0/123 (0%)
Nongenotoxic Hepatocarcinogenicity Biomarker Panel	0.00912	9.09	11/22 (50%)	0/22 (0%)	10/22 (45%)	1/22 (5%)
Increases Renal Damage	0.016218	3.7	38/81 (47%)	0/81 (0%)	36/81 (44%)	7/81 (9%)
NRF2-mediated Oxidative Stress Response	0.019498	2.14	99/234 (42%)	0/234 (0%)	103/234 (44%)	32/234 (14%)
TGF-β Signaling	0.021878	3.33	54/90 (60%)	0/90 (0%)	35/90 (39%)	1/90 (1%)

Table 5. Ingenuity toxicity list secondary to keratinocytes treatment with 20,23(OH)$_2$D3 in humans for 6 h. Nuclear receptors are marked in bold.

Ingenuity Toxicity Lists	*p*-Value	Overlap (%)	Downregulated	No Change	Upregulated	No Overlap with Dataset
Cytochrome P450 Panel—Substrate is a Vitamin (Human)	0.007244	16.7	2/6 (33%)	0/6 (0%)	4/6 (67%)	0/6 (0%)
Aryl Hydrocarbon Receptor Signaling	0.016218	1.24	71/161 (44%)	0/161 (0%)	75/161 (47%)	15/161 (9%)
Cytochrome P450 Panel—Substrate is a Sterol (Human)	0.016982	7.14	5/14 (36%)	0/14 (0%)	9/14 (64%)	0/14 (0%)
Cytochrome P450 Panel—Substrate is a Xenobiotic (Human)	0.021878	5.56	7/18 (39%)	0/18 (0%)	9/18 (50%)	2/18 (11%)
Nongenotoxic Hepatocarcinogenicity Biomarker Panel	0.026303	4.55	12/22 (55%)	0/22 (0%)	9/22 (41%)	1/22 (5%)
Cytochrome P450 Panel—Substrate is a Xenobiotic (Mouse)	0.0302	4	5/25 (20%)	0/25 (0%)	7/25 (28%)	13/25 (52%)
Cytochrome P450 Panel—Substrate is a Xenobiotic (Rat)	0.030903	3.85	5/26 (19%)	0/26 (0%)	7/26 (27%)	14/26 (54%)
Xenobiotic Metabolism Signaling	0.063096	0.595	155/336 (46%)	0/336 (0%)	139/336 (41%)	42/336 (13%)
VDR/RXR Activation	0.091201	1.28	34/78 (44%)	0/78 (0%)	43/78 (55%)	1/78 (1%)
TR/RXR Activation	0.097724	1.18	39/85 (46%)	0/85 (0%)	46/85 (54%)	0/85 (0%)
Hepatic Fibrosis	0.114025	1.01	49/99 (49%)	0/99 (0%)	47/99 (47%)	3/99 (3%)
Increases Liver Hyperplasia/ Hyperproliferation	0.116145	0.99	39/101 (39%)	0/101 (0%)	52/101 (51%)	10/101 (10%)

Table 5. *Cont.*

Ingenuity Toxicity Lists	p-Value	Overlap (%)	Downregulated	No Change	Upregulated	No Overlap with Dataset
Renal Necrosis/Cell Death	0.12388	0.399	224/501 (45%)	1/501 (0%)	258/501 (51%)	18/501 (4%)
Fatty Acid Metabolism	0.133352	0.855	57/117 (49%)	0/117 (0%)	39/117 (33%)	21/117 (18%)
Cardiac Fibrosis	0.209894	0.521	89/192 (46%)	0/192 (0%)	87/192 (45%)	16/192 (8%)
Liver Proliferation	0.24322	0.441	98/227 (43%)	0/227 (0%)	118/227 (52%)	11/227 (5%)

Table 6. Categories of biological functions with diseases or function annotation activated by 1,25(OH)$_2$D3 in human epidermal keratinocytes after 6 h of treatment.

Categories of Biological Function	Diseases or Functions Annotation	p-Value	Activation z-Score	# of Genes
Cancer, Organismal Injury and Abnormalities	growth of tumor	1.5×10^{-12}	0.033	31
Cellular Movement	cell movement	4.5×10^{-12}	1.845	52
Cancer, Cellular Development, Cellular Growth and Proliferation, Organismal Injury and Abnormalities, Tumor Morphology	proliferation of tumor cells	7.5×10^{-12}	−0.27	23
Cellular Movement	migration of cells	1.3×10^{-11}	1.801	48
Cellular Growth and Proliferation	proliferation of cells	4.2×10^{-11}	0.347	70
Carbohydrate Metabolism	metabolism of polysaccharide	4.4×10^{-11}	0.755	16
Cell Death and Survival	apoptosis of tumor cell lines	8.3×10^{-11}	1.089	36
Cellular Movement	invasion of cells	8.7×10^{-11}	0.571	30
Inflammatory Response	inflammatory response	1.4×10^{-10}	0.766	28
Cellular Development	differentiation of cells	1.5×10^{-10}	2.774	51
Cell Death and Survival	cell survival	3.1×10^{-10}	2.346	38
Cell Death and Survival	apoptosis	5.7×10^{-10}	1.307	55
Cell Death and Survival	necrosis	6.3×10^{-10}	1.7	54
Cell Death and Survival	cell viability	6.4×10^{-10}	2.547	36
Tissue Morphology	quantity of cells	7.1×10^{-10}	1.065	43
Cardiovascular System Development and Function, Organismal Development	vasculogenesis	9.4×10^{-10}	0.844	26
Carbohydrate Metabolism	synthesis of polysaccharide	9.6×10^{-10}	0.297	13
Cellular Growth and Proliferation, Tissue Development	proliferation of connective tissue cells	1.2×10^{-9}	1.232	23
Cellular Movement	cell movement of tumor cell lines	1.2×10^{-9}	0.955	28
Cell Death and Survival	cell death of tumor cell lines	1.2×10^{-9}	0.81	39
Cellular Development, Cellular Growth and Proliferation	proliferation of tumor cell lines	1.9×10^{-9}	0.324	39
Organismal Survival	morbidity or mortality	2.3×10^{-9}	−1.006	51
Embryonic Development, Organismal Development	development of body trunk	2.7×10^{-9}	0.06	32
Cell Death and Survival	cell death	3.1×10^{-9}	1.556	62
Cancer, Organismal Injury and Abnormalities	growth of malignant tumor	3.3×10^{-9}	0.518	19
Cellular Development, Cellular Growth and Proliferation, Connective Tissue Development and Function, Tissue Development	proliferation of fibroblasts	4.0×10^{-9}	0.604	17

Table 6. *Cont.*

Categories of Biological Function	Diseases or Functions Annotation	*p*-Value	Activation z-Score	# of Genes
Cellular Function and Maintenance, Hematological System Development and Function	function of myeloid cells	4.5×10^{-9}		14
Cell Signaling, Small Molecule Biochemistry	synthesis of nitric oxide	4.7×10^{-9}	0.89	15
Dermatological Diseases and Conditions	psoriasis	5.0×10^{-9}		22

Table 7. Categories of biological functions with diseases or function annotation activated by 20,23(OH)$_2$D3 in human epidermal keratinocytes after 6 h of treatment.

Categories of Biological Function	Diseases or Functions Annotation	*p*-Value	# of Genes
Cancer, Organismal Injury and Abnormalities, Respiratory Disease	carcinoma in lung	6.5×10^{-5}	8
Vitamin and Mineral Metabolism	metabolism of vitamin	0.000254	3
Developmental Disorder, Skeletal and Muscular Disorders	hypertrophy of smooth muscle	0.000325	2
Cancer, Organismal Injury and Abnormalities, Respiratory Disease	non-small cell lung cancer	0.000334	7
Infectious Diseases	internalization of virus	0.000355	2
Cancer, Organismal Injury and Abnormalities	adenocarcinoma	0.000603	20
Cancer, Organismal Injury and Abnormalities, Reproductive System Disease	prostate cancer	0.000618	7
Cancer, Gastrointestinal Disease, Hepatic System Disease, Organismal Injury and Abnormalities	liver adenoma	0.000692	2
Cancer, Endocrine System Disorders, Organismal Injury and Abnormalities	endocrine gland tumor	0.000718	9
Cell Death and Survival	apoptosis of germ cells	0.000799	3
Lipid Metabolism, Small Molecule Biochemistry, Vitamin and Mineral Metabolism	catabolism of terpenoid	0.000828	2
Cancer, Organismal Injury and Abnormalities	epithelial cancer	0.000989	23
Endocrine System Development and Function, Lipid Metabolism, Small Molecule Biochemistry, Vitamin and Mineral Metabolism	synthesis of estrogen	0.00114	2
Ophthalmic Disease, Organismal Injury and Abnormalities	age-related macular degeneration type 6	0.00122	1
Cell Cycle	arrest in sub-G1 phase of endometrial cancer cell lines	0.00122	1
Cell Morphology, Connective Tissue Development and Function	blebbing of pulmonary fibroblasts	0.00122	1
Organismal Injury and Abnormalities	calcification of uterus	0.00122	1
Cell Cycle, Cell Death and Survival	chromosome condensation of pulmonary fibroblasts	0.00122	1

Table 7. *Cont.*

Categories of Biological Function	Diseases or Functions Annotation	*p*-Value	# of Genes
Cell-To-Cell Signaling and Interaction, Inflammatory Response	cytotoxic reaction of bone marrow cells	0.00122	1
Tissue Morphology	deficiency of mast cells	0.00122	1
Cell Cycle	delay in G1/S phase transition of hepatoma cell lines	0.00122	1
Embryonic Development, Organ Development, Organismal Development, Tissue Development, Visual System Development and Function	development of outflow pathway	0.00122	1
Embryonic Development, Organ Development, Organismal Development, Reproductive System Development and Function, Tissue Development	development of placenta decidua	0.00122	1
Embryonic Development, Organ Development, Organismal Development, Reproductive System Development and Function, Tissue Development	development of placental spongiotrophoblast layer	0.00122	1
Cardiovascular System Development and Function, Tissue Morphology	diameter of portal vein	0.00122	1
Cardiovascular System Development and Function, Tissue Morphology	diameter of umbilical vein	0.00122	1
Hereditary Disorder, Ophthalmic Disease, Organismal Injury and Abnormalities	digenic early-onset glaucoma	0.00122	1
Cancer, Organismal Injury and Abnormalities, Reproductive System Disease	estrogen receptor positive endometrial cancer	0.00122	1
Connective Tissue Disorders, Organismal Injury and Abnormalities	fibrosis of submucosa	0.00122	1
Digestive System Development and Function, Embryonic Development, Organ Development, Organismal Development, Tissue Development	formation of salivary duct	0.00122	1
Cardiovascular System Development and Function, Embryonic Development, Lymphoid Tissue Structure and Development, Organ Development, Organismal Development, Respiratory System Development and Function, Tissue Development	formation of tracheal duct	0.00122	1
Cancer, Gastrointestinal Disease, Organismal Injury and Abnormalities	hyperplasia of pylorus	0.00122	1
Cancer, Cardiovascular Disease, Organismal Injury and Abnormalities	hyperplasia of vasculature	0.00122	1
Developmental Disorder, Gastrointestinal Disease	hypertrophy of gastric epithelium	0.00122	1
Dermatological Diseases and Conditions, Developmental Disorder	hypertrophy of skin	0.00122	1

Because of the unexpected differences between 1,25$(OH)_2$D3 and 20,23$(OH)_2$D3, the 6 h incubation experiment was repeated in a similar manner as shown in Figure 2 and microarray analyses were performed using Illumina's HumanWG-6_V2 (Platform GPL13376) chip/array. Average signal values for filtered gene clusters with FC $\geq \pm 1.5$ are shown in Supplemental excel file #2. The heat maps corresponding to relative gene expression and Venn diagrams are shown in Figure 3C. Again, for a 2-fold cut-off value there was only one common gene (*CYP24A1*) whose expression was stimulated by both 1,25$(OH)_2$D3 (80-fold) and 20,23$(OH)_2$D3 (2.9-fold). For FC $\geq \pm 1.5$ there were 11 common genes upregulated and 4 downregulated. Again, ingenuity pathway analysis showed that VDR/RXR was the top canonical pathway induced by 1,25$(OH)_2$D3, followed by the role of osteoblasts, osteoclasts and chondrocytes in rheumatoid arthritis. As before, other nuclear receptor signaling pathways included LXR/RXR, GR and AhR. For 20,23$(OH)_2$D3 the top nuclear receptor signaling pathways were again AhR and VDR/RXR. Of note, this microarray showed that 20,23$(OH)_2$D3 upregulated two genes downstream of AhR signaling, *CYP1A1* and *CYP1B1*, by factors of 2.4 and 2.6, respectively. This stimulation was confirmed by qPCR (Figure 3D). VDR/RXR was identified as the top toxicity pathway for 1,25$(OH)_2$D3 and AhR for 20,23$(OH)_2$D3.

More robust data were obtained with 24 h of treatment for which the average signal values for filtered gene clusters with FC $\geq \pm 1.5$ are shown in Supplemental excel file #3. Because of the large number of genes affected (Table 1), the heat map of differentially expressed genes and Venn diagrams were generated using the 4-FC value which show three overlapping genes (*CYP24A1*, *MMP3* and *SERPINB1*) as well as distinct gene expression patterns (Figure 4). For FC $\geq \pm 1.5$, 93 and 72 common genes were up- and downregulated, respectively. Ingenuity pathway analysis using FC $\geq \pm 2.0$ was consistent with results obtained after 6 h of treatment. Again, the top canonical pathway for 1,25$(OH)_2$D3 was VDR/RXR (Supplemental Figure S1B) followed by MIF-related glucocorticoid regulation and regulation of the innate immunity system (Table 8). AhR signaling was also listed. The top canonical pathways induced by 20,23$(OH)_2$D3 were AhR signaling (Supplemental Figure S2B) and the cholesterol biosynthesis pathway (Table 9). Interestingly, the involvement of a second nuclear receptor complex was emphasized by VDR/RXR activation (Supplemental Figure S3B), with p53 signaling also being listed. The latter is consistent with the photoprotective properties of 20,23$(OH)_2$D3 and activation of p53 by its direct precursor, 20(OH)D3 [23]. The top affected toxicity pathways for 1,25$(OH)_2$D3 included VDR/RXR, xenobiotic metabolism, cardiac fibrosis and cytochrome P450s (Table 10). AhR signaling was also listed. For 20,23$(OH)_2$D3, AhR signaling was again listed as the top toxicity pathway followed by cholesterol synthesis, p53 signaling and again VDR/RXR (Table 11). The top upstream gene regulation pathways for 1,25$(OH)_2$D3 included vitamin D3-VDR-RXR, calcitriol, dexamethasone, progesterone and β-estradiol, while for 20,23$(OH)_2$D3, included TP53 (p53 tumor suppressor), β-estradiol, lipopolysaccharide, TNF (tumor necrosis factor) and TGF β1 (transforming growth factor-β1) (not shown).

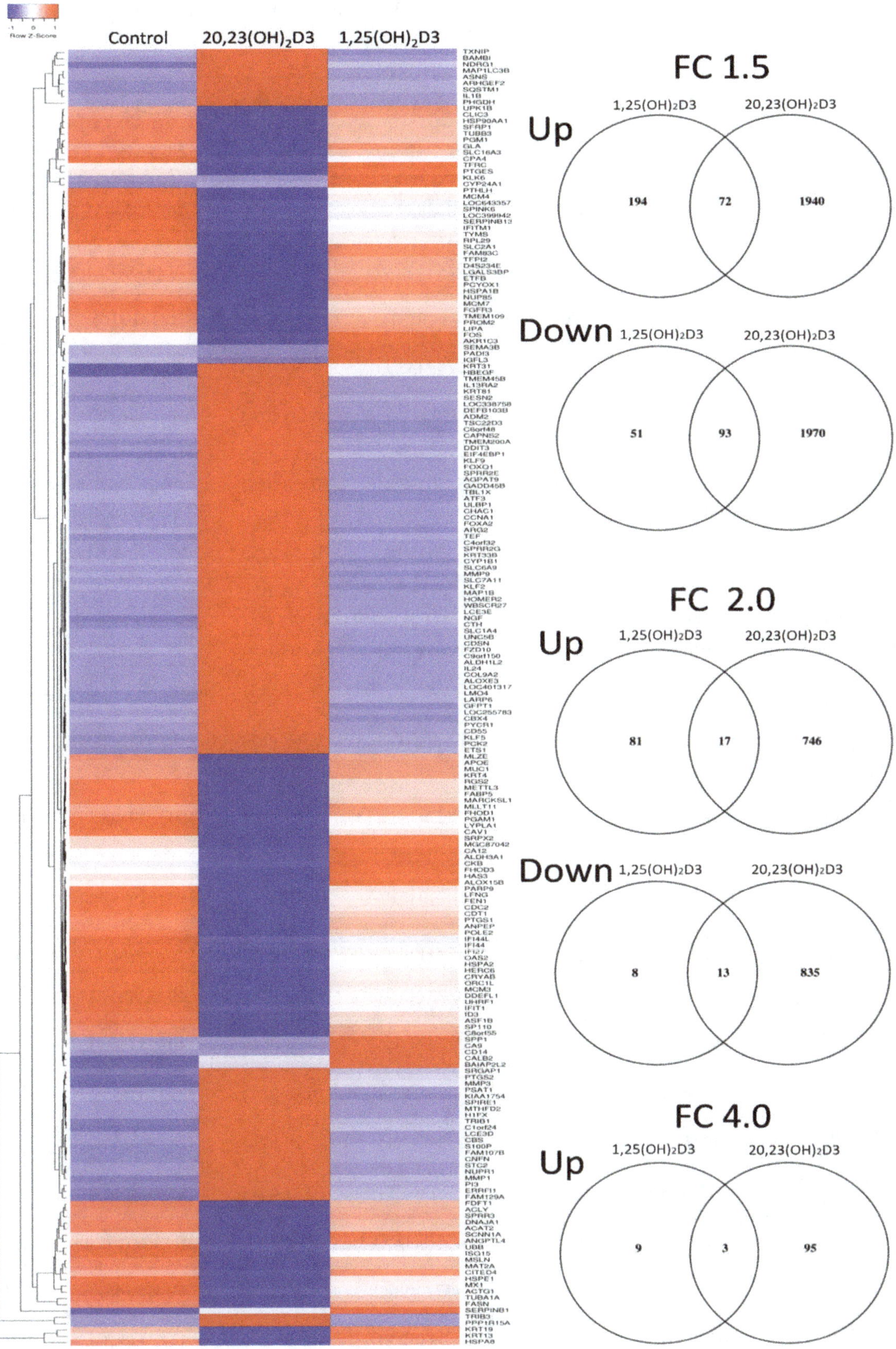

Figure 4. Heat map of gene expression pattern in human epidermal keratinocytes treated with 10^{-7} M of 1,25(OH)$_2$D3 or 20,23(OH)$_2$D3 for 24 h. On the right are the corresponding Venn diagrams for FC $\geq$ 4, 2 and 1.5.

Table 8. Canonical pathways activated by 1,25(OH)$_2$D3 in human epidermal keratinocytes after 24 h of treatment. Nuclear receptors are marked in bold.

Ingenuity Canonical Pathways	*p*-Value	Overlap (%)	Downregulated	No Change	Upregulated	No Overlap with Dataset
VDR/RXR Activation	7.9×10^{-15}	15.4	23/78 (29%)	0/78 (0%)	54/78 (69%)	1/78 (1%)
MIF-mediated Glucocorticoid Regulation	2.6×10^{-5}	12.1	12/33 (36%)	0/33 (0%)	20/33 (61%)	1/33 (3%)
MIF Regulation of Innate Immunity	6.3×10^{-5}	9.76	19/41 (46%)	0/41 (0%)	21/41 (51%)	1/41 (2%)
α-tocopherol Degradation	0.000162181	50	0/4 (0%)	0/4 (0%)	4/4 (100%)	0/4 (0%)
Antioxidant Action of Vitamin C	0.000177828	5.05	43/99 (43%)	0/99 (0%)	50/99 (51%)	6/99 (6%)
Retinoate Biosynthesis I	0.000691831	9.09	9/33 (27%)	0/33 (0%)	20/33 (61%)	4/33 (12%)
Coagulation System	0.000831764	8.57	17/35 (49%)	0/35 (0%)	18/35 (51%)	0/35 (0%)
Estrogen Biosynthesis	0.001047129	7.89	18/38 (47%)	0/38 (0%)	19/38 (50%)	1/38 (3%)
iNOS Signaling	0.00162181	6.82	17/44 (39%)	0/44 (0%)	26/44 (59%)	1/44 (2%)
Role of IL-17A in Arthritis	0.002884032	5.56	27/54 (50%)	0/54 (0%)	27/54 (50%)	0/54 (0%)
Parkinson's Signaling	0.003162278	12.5	9/16 (56%)	0/16 (0%)	7/16 (44%)	0/16 (0%)
LXR/RXR Activation	0.003890451	3.31	61/121 (50%)	0/121 (0%)	60/121 (50%)	0/121 (0%)
CD40 Signaling	0.004897788	4.62	31/65 (48%)	0/65 (0%)	33/65 (51%)	1/65 (2%)
IL-10 Signaling	0.005495409	4.41	32/68 (47%)	0/68 (0%)	35/68 (51%)	1/68 (1%)
Role of MAPK Signaling in the Pathogenesis of Influenza	0.005754399	4.35	27/69 (39%)	0/69 (0%)	39/69 (57%)	3/69 (4%)
LPS/IL-1 Mediated Inhibition of RXR Function	0.006025596	2.28	102/219 (47%)	0/219 (0%)	105/219 (48%)	12/219 (5%)
Role of Osteoblasts, Osteoclasts and Chondrocytes in Rheumatoid Arthritis	0.006025596	2.28	111/219 (51%)	0/219 (0%)	103/219 (47%)	5/219 (2%)
IL-17 Signaling	0.006456542	4.17	33/72 (46%)	0/72 (0%)	39/72 (54%)	0/72 (0%)
LPS-stimulated MAPK Signaling	0.00676083	4.11	33/73 (45%)	0/73 (0%)	40/73 (55%)	0/73 (0%)
Toll-like Receptor Signaling	0.007079458	4.05	32/74 (43%)	0/74 (0%)	40/74 (54%)	2/74 (3%)
BMP signaling pathway	0.007585776	3.95	43/76 (57%)	0/76 (0%)	31/76 (41%)	2/76 (3%)
Intrinsic Prothrombin Activation Pathway	0.01023293	6.9	12/29 (41%)	0/29 (0%)	16/29 (55%)	1/29 (3%)
4-1BB Signaling in T Lymphocytes	0.011481536	6.45	19/31 (61%)	0/31 (0%)	12/31 (39%)	0/31 (0%)
Acute Phase Response Signaling	0.012302688	2.37	76/169 (45%)	0/169 (0%)	91/169 (54%)	2/169 (1%)
Endothelin-1 Signaling	0.013182567	2.33	89/172 (52%)	0/172 (0%)	77/172 (45%)	6/172 (3%)
Inhibition of Angiogenesis by TSP1	0.013803843	5.88	21/34 (62%)	0/34 (0%)	11/34 (32%)	2/34 (6%)
Xenobiotic Metabolism Signaling	0.014454398	1.85	127/271 (47%)	0/271 (0%)	128/271 (47%)	16/271 (6%)
IL-17A Signaling in Fibroblasts	0.014454398	5.71	15/35 (43%)	0/35 (0%)	20/35 (57%)	0/35 (0%)
Interferon Signaling	0.015488166	5.56	28/36 (78%)	0/36 (0%)	8/36 (22%)	0/36 (0%)

Table 8. *Cont.*

Ingenuity Canonical Pathways	*p*-Value	Overlap (%)	Downregulated	No Change	Upregulated	No Overlap with Dataset
Thyroid Hormone Biosynthesis	0.015848932	33.3	1/3 (33%)	0/3 (0%)	2/3 (67%)	0/3 (0%)
April Mediated Signaling	0.016982437	5.26	18/38 (47%)	0/38 (0%)	20/38 (53%)	0/38 (0%)
Inhibition of Matrix Metalloproteases	0.017782794	5.13	17/39 (44%)	0/39 (0%)	21/39 (54%)	1/39 (3%)
RAR Activation	0.018197009	2.11	87/190 (46%)	0/190 (0%)	99/190 (52%)	4/190 (2%)
Thrombin Signaling	0.018620871	2.09	90/191 (47%)	0/191 (0%)	96/191 (50%)	5/191 (3%)
B Cell Activating Factor Signaling	0.018620871	5	21/40 (53%)	0/40 (0%)	19/40 (48%)	0/40 (0%)
Dermatan Sulfate Biosynthesis (Late Stages)	0.022387211	4.55	16/44 (36%)	0/44 (0%)	26/44 (59%)	2/44 (5%)
IL-6 Signaling	0.023442288	2.59	52/116 (45%)	0/116 (0%)	64/116 (55%)	0/116 (0%)
p38 MAPK Signaling	0.023988329	2.56	52/117 (44%)	0/117 (0%)	62/117 (53%)	3/117 (3%)

Table 9. Canonical pathways activated by 20,23(OH)$_2$D3 in human epidermal keratinocytes after 24 h of treatment. Nuclear receptors are marked in bold.

Ingenuity Canonical Pathways	*p*-Value	Overlap (%)	Downregulated	No Change	Upregulated	No Overlap with Dataset
Aryl Hydrocarbon Receptor Signaling	9.5×10^{-10}	22.9	80/140 (57%)	0/140 (0%)	54/140 (39%)	6/140 (4%)
Superpathway of Cholesterol Biosynthesis	9.1×10^{-9}	46.4	22/28 (79%)	0/28 (0%)	4/28 (14%)	2/28 (7%)
Cell Cycle Control of Chromosomal Replication	6.3×10^{-8}	44.4	21/27 (78%)	0/27 (0%)	6/27 (22%)	0/27 (0%)
Mismatch Repair in Eukaryotes	2.3×10^{-7}	56.2	15/16 (94%)	0/16 (0%)	1/16 (6%)	0/16 (0%)
Unfolded protein response	3.5×10^{-7}	29.6	24/54 (44%)	0/54 (0%)	29/54 (54%)	1/54 (2%)
Fatty Acid α-oxidation	1.5×10^{-6}	47.4	10/19 (53%)	0/19 (0%)	6/19 (32%)	3/19 (16%)
Ethanol Degradation IV	6.8×10^{-6}	40.9	17/22 (77%)	0/22 (0%)	2/22 (9%)	3/22 (14%)
Cholesterol Biosynthesis I	7.9×10^{-6}	53.8	12/13 (92%)	0/13 (0%)	1/13 (8%)	0/13 (0%)
p53 Signaling	8.3×10^{-6}	20.4	53/98 (54%)	0/98 (0%)	45/98 (46%)	0/98 (0%)
VDR/RXR Activation	1.5×10^{-5}	21.8	26/78 (33%)	0/78 (0%)	51/78 (65%)	1/78 (1%)
GADD45 Signaling	1.7×10^{-5}	42.1	14/19 (74%)	0/19 (0%)	5/19 (26%)	0/19 (0%)
Putrescine Degradation III	2.8×10^{-5}	40	12/20 (60%)	0/20 (0%)	5/20 (25%)	3/20 (15%)
Histamine Degradation	4.5×10^{-5}	43.8	10/16 (63%)	0/16 (0%)	3/16 (19%)	3/16 (19%)
Dopamine Degradation	4.7×10^{-5}	33.3	16/27 (59%)	0/27 (0%)	6/27 (22%)	5/27 (19%)
Tryptophan Degradation X (Mammalian, via Tryptamine)	6.2×10^{-5}	36.4	13/22 (59%)	0/22 (0%)	5/22 (23%)	4/22 (18%)

Table 9. *Cont.*

Ingenuity Canonical Pathways	*p*-Value	Overlap (%)	Downregulated	No Change	Upregulated	No Overlap with Dataset
Xenobiotic Metabolism Signaling	9.3×10^{-5}	13.3	131/271 (48%)	0/271 (0%)	124/271 (46%)	16/271 (6%)
Oxidative Ethanol Degradation III	0.000109648	38.9	13/18 (72%)	0/18 (0%)	2/18 (11%)	3/18 (17%)
Mevalonate Pathway I	0.000112202	46.2	8/13 (62%)	0/13 (0%)	3/13 (23%)	2/13 (15%)
Estrogen-mediated S-phase Entry	0.000125893	33.3	18/24 (75%)	0/24 (0%)	6/24 (25%)	0/24 (0%)
Hereditary Breast Cancer Signaling	0.000165959	16.3	77/129 (60%)	0/129 (0%)	45/129 (35%)	7/129 (5%)
Glucocorticoid Receptor Signaling	0.000269153	12.7	122/275 (44%)	0/275 (0%)	147/275 (53%)	6/275 (2%)
Adipogenesis pathway	0.000371535	15.7	66/127 (52%)	0/127 (0%)	55/127 (43%)	6/127 (5%)
Interferon Signaling	0.000537032	25	24/36 (67%)	0/36 (0%)	12/36 (33%)	0/36 (0%)
Superpathway of Serine and Glycine Biosynthesis I	0.000630957	57.1	3/7 (43%)	0/7 (0%)	4/7 (57%)	0/7 (0%)
Superpathway of Geranylgeranyldi phosphate Biosynthesis I (via Mevalonate)	0.000630957	35.3	11/17 (65%)	0/17 (0%)	4/17 (24%)	2/17 (12%)
Semaphorin Signaling in Neurons	0.000758578	20.8	27/53 (51%)	0/53 (0%)	24/53 (45%)	2/53 (4%)
Glutaryl-CoA Degradation	0.000776247	41.7	7/12 (58%)	0/12 (0%)	4/12 (33%)	1/12 (8%)
Pancreatic Adenocarcinoma Signaling	0.000794328	16	53/106 (50%)	0/106 (0%)	53/106 (50%)	0/106 (0%)
Role of CHK Proteins in Cell Cycle Checkpoint Control	0.001047129	20	35/55 (64%)	0/55 (0%)	20/55 (36%)	0/55 (0%)
Glycolysis I	0.001096478	28	20/25 (80%)	0/25 (0%)	4/25 (16%)	1/25 (4%)
NRF2-mediated Oxidative Stress Response	0.001230269	13.3	89/180 (49%)	0/180 (0%)	87/180 (48%)	4/180 (2%)
HIF1α Signaling	0.001412538	15.7	52/102 (51%)	0/102 (0%)	48/102 (47%)	2/102 (2%)
Aldosterone Signaling in Epithelial Cells	0.001548817	13.8	82/152 (54%)	0/152 (0%)	67/152 (44%)	3/152 (2%)
Serotonin Degradation	0.001737801	17.9	38/67 (57%)	0/67 (0%)	16/67 (24%)	13/67 (19%)

Table 10. Toxicity-related pathways identified by Ingenuity in human keratinocytes treated with $1{,}25(OH)_2D3$ for 24 h. Nuclear receptors are marked in bold.

Ingenuity Toxicity Lists	*p*-Value	Overlap (%)	Downregulated	No Change	Upregulated	No Overlap with Dataset
VDR/RXR Activation	7.9×10^{-15}	15.4	23/78 (29%)	0/78 (0%)	54/78 (69%)	1/78 (1%)
Xenobiotic Metabolism Signaling	0.00040738	2.38	144/336 (43%)	0/336 (0%)	150/336 (45%)	42/336 (13%)
Cardiac Fibrosis	0.000537032	3.12	85/192 (44%)	0/192 (0%)	91/192 (47%)	16/192 (8%)
Cytochrome P450 Panel—Substrate is an Eicosanoid (Human)	0.000562341	28.6	1/7 (14%)	0/7 (0%)	6/7 (86%)	0/7 (0%)
Cytochrome P450 Panel—Substrate is a Fatty Acid (Human)	0.001202264	20	3/10 (30%)	0/10 (0%)	7/10 (70%)	0/10 (0%)

Table 10. *Cont.*

Ingenuity Toxicity Lists	*p*-Value	Overlap (%)	Downregulated	No Change	Upregulated	No Overlap with Dataset
Cardiac Hypertrophy	0.00128825	2	193/401 (48%)	0/401 (0%)	185/401 (46%)	23/401 (6%)
Liver Proliferation	0.00128825	2.64	103/227 (45%)	0/227 (0%)	113/227 (50%)	11/227 (5%)
Hepatic Fibrosis	0.001862087	4.04	49/99 (49%)	1/99 (1%)	46/99 (46%)	3/99 (3%)
LXR/RXR Activation	0.004073803	3.25	62/123 (50%)	0/123 (0%)	61/123 (50%)	0/123 (0%)
Renal Necrosis/Cell Death	0.005011872	1.6	238/501 (48%)	0/501 (0%)	245/501 (49%)	18/501 (4%)
LPS/IL-1 Mediated Inhibition of RXR Function	0.010715193	1.99	107/251 (43%)	0/251 (0%)	110/251 (44%)	34/251 (14%)
Positive Acute Phase Response Proteins	0.010964782	6.67	11/30 (37%)	0/30 (0%)	19/30 (63%)	0/30 (0%)
Liver Necrosis/Cell Death	0.016218101	1.79	118/279 (42%)	0/279 (0%)	149/279 (53%)	12/279 (4%)
RAR Activation	0.018197009	2.11	87/190 (46%)	0/190 (0%)	99/190 (52%)	4/190 (2%)
Increases Liver Damage	0.019054607	2.8	46/107 (43%)	0/107 (0%)	58/107 (54%)	3/107 (3%)
Fatty Acid Metabolism	0.023988329	2.56	48/117 (41%)	0/117 (0%)	48/117 (41%)	21/117 (18%)
Increases Liver Hepatitis	0.030902954	3.85	22/52 (42%)	0/52 (0%)	29/52 (56%)	1/52 (2%)

Table 11. Toxicity-related pathways identified by Ingenuity in human keratinocytes treated with 20,23(OH)$_2$D3 for 24 h. Nuclear receptors are marked in bold.

Ingenuity Toxicity Lists	*p*-Value	Overlap (%)	Downregulated	No Change	Upregulated	No Overlap with Dataset
Aryl Hydrocarbon Receptor Signaling	2.6×10^{-9}	21.1	90/161 (56%)	0/161 (0%)	56/161 (35%)	15/161 (9%)
Cholesterol Biosynthesis	1.1×10^{-8}	62.5	13/16 (81%)	0/16 (0%)	3/16 (19%)	0/16 (0%)
Renal Necrosis/Cell Death	1.9×10^{-7}	13.2	228/501 (46%)	0/501 (0%)	255/501 (51%)	18/501 (4%)
Primary Glomerulonephritis Biomarker Panel (Human)	1.7×10^{-6}	63.6	5/11 (45%)	0/11 (0%)	6/11 (55%)	0/11 (0%)
p53 Signaling	2.6×10^{-6}	21.2	54/99 (55%)	0/99 (0%)	45/99 (45%)	0/99 (0%)
VDR/RXR Activation	1.5×10^{-5}	21.8	26/78 (33%)	0/78 (0%)	51/78 (65%)	1/78 (1%)
Liver Proliferation	3.0×10^{-5}	14.5	96/227 (42%)	0/227 (0%)	120/227 (53%)	11/227 (5%)
Cardiac Hypertrophy	5.1×10^{-5}	12.2	176/401 (44%)	0/401 (0%)	202/401 (50%)	23/401 (6%)
Liver Necrosis/Cell Death	7.8×10^{-5}	13.3	117/279 (42%)	0/279 (0%)	150/279 (54%)	12/279 (4%)
Oxidative Stress	0.000380189	21.1	39/57 (68%)	0/57 (0%)	17/57 (30%)	1/57 (2%)
Mechanism of Gene Regulation by Peroxisome Proliferators via PPARα	0.000645654	16.8	38/95 (40%)	0/95 (0%)	56/95 (59%)	1/95 (1%)
Xenobiotic Metabolism Signaling	0.000794328	11.6	152/336 (45%)	0/336 (0%)	142/336 (42%)	42/336 (13%)
Increases Renal Proliferation	0.002398833	13.9	68/137 (50%)	0/137 (0%)	62/137 (45%)	7/137 (5%)
Fatty Acid Metabolism	0.002398833	14.5	65/117 (56%)	0/117 (0%)	31/117 (26%)	21/117 (18%)

Table 11. *Cont.*

Ingenuity Toxicity Lists	*p*-Value	Overlap (%)	Downregulated	No Change	Upregulated	No Overlap with Dataset
Increases Liver Steatosis	0.003890451	15.7	32/83 (39%)	0/83 (0%)	48/83 (58%)	3/83 (4%)
Decreases Depolarization of Mitochondria and Mitochondrial Membrane	0.004570882	25	18/24 (75%)	0/24 (0%)	5/24 (21%)	1/24 (4%)
Cell Cycle: G1/S Checkpoint Regulation	0.004677351	16.7	35/66 (53%)	0/66 (0%)	28/66 (42%)	3/66 (5%)

Tables 12 and 13 show some similarities and differences with dermatological diseases and conditions; with cancer, organismal injury and abnormalities being the main diseases affected by 20,23(OH)$_2$D3 and 1,25(OH)$_2$D3. With regard to molecular and cellular functions, cellular growth and proliferation, cell death and survival, cellular movement and cell cycle were the major functions for 20,23(OH)$_2$D3, and cellular movement, cell signaling, small molecule biochemistry, lipid metabolism and cellular development for 1,25(OH)$_2$D3. Among the 25 networks activated by 20,23(OH)$_2$D3, the top five included: (1) connective tissue disorders, neurological diseases, organismal injuries and abnormalities, (2) RNA post-transcriptional modification, carbohydrate metabolism and lipid metabolism, (3) connective tissue, developmental, skeletal and muscular disorders, (4) cellular movement, endocrine system disorders, gastrointestinal diseases and (5) nucleic acid metabolism, small molecules biochemistry and dermatological diseases and conditions. Among the 15 networks activated by 1,25(OH)$_2$D3, the top five included: (1) cancer, organismal functions, organismal injuries and abnormalities, (2) cell-to-cell signaling and interaction, cellular assembly and organization, cellular development, (3) cellular growth and proliferation, tissue development and cancer, (4) molecular transport, carbohydrate and lipid metabolism and (5) protein degradation, protein synthesis, cellular assembly and organization.

Table 12. Categories of biological functions with diseases or function annotation activated by 1,25(OH)$_2$D3 in human epidermal keratinocytes after 24 of treatment.

Categories of Biological Function	Diseases or Functions Annotation	*p*-Value	Activation z-Score	# of Genes
Cancer, Organismal Injury and Abnormalities	benign neoplasia	1.0×10^{-9}	0.927	26
Dermatological Diseases and Conditions	psoriasis	2.6×10^{-9}		20
Cardiovascular System Development and Function, Cellular Movement	cell movement of endothelial cells	8.8×10^{-9}	1.37	15
Cancer, Cellular Movement, Organismal Injury and Abnormalities, Tumor Morphology	invasion of tumor cells	1.2×10^{-8}	1.596	11
Cell Signaling, Small Molecule Biochemistry	synthesis of nitric oxide	1.9×10^{-8}	−0.217	13
Cardiovascular System Development and Function, Cellular Movement	homing of endothelial cells	3.2×10^{-8}	1.597	7
Cancer, Organismal Injury and Abnormalities, Tumor Morphology	invasion of tumor	3.4×10^{-8}	1.63	12
Lipid Metabolism, Small Molecule Biochemistry	metabolism of eicosanoid	3.4×10^{-8}	2.747	12

Table 12. *Cont.*

Categories of Biological Function	Diseases or Functions Annotation	*p*-Value	Activation z-Score	# of Genes
Cardiovascular Disease, Hematological Disease	Thrombosis	5.9×10^{-8}	−0.946	10
Organismal Injury and Abnormalities	Fibrosis	1.1×10^{-7}	−1.401	17
Lipid Metabolism, Small Molecule Biochemistry	metabolism of prostaglandin	1.2×10^{-7}	2.589	10
Immunological Disease	hypersensitive reaction	1.5×10^{-7}	0.914	15
Cardiovascular System Development and Function, Organismal Development	vasculogenesis	1.6×10^{-7}	1.825	20
Inflammatory Response	inflammation of organ	1.8×10^{-7}	−0.022	26
Dermatological Diseases and Conditions, Inflammatory Disease, Inflammatory Response	Dermatitis	1.8×10^{-7}	−0.355	15
Cardiovascular System Development and Function, Organismal Development	vascularization of hindlimb	$2.3 X 10^{-7}$	1.994	4
Cellular Movement	homing	3.4×10^{-7}	1.468	17
Cancer, Cellular Development, Cellular Growth and Proliferation, Organismal Injury and Abnormalities, Tumor Morphology	proliferation of tumor cells	5.4×10^{-7}	−0.189	15
Cancer, Organismal Injury and Abnormalities	growth of tumor	6.0×10^{-7}	0.402	20
Cellular Movement	invasion of cells	6.3×10^{-7}	1.731	21

Table 13. Categories of biological functions with diseases or function annotation activated by 20,23(OH)$_2$D3 in human epidermal keratinocytes after 24 h of treatment.

Categories of Biological Function	Diseases or Functions Annotation	*p*-Value	Activation z-Score	# of Genes
Cellular Growth and Proliferation	proliferation of cells	7.0×10^{-33}	−3.052	551
Dermatological Diseases and Conditions	psoriasis	4.6×10^{-29}		142
Cell Death and Survival	cell death	1.2×10^{-27}	1.116	493
Cell Death and Survival	necrosis	1.9×10^{-26}	1.15	400
Cell Death and Survival	apoptosis	1.9×10^{-25}	0.619	405
Cell Death and Survival	cell death of tumor cell lines	7.2×10^{-25}	0.971	266
Cell Death and Survival	apoptosis of tumor cell lines	7.6×10^{-23}	0.672	219
Cellular Movement	cell movement	1.3×10^{-22}	−0.187	334
Cellular Movement	migration of cells	6.7×10^{-21}	−0.554	301
Cancer, Organismal Injury and Abnormalities	abdominal neoplasm	8.7×10^{-20}	−1.733	1030
Infectious Diseases	Viral Infection	1.2×10^{-19}	0.737	261
Cancer, Organismal Injury and Abnormalities	tumorigenesis of tissue	6.5×10^{-19}	−0.349	1047
Cancer, Organismal Injury and Abnormalities	abdominal cancer	2.3×10^{-18}	−1.938	1014
Cancer, Organismal Injury and Abnormalities	cancer	4.2×10^{-18}	1.528	1215
Cancer, Organismal Injury and Abnormalities	neoplasia of epithelial tissue	2.3×10^{-17}	−0.365	1026

Table 13. *Cont.*

Categories of Biological Function	Diseases or Functions Annotation	*p*-Value	Activation z-Score	# of Genes
Cellular Development, Cellular Growth and Proliferation	proliferation of tumor cell lines	3.0×10^{-17}	−2.431	245
Cancer, Organismal Injury and Abnormalities	benign neoplasia	3.5×10^{-17}	−0.029	165
Cell Death and Survival	cell survival	4.7×10^{-17}	−0.537	225
Cancer, Organismal Injury and Abnormalities	advanced stage solid tumor	7.1×10^{-17}	−0.397	106

Because of the unexpected finding that AhR signaling represented the top regulatory pathway activated by 20,23$(OH)_2$D3, and is validated by qPCR analysis of *CYP1A1* and *CYP1B1* genes expression (Figure 3D), we examined whether 20(OH)D3, which is the precursor to 20,23$(OH)_2$D3, and 17,20,23$(OH)_2$D3 and 1,20$(OH)_2$D3, which are downstream metabolites (see Figure 1), also affected the expression of genes linked to AhR in HaCaT keratinocytes. Figure 5A shows that 20(OH)D3 stimulated the expression of *CYP1A1* and *CYP1B1* in a dose-dependent fashion, with a stimulatory effect also seen for the *AhR* gene. 17,20,23$(OH)_3$D3 (1 μM) could also stimulate *CYPA1, CYP1B1* and *AhR* expression, while 1,20$(OH)_2$D3 had only a small effect on *CYPB1* and no effect on *CYP1A1* and *AhR*. Finally, we used a Human AhR Reporter Assay System (INDIGO, Biosciences) to analyze the effect of several D3-hydroxyderivatives on AhR-mediated transactivation. The kit contains AhR Reporter Cells that contain the luciferase reporter gene functionally linked to an AhR-responsive promoter, which provides a sensitive surrogate measure of the changes in AhR-mediated activation of luciferase reporter. Figure 6 shows that there was marked activation of AhR activity by 20,23$(OH)_2$D3 with weaker but significant activation by 20(OH)D3 or 1,25$(OH)_2$D3. Thus, the functional studies support the microarray analysis indicating that hydroxyderivatives of D3 can act on AhR. This finding can be explained by the promiscuous nature of AhR and its activity [85].

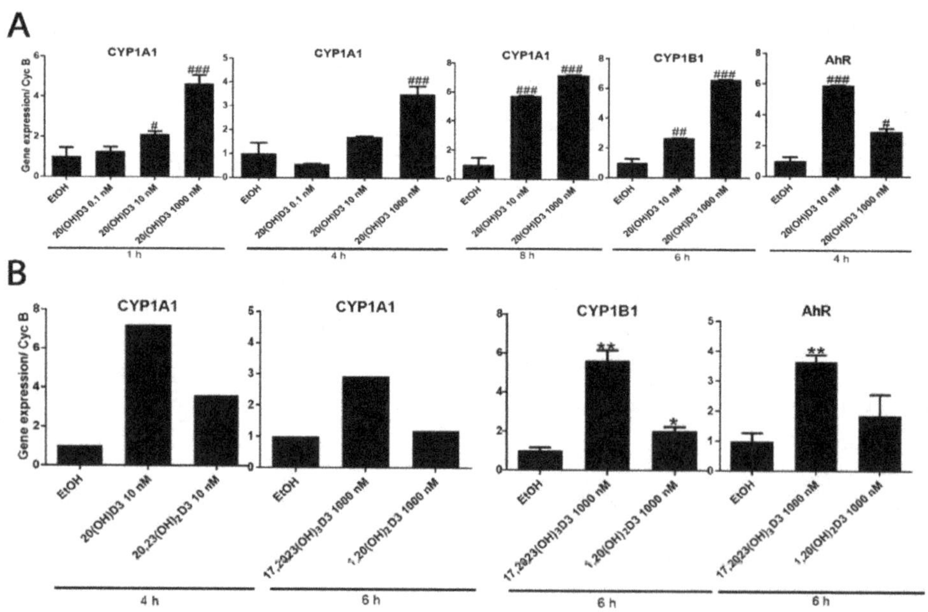

Figure 5. Changes in CYP1A1, CYP1B1 and AhR gene expression in HaCaT keratinocytes treated with vitamin D3 hydroxyderivatives as a function of the time of treatment. **A.** Dose-dependent effect of 20(OH)D3 on the gene expression. Data represent means ± SD ($n = 3$) where $^{\#}$ $p < 0.05$, $^{\#\#}$ $p < 0.01$ and $^{\#\#\#}$ $p < 0.001$ at one-way ANOVA test. **B.** Effect of 1,25$(OH)_2$D3 and 20,23$(OH)_2$D3 on the gene expression as indicated. Data represent means ($n = 2$) for CYP1A1, or means ± SD ($n = 3$) for CYP1B1 and AhR where * $p < 0.05$, ** $p < 0.01$, at student *t*-test.

An additional mechanistic insight into the above interactions was provided by modeling using the crystal structure of the ligand-binding domain (LBD) of human AhR. The presently available crystal structure of the human AhR (PDB: 5NJ8) is missing the LBD region. A model of the human AhR LBD with bound 20S,23S$(OH)_2$D3 was developed as described under Methods. Briefly, the final model was based on the homology modelling template of C-terminal Per-ARNT-Sim domain of Hypoxia-Inducible Factor-2α, PDB entry code 3H82. The sequence identity between human AhR and the modelled sequence is 27%; the alignment is shown in Supplemental Figure S4. Short molecular dynamic simulation runs were performed on selected docked poses of 20S,23R/S$(OH)_2$D3 epimers in order to identify binding modes most favorably accommodated in the binding site of the homology model. The selected complex with 20S,23S$(OH)_2$D3 was simulated for 100 ns to allow for local structural adjustments of flexible regions to the presence of the vitamin D3 scaffold. The final conformer obtained is referred to as the 'refined AhR model'. Further ligand-induced effects were explored through a 250 ns simulation production run starting with this model. Over the first 130 ns the ligand-induced conformational changes were in the vicinity of F295 and S320. The latter is in a flexible region with two adjacent glycine residues while F295 is part of a loop structure 'covering' the binding pocket. The conformation adopted by 130 ns in these regions were maintained for the rest of the simulation time, likely stabilized by a hydrogen bonding network that formed, involving ligand hydroxyl groups, T289, S320 side chains and the backbone of F295 as shown in a representative simulation snapshot at 230 ns in Figure 7. Interactions of this network link the more rigid beta-sheet structure of the pocket containing T289 with two loop regions. The flexible 'belt' between G309-H326 includes a short helical segment near S320 that also shifted due to the presence of the ligand. This binding mode also changes the preferred orientation of H291 which by 130 ns simulation time forms a stable hydrogen bond with the backbone carbonyl of K292, an interaction not present in the initial or refined AhR models. Alanine mutation of T281, H285 of mouse AhR corresponding to the human residues T289 and H291 was shown to dramatically decrease Hsp90 binding [86]. Figure 7 illustrates that differences in the structural fold of AhR between the homology model, the refined AhR model and the simulation conformer are mainly within loops and the flexible 'belt' region.

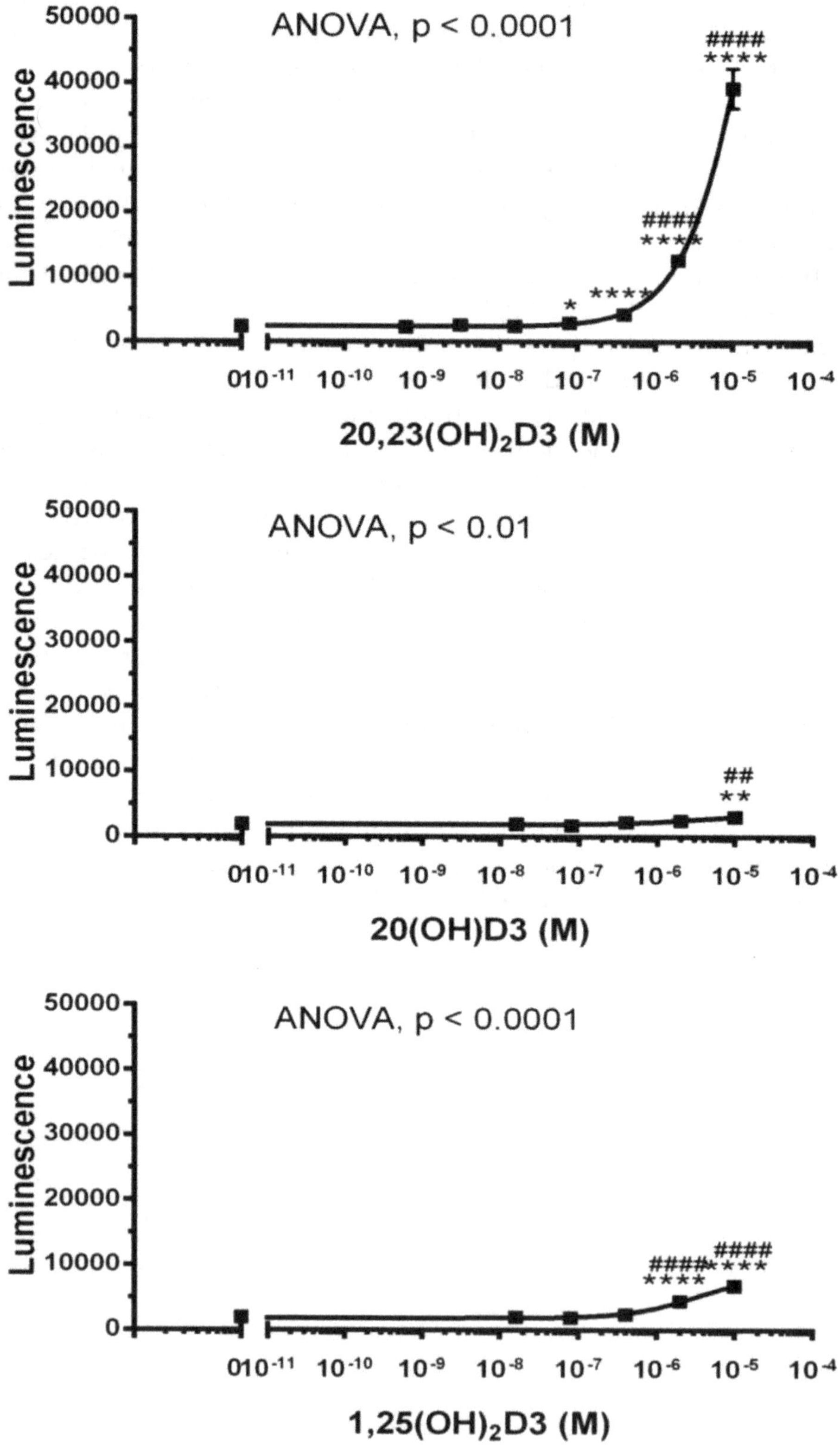

Figure 6. Stimulation of AhR activity by 20(OH)D3, 22,23$(OH)_2$D3, and 1,25$(OH)_2$D3. The assays for 22,23$(OH)_2$D3 were performed in quadruplicate, while for 20(OH)D3 and 1,25$(OH)_2$D3 in triplicate. Data represent means ± SD where * $p < 0.05$, ** $p < 0.01$ and **** $p < 0.0001$ at student *t*-test; ## $p < 0.01$ and #### $p < 0.0001$ at one-way ANOVA test.

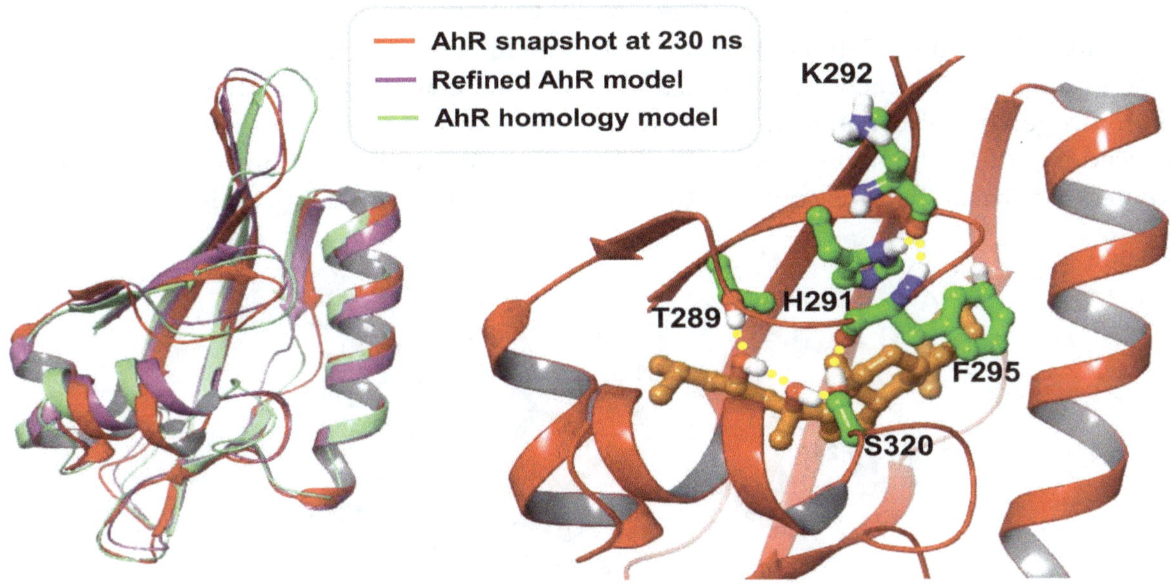

Figure 7. Structural fold of AhR models. To the left: Superimposed are the initial homology model, the refined AhR model and a molecular dynamic simulation snapshot at 230 ns. To the right: Close-up view of the simulation snapshot at 230 ns, displaying the ligand and AhR residues involved in an interaction network, as discussed in the text. 20*S*,23*S*$(OH)_2$D3 is shown with carbon atoms colored light brown, AhR residue carbons colored green; all other atoms are colored by atom type (O: red, N: blue, S: yellow). Hydrogen bonding interactions are indicated with yellow spheres.

The proposed binding model of 20S,23S$(OH)_2$D3 is shown in Figure 8A through a representative simulation conformer at 230 ns. Figure 8B shows the fraction of simulation time during which interactions are present with each AhR residue, as averaged over 130—250 ns. The most stable polar interactions are hydrogen bonding between 23-OH and T289 at 90% and between 3-OH and S336 at 85%, with S346 also contributing 26% of the simulation time. These interactions anchor the two end regions of the scaffold in the pocket. 20-OH is hydrogen bonding with S320 for 39% of the stimulation time. Due to intra-molecular hydrogen bonding between the ligand hydroxyls, the 20-OH group is positioned to act as a hydrogen bond donor to S320, which allows S320 to interact with F295. This interaction is likely important for these loop conformational changes and their effect on H291. Ligand–protein contacts versus simulation time are shown in Supplemental Figure S5.

Loop conformational changes induced by 20S,23S$(OH)_2$D3 are likely specific to this ligand. Therefore, for docking other vitamin D3 analogs the refined AhR model was utilized, applying the Induced Fit method. As shown in Table 14, Glide XP docking scores of three analogs are notably lower compared to other compounds within this set, 20(OH)D3, 1,25$(OH)_2$D3 and 1,20$(OH)_2$D3. Docked poses of all analogues are very similar, and also closely overlap with 20S,23S$(OH)_2$D3 in the refined AhR model. Docked poses for all analogs are displayed in Figure 9, along with the binding mode of 20S,23S$(OH)_2$D3 for comparison. Residues from Induced Fit structures contributing to polar interactions with ligands are shown only; all residues in proximity of docked ligands are included in Supplemental Figure S6. Docked Vitamin D3 analogs share similar hydrogen bonding interactions through hydroxyl groups: 1-OH interacts with S365, 3-OH with S336 and possibly S346, 17-OH and 20-OH with S320, 23-OH with T289. Docking results predict that 25-OH interacts with T289. A short, 20 ns molecular dynamic simulation was performed on 20(OH)D3, 1,25$(OH)_2$D3, 17,20,23S$(OH)_3$D3, starting with docked poses. The ligands maintained the binding mode and predicted interactions during simulation except for 1,25$(OH)_2$D3. Therefore, simulation of the latter was extended another 50 ns, during which the pose of 1,25$(OH)_2$D3 shifted, disrupting hydrogen bonding between 3-OH and S336 that was only present for 35% of simulation time. In comparison, in the case of 20(OH)D3 and 17,20,23S$(OH)_3$D3 the same interaction was present 85% and 66% of time, respectively. Due to mobility of the aliphatic chain in the binding site, 25-OH formed contacts with T289 30% and Y310 37% of the simulation time. 1,25$(OH)_2$D3 may have a distinct binding mode and interaction with AhR than the other analogs. Interactions of 17,20,23S$(OH)_3$D3 are analogous to those of 20*S*,23*S*$(OH)_2$D3. However, hydrogen bonding between 17-OH with S320 may interfere with structural changes such as those induced by 20*S*,23*S*$(OH)_2$D3 during the 250 ns simulation production run. While 20(OH)D3 is also predicted to form analogous contacts, the absence of 23(OH) interactions is likely significant.

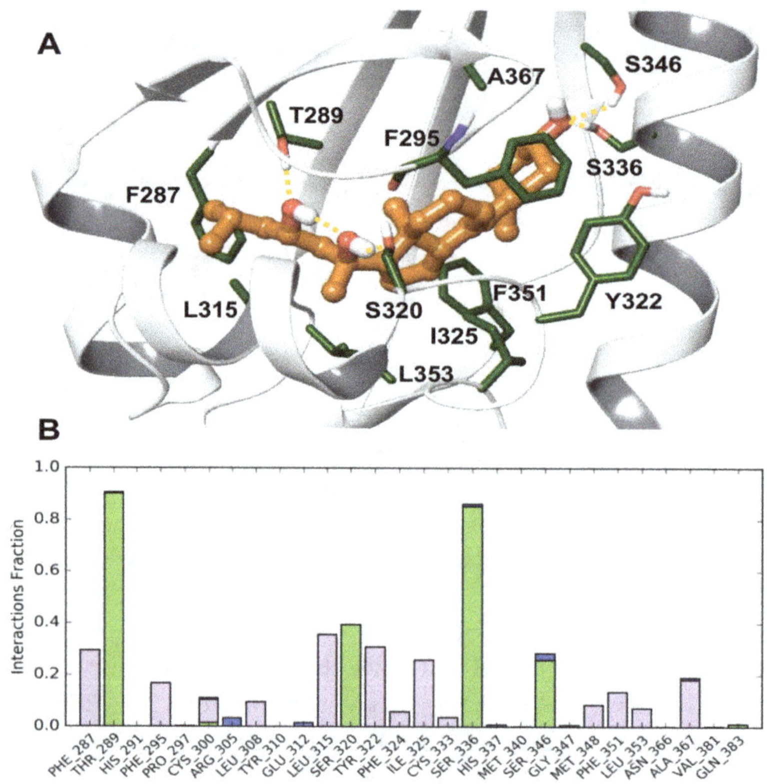

Figure 8. (**A**) The proposed binding model 20*S*,23*S*$(OH)_2$D3 at human AhR. (**A**) Representative simulation snapshot at 230 ns. Shown residues contribute to the binding of the ligand over simulation time. (**B**) Fraction of simulation time during which interactions are present with each AhR residue, averaged over 130–250 ns of the simulation production run.

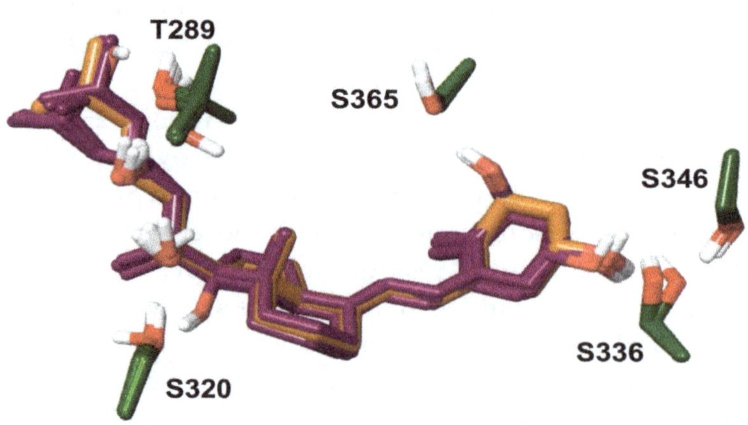

Figure 9. Induced Fit docked vitamin D3 analogs displayed simultaneously. The pose of 20*S*,23*S*$(OH)_2$D3 from the refined AhR model is shown for comparison, with carbon atoms colored light brown. Only AhR residues involved in polar interactions are shown.

Table 14. Glide XP scores of vitamin D3 analogs docked into the refined human AhR LBD model.

Compound	Score	Compound	Score
20*S*OHD3	−13.3	1,20*S*,23*S*$(OH)_3$D3	−16.1
1,25$(OH)_2$D3	−13.1	1,20*S*,23*R*$(OH)_3$D3	−16.4
20*S*,23*S*$(OH)_2$D3	−15.1	17,20*S*,23*S*$(OH)_3$D3	−14.9
20*S*,23*R*$(OH)_2$D3	−15.7	17,20*S*,23*R*$(OH)_3$D3	−15.4
1,20*S*$(OH)_2$D3	−13.0		

Modelling Conclusions

Molecular dynamic simulation of the developed AhR-20*S*,23*S*$(OH)_2$D3 model predicts strong hydrogen bonding interactions between this ligand and T289, S336. A hydrogen bond formed with S320 is also well maintained during simulation. A number of AhR residues have favorable non-polar contacts with the ligand (Figure 8). The simulation trajectory predicts that ligand-specific interactions induce a conformational change in the region in the vicinity of S320 and F295, also leading to a distinct position and interaction of H291. The interaction network that forms during simulation due to the ligand links the beta-sheet structure of the pocket with two loops, restraining the conformation of flexible regions in the binding site. The presented model is also consistent with the observed effect of 20*S*,23*S*$(OH)_2$D3 on AhR since, in particular, T289 and H291 are essential residues for Hsp90 binding.

Docking of a set of D3 analogs predicts ligand binding modes close to that of 20*S*,23*S*$(OH)_2$D3, as well as analogous interactions with AhR. Short simulation runs of docked poses of 20(OH)D3 and 17,20,23*S*$(OH)_3$D3 predict stability of the starting ligand poses. While forming interactions analogous to those of 20*S*,23*S*$(OH)_2$D3, these two analogs lack features that contribute to the induced effects of 20*S*,23*S*$(OH)_2$D3 during simulation. The 20(OH)D3 analog lacks hydrogen bonding through 23-OH and in the case of 17,20,23*S*$(OH)_3$D3 the 17-OH group may interfere with the interactions between S320 and the F295 backbone. Stability of the docked pose of 1,25$(OH)_2$D3 was also explored through molecular dynamic simulation. Shifting and fluctuations of 1,25$(OH)_2$D3 over simulation time suggests that this ligand would not adopt a binding mode close to that of 20*S*,23*S*$(OH)_2$D3 in the AhR binding site. Thus, modelling predictions are consistent with the distinct effects of these D3 analogs on AhR.

3. Materials and Methods

3.1. Materials

Vitamin D3 (D3) and 1,25$(OH)_2$D3 were purchased from Sigma-Aldrich (St. Louis, MO, USA). 20,23$(OH)_2$D3 was produced by hydroxylation of D3 by CYP11A, extracted with dichloromethane and purified as described in References [14,66]. 20*S*-Hydroxyvitamin D3 (20(OH)D3, 1α,20*S*-dihydroxyvitamin D3 (1,20$(OH)_2$D3) and 17,20S,23*S*-trihydroxyvitamin D3 (17,20,23$(OH)_3$D3) were also synthesized using CYP11A1 as described before [66,87]. An extinction coefficient of 18,000 M^{-1} cm^{-1} at 263 nm was used to quantify concentrations of 20,23$(OH)_2$D3 [88] and the secosteroids were divided, dried and stored at −80 °C until use. Secosteroids were dissolved in ethanol prior to experiments to obtain stock solutions of 10^{-4} M.

The structures of the secosteroids tested and the routes of enzymatic synthesis that include C25 and C1 hydroxylation for 1,25$(H)_2$D3 [5], and the sequential hydroxylation of the D3 side chain by CYP11A1 producing 20,23$(OH)_2$D3 and 17,20.23$(OH)_3$D3 [14,66], are shown in Figure 1.

3.2. Cell Culture

Neonatal foreskins of African American [79] donors were used to isolate neonatal human epidermal keratinocytes (HEK) following standard protocols described previously [69,89]. The use of human tissues were approved both by the IRB at the UTHSC as an exempt protocol #4 and by the IRB at the University of Alabama Birmingham, as they are not subject to FDA regulation and not Human Subject Research. Cells were grown in keratinocyte basal medium (KBM) supplemented with keratinocyte growth factors (KGF) (Lonza, Walkersville, MD, USA) on collagen coated plates [68] and second and third passages were used for the experiments [69]. Human epidermal HaCaT keratinocytes were cultured in Dulbecco's Modified Eagle Medium (DMEM) supplemented with glucose, L-glutamine, pyridoxine hydrochloride (Cell Grow), 5% fetal bovine serum (FBS) (Atlanta Biologicals, Flowery Branch, GA, USA) and 1% penicillin/streptomycin/amphotericin antibiotic solution (Thermo Fisher Scientific, Waltham, MA, USA). Human cells were cultured at 37 °C, with a CO_2 concentration of 5%, 100% humidity, and media were changed every second and/or third day.

Prior to treatment with secosteroids, HaCaT cells were serum deprived for 24 h and the medium was changed to DMEM medium containing 5% charcoal-treated FBS (ctFBS) (Atlanta Biologicals, Flowery Branch, GA, USA) to which D3 hydroxymetabolites from the stock solutions were added. For epidermal neonatal keratinocytes, the KBM with KGF was supplemented with 0.5% bovine serum albumin (BSA) prior to the addition of D3 derivatives.

3.3. Microarray Assays

Petri dishes (100 mm in diameter) were seeded with human neonatal keratinocytes that were combined from five different black donors at either passage 2 or 3. After reaching 70–80% of confluence, cells were treated with 10^{-7} M of either 20,23(OH)$_2$D3 or 1,25(OH)$_2$D3, or with 0.1% ethanol (EtOH) as a solvent control for 6 or 24 h. After, these cells were isolated from three plates per each experimental condition and combined for passage 2 and 3, separately (Figure 2).

The RNA from HEK treated with either 20,23(OH)$_2$D3 or 1,25(OH)$_2$D3, or 0.1% ethanol control, was isolated using the Absolutely RNA Miniprep Kit (Qiagen, Germantown, MD, USA). High purity RNA samples were subjected to microarray analysis at the Molecular Resources Center at the UTHSC. Expression profiling was accomplished using whole-genome gene expression direct hybridization assay using Illumina's HumanWG-6_V2 (Platform GPL13376) chip/array (Illumina, San Diego, CA, USA). Each array contains full-length 50-mer probes representing more than 22,000 well-annotated RefSeq transcripts, including up-to-date genes derived from the National Center for Biotechnology Information Reference Sequence (NCBI RefSeq) database. Initially, 250 ng total RNA was converted to cDNA, followed by an in vitro transcription step to generate labeled cRNA following the manufacturer's recommendations (Applied Biosystems, Foster City, CA, USA).

The labeled probes were then mixed with hybridization reagents and hybridized overnight to the Human BeadChips. Following washing and staining, the BeadChips were imaged using the Illumina BeadArray Reader to measure fluorescence intensity at each probe. The intensity of the signal corresponds to the quantity of the respective mRNA in the original sample.

3.4. Bioinformatics Analysis

For generating networks, a data set containing gene identifiers and corresponding expression values was uploaded into the application. Each identifier was mapped to its corresponding object in Ingenuity's Knowledge Base. A FC of ± 2 or ± 1.5, where indicated, was set to identify molecules whose expression was significantly differentially regulated. These molecules, called Network Eligible molecules, were overlaid onto a global molecular network developed from information contained in Ingenuity's Knowledge Base. Networks of Network Eligible Molecules were then algorithmically generated based on their connectivity. The Functional Analysis identified the biological functions and/or diseases that were most significant to the entire data set. Molecules from the dataset that met the FC cutoff of ± 2 or ± 1.5 and were associated with biological functions and/or diseases in Ingenuity's Knowledge Base were considered for the analysis. Right-tailed Fisher's exact test was used to calculate a p-value determining the probability that each biological function and/or disease assigned to that data set is due to chance alone.

3.5. *Real-Time Reverse Transcription Polymerase Chain Reaction (qRT-PCR)*

Semiconfluent cultures of human neonatal keratinocytes or HaCaT cells were treated for 6 h, 24 h or as indicated in the figure legends with vitamin D3 hydroxyderivatives or ethanol, and RNA isolated as described above. Reverse transcription was done using the Transcriptor First Strand cDNA Synthesis Kit (Applied Biosystems, Foster City, CA, USA) with 100 ng RNA per reaction. qRT-PCR was performed using cDNA diluted 10-fold in sterile water and a TaqMan PCR Master Mix. Reactions (in triplicate) were performed at 50 °C for 2 min, 95 °C for 10 min and then 50 cycles of 95 °C for 15 s and 60 °C for 1 min. The primers and probes were designed with the universal probe library (Roche). Data were collected on a Roche Light Cycler 480. The amount of amplified product for each gene was compared to that of Cyclophilin B or GAPDH using a comparative C_T ($\Delta\Delta C_T$) method. Supplemental Table S1 lists the primers used for qRT-PCR amplifications.

3.6. *Interaction of Hydroxyvitamin D Derivatives with AhR*

Interaction of 20(OH)D3, 20,23(OH)$_2$D3 and 1,25(OH)$_2$D3 with AhR was evaluated using the Human AhR Reporter Assay System (INDIGO Biosciences, State College, PA, USA) according to the manufacture's protocol. Briefly, AhR reporter cells were recovered on a 96-well plate frame using the cell recovery medium for 5 h, followed by treatment with vitamin D3 hydroxyderivatives in the compound screening medium for 22 h. After removing the media from the wells, luciferase detection reagent was added to the wells and luminescence was measured using a Cytation 5 Cell Imaging Multi-Mode Reader (Winooski, VT, USA).

3.7. *Statistical Analyses*

Data are presented as means $\pm$ SD (n = 3–4), and were analyzed with a Student's *t*-test (for two groups) or ANOVA using Prism 4.00 (GraphPad Software, San Diego, CA, USA). Statistically significant differences are denoted with asterisks for *t*-tests or for one way ANOVA with # as indicated in the figure legends.

3.8. *Data Deposition*

The data reported in this paper have been deposited in the Gene Expression Omnibus (GEO) database, https://www.ncbi.nlm.nih.gov/geo (accession no. GEO: GSE117351).

3.9. *Development of a Human AhR LBD Model Complexed with 20S,23S(OH)$_2$D3*

The strategy applied utilized tools implemented in the Schrödinger software package, version 2017-4 (Schrödinger, LLC, New York, NY, USA). Homology modelling of the human AhR ligand-binding domain was based on crystal structures of the C-terminal Per-ARNT-Sim domain of Hypoxia-Inducible Factor-2α (HIF-2α PAS-B), PDB entry codes 3H82 and 4XT2. Based on the two templates, two homology models were built using the energy-based homology model building method in Schrödinger. The sequence identity is 27% between human AhR and template sequences in the modelled LBD region. The sequence alignment is shown in Supplemental Figure S4. Residues were numbered according to the human AhR sequence (Uniprot ID P35869). Co-crystallized ligands were included. Modeled loops that contained gaps in the sequence alignment were refined through default loop refinement options. The models were relaxed through restrained energy minimization in Protein Preparation Wizard (OPLS3 force field).

Initial binding mode hypotheses were generated through docking 20*S*,23*R*/*S*(OH)$_2$D3 into the two obtained AhR models. Out of the top scoring poses at both AhR models, eight were selected for protein-ligand complex refinement (Prime tool in Schrödinger software), followed by a 10 ns molecular dynamic simulation run for each complex using Desmond. Four poses induced distortions in rigid, AhR beta-sheet/helical backbone structures within 10 ns simulation and were not considered further. Out of the remaining poses, the most favorable contacts were formed by two similar poses of the epimers: 20*S*,23*S*/*R*$(OH)_2$D3. Simulation of these poses was extended to 20 ns, which suggested that 20*S*,23*S*$(OH)_2$D3 is more favorably accommodated than its *R* epimer. The 20*S*,23*S*$(OH)_2$D3 complex conformer at 20 ns showed an overall RMSD (root-mean-square deviation) of 1.48 from its homology modelling template (PDB: 3H82). In order to allow flexible regions to adjust to the presence of the bound vitamin D3 scaffold, the model was further simulated for 100 ns or for 230 or 25 ns as indicated. The final conformer was relaxed through restrained energy minimization and is referred to as the 'refined AhR model'. The overall RMSD of this model from its homology modelling template (PDB: 3H82) is 1.58, suggesting stability of the AhR structure over simulation time. The model structure contains only two residues with backbone dihedrals in disallowed regions, both of which are glycines: Gly309 and Gly374.

3.10. Docking Method

The induced Fit docking method was used as implemented in Schrödinger, version 2017-4 (Schrödinger, LLC, New York, NY, USA). This method combines Prime tools and Glide docking, taking into account the flexibility of residues in proximity to the ligand. 20,23$(OH)_2$D3 was Induced Fit docked into the two human AhR homology models using default parameters except optimization of side chains was extended to 6 Å around the ligand and Glide re-docking was done in extra-precision mode. Docking of vitamin D3 analogs into the refined AhR model also utilized Induced Fit with default options, except that van der Waals scaling parameters for docking were set to 1.0 for both protein and ligand (no scaling), and re-docking was done in extra-precision mode.

3.11. Molecular Dynamic Simulation Method

Molecular dynamic simulations were performed using Desmond (Schrödinger, LLC, New York, NY, USA) with the OPLS3 force field. Structures were solved in TIP3P explicit waters with boundary conditions in a 10 Å buffered orthorhombic system. Counter-ions were added. The NPT ensemble was employed with temperature fixed at 300 K and pressure at 1.01 bar. The cutoff radius for Coulombic interactions was set to 10 Å. The trajectory was recorded at 10 ps intervals.

4. Conclusions

Gene expression profile analysis demonstrated that 20,23$(OH)_2$D3 and 1,25$(OH)_2$D3 induce distinct and overlapping gene expression patterns in keratinocytes linked to the activation of common (VDR-dependent) and distinct (involving other nuclear receptors) signal transduction pathways. Taking into consideration the strong chemical similarity between 20,23$(OH)_2$D3 and 1,25$(OH)_2$D3 (Figure 1), the marked differences in gene expression panels (Table 1, Figures 3 and 4) were unexpected. This is because our previous studies predominantly showed phenotypic similarities between the effects of both dihydroxy-vitamin D3 species, such as regulation of cell proliferation and differentiation, and anti-inflammatory, photoprotective and anticancer functions, with only a couple of notable differences where 20,23$(OH)_2$D3 displayed no calcemic effects and poor activation of CYP24A1. These predominantly overlapping effects are most likely secondary to the redundancy of downstream phenotypic regulators and intercommunication between distinct transduction pathways at the cell or organ levels. The similarities are likely related to the activation of the VDR. The most significant and unexpected finding is the identification of AhR as the major receptor for 20,23$(OH)_2$D3, which also appears to be activated by other CYP11A1-derived vitamin D3 derivatives, and possibly by 1,25$(OH)_2$D3 to some extent, as predicted by molecular modeling. The future challenge is to precisely define the interaction of different vitamin D3 hydroxyderivatives with the ligand binding domain of AhR and how it is affected by the location of the OH-group on the side chain or at C1α, and how the activation of downstream signal transduction pathways occurs.

Author Contributions: A.T.S. designed experiments, analyzed data and wrote the manuscript. T.-K.K. performed the main experiments, took part in data analysis and preparation of the manuscript. Z.J. performed the main experiments, took part in data analysis and preparation of the manuscript. A.A.B. performed experiments, took part in data analysis and preparation of the manuscript. M.A.Ż. performed the experiments, took part in data analysis and preparation of the manuscript. H.X. took part in data analysis and preparation of the manuscript. T.R.S. performed bioinformatics analysis and took part in preparation of the manuscript. R.C.T. took part in data analysis and preparation of the manuscript. A.M.J. took part in data analysis and preparation of the manuscript. D.K.C. performed bioinformatics analysis and took part in preparation of the manuscript.

Acknowledgments: We thank Quynh Tran for initial normalization of the microarray data.

Abbreviations

1,20(OH)$_2$D3	1,20-dihyhydroxyvitamin D3
17,20,23(OH)$_2$D3	17,20,23-trihyhydroxyvitamin D3
1α,25(OH)$_2$D3	1α,25-dihydroxyvitamin D3
20(OH)D3	20-hydroxyvitamin D3
20,23(OH)$_2$D3	20,23-dihyhydroxyvitamin D3
25(OH)D3	25-hydroxyvitamin D3
7-DHC	7-dehydrocholesterol
AA	African-American
AhR	aryl hydrocarbon receptor
GR	glucocorticoid receptor
LBD	ligand binding domain
LXR	liver X receptor
PPAR	peroxisome proliferator-activated receptor
RAR	retinoic acid receptor
RXR	retinoid X receptor
VDR	vitamin D receptor
UVB	ultraviolet B radiation

References

1. Holick, M.F. Vitamin D: A millenium perspective. *J. Cell. Biochem.* **2003**, *88*, 296–307. [CrossRef] [PubMed]
2. Wacker, M.; Holick, M.F. Sunlight and vitamin D: A global perspective for health. *Dermato-Endocrinology* **2013**, *5*, 51–108. [CrossRef] [PubMed]
3. Holick, M.F. Vitamin D deficiency. *N. Engl. J. Med.* **2007**, *357*, 266–281. [CrossRef] [PubMed]
4. Zhu, J.; DeLuca, H.F. Vitamin d 25-hydroxylase—Four decades of searching, are we there yet? *Arch. Biochem. Biophys.* **2012**, *523*, 30–36. [CrossRef] [PubMed]
5. Jones, G.; Prosser, D.E.; Kaufmann, M. Cytochrome P450-mediated metabolism of vitamin D. *J. Lipid Res.* **2014**, *55*, 13–31. [CrossRef] [PubMed]
6. Christakos, S.; Dhawan, P.; Verstuyf, A.; Verlinden, L.; Carmeliet, G. Vitamin D: Metabolism, molecular mechanism of action, and pleiotropic effects. *Physiol. Rev.* **2016**, *96*, 365–408. [CrossRef] [PubMed]
7. Adams, J.S.; Hewison, M. Extrarenal expression of the 25-hydroxyvitamin D-1-hydroxylase. *Arch. Biochem. Biophys.* **2012**, *523*, 95–102. [CrossRef] [PubMed]
8. Slominski, A.T.; Li, W.; Kim, T.K.; Semak, I.; Wang, J.; Zjawiony, J.K.; Tuckey, R.C. Novel activities of CYP11A1 and their potential physiological significance. *J. Steroid Biochem. Mol. Biol.* **2015**, *151*, 25–37. [CrossRef] [PubMed]
9. Tuckey, R.C. Progesterone synthesis by the human placenta. *Placenta* **2005**, *26*, 273–281. [CrossRef] [PubMed]
10. Miller, W.L.; Auchus, R.J. The molecular biology, biochemistry, and physiology of human steroidogenesis and its disorders. *Endocr. Rev.* **2011**, *32*, 81–151. [CrossRef] [PubMed]

11. Guryev, O.; Carvalho, R.A.; Usanov, S.; Gilep, A.; Estabrook, R.W. A pathway for the metabolism of vitamin D3: Unique hydroxylated metabolites formed during catalysis with cytochrome P450scc (CYP11A1). *Proc. Natl. Acad. Sci. USA* **2003**, *100*, 14754–14759. [CrossRef] [PubMed]
12. Slominski, A.; Zjawiony, J.; Wortsman, J.; Semak, I.; Stewart, J.; Pisarchik, A.; Sweatman, T.; Marcos, J.; Dunbar, C.; R, C.T. A novel pathway for sequential transformation of 7-dehydrocholesterol and expression of the P450scc system in mammalian skin. *Eur. J. Biochem.* **2004**, *271*, 4178–4188. [CrossRef] [PubMed]
13. Slominski, A.; Semak, I.; Zjawiony, J.; Wortsman, J.; Li, W.; Szczesniewski, A.; Tuckey, R.C. The cytochrome P450scc system opens an alternate pathway of vitamin D3 metabolism. *FEBS J.* **2005**, *272*, 4080–4090. [CrossRef] [PubMed]
14. Tuckey, R.C.; Li, W.; Zjawiony, J.K.; Zmijewski, M.A.; Nguyen, M.N.; Sweatman, T.; Miller, D.; Slominski, A. Pathways and products for the metabolism of vitamin D3 by cytochrome P450scc. *FEBS J.* **2008**, *275*, 2585–2596. [CrossRef] [PubMed]
15. Slominski, A.; Semak, I.; Wortsman, J.; Zjawiony, J.; Li, W.; Zbytek, B.; Tuckey, R.C. An alternative pathway of vitamin D metabolism. Cytochrome P450scc (CYP11A1)-mediated conversion to 20-hydroxyvitamin D2 and 17,20-dihydroxyvitamin D2. *FEBS J.* **2006**, *273*, 2891–2901. [CrossRef] [PubMed]
16. Nguyen, M.N.; Slominski, A.; Li, W.; Ng, Y.R.; Tuckey, R.C. Metabolism of vitamin D2 to 17,20,24-trihydroxyvitamin D2 by cytochrome P450scc (CYP11A1). *Drug Metab. Dispos.* **2009**, *37*, 761–767. [CrossRef] [PubMed]
17. Lin, Z.; Marepally, S.R.; Ma, D.; Myers, L.K.; Postlethwaite, A.E.; Tuckey, R.C.; Cheng, C.Y.; Kim, T.K.; Yue, J.; Slominski, A.T.; et al. Chemical synthesis and biological activities of 20s,24s/r-dihydroxyvitamin D3 epimers and their 1alpha-hydroxyl derivatives. *J. Med. Chem.* **2015**, *58*, 7881–7887. [CrossRef] [PubMed]
18. Slominski, A.T.; Kim, T.K.; Shehabi, H.Z.; Semak, I.; Tang, E.K.; Nguyen, M.N.; Benson, H.A.; Korik, E.; Janjetovic, Z.; Chen, J.; et al. In vivo evidence for a novel pathway of vitamin D(3) metabolism initiated by P450scc and modified by CYP27B1. *FASEB J.* **2012**, *26*, 3901–3915. [CrossRef] [PubMed]
19. Slominski, A.T.; Kim, T.K.; Shehabi, H.Z.; Tang, E.K.; Benson, H.A.; Semak, I.; Lin, Z.; Yates, C.R.; Wang, J.; Li, W.; et al. In vivo production of novel vitamin D2 hydroxy-derivatives by human placentas, epidermal keratinocytes, Caco-2 colon cells and the adrenal gland. *Mol. Cell. Endocrinol.* **2014**, *383*, 181–192. [CrossRef] [PubMed]
20. Slominski, A.T.; Kim, T.K.; Li, W.; Tuckey, R.C. Classical and non-classical metabolic transformation of vitamin D in dermal fibroblasts. *Exp. Dermatol.* **2016**, *25*, 231–232. [CrossRef] [PubMed]
21. Slominski, A.T.; Zmijewski, M.A.; Semak, I.; Sweatman, T.; Janjetovic, Z.; Li, W.; Zjawiony, J.K.; Tuckey, R.C. Sequential metabolism of 7-dehydrocholesterol to steroidal 5,7-dienes in adrenal glands and its biological implication in the skin. *PLoS ONE* **2009**, *4*, e4309. [CrossRef] [PubMed]
22. Slominski, A.T.; Kim, T.K.; Chen, J.; Nguyen, M.N.; Li, W.; Yates, C.R.; Sweatman, T.; Janjetovic, Z.; Tuckey, R.C. Cytochrome P450scc-dependent metabolism of 7-dehydrocholesterol in placenta and epidermal keratinocytes. *Int. J. Biochem. Cell Biol.* **2012**, *44*, 2003–2018. [CrossRef] [PubMed]
23. Slominski, A.T.; Janjetovic, Z.; Kim, T.K.; Wasilewski, P.; Rosas, S.; Hanna, S.; Sayre, R.M.; Dowdy, J.C.; Li, W.; Tuckey, R.C. Novel non-calcemic secosteroids that are produced by human epidermal keratinocytes protect against solar radiation. *J. Steroid Biochem. Mol. Biol.* **2015**, *148*, 52–63. [CrossRef] [PubMed]
24. Slominski, A.T.; Kim, T.K.; Li, W.; Postlethwaite, A.; Tieu, E.W.; Tang, E.K.; Tuckey, R.C. Detection of novel CYP11A1-derived secosteroids in the human epidermis and serum and pig adrenal gland. *Sci. Rep.* **2015**, *5*, 14875. [CrossRef] [PubMed]
25. DeLuca, H.F. Overview of general physiologic features and functions of vitamin D. *Am. J. Clin. Nutr.* **2004**, *80*, 1689S–1696S. [CrossRef] [PubMed]
26. Holick, M.F. Vitamin D and bone health. *J. Nutr.* **1996**, *126*, 1159S–1164S. [CrossRef] [PubMed]
27. Bikle, D.D. Vitamin D: An ancient hormone. *Exp. Dermatol.* **2011**, *20*, 7–13. [CrossRef] [PubMed]
28. Pike, J.W.; Christakos, S. Biology and mechanisms of action of the vitamin D hormone. *Endocrinol. Metab. Clin. N. Am.* **2017**, *46*, 815–843. [CrossRef] [PubMed]
29. Van Driel, M.; van Leeuwen, J. Vitamin D endocrinology of bone mineralization. *Mol. Cell. Endocrinol.* **2017**, *453*, 46–51. [CrossRef] [PubMed]
30. Hewison, M. An update on vitamin D and human immunity. *Clin. Endocrinol.* **2012**, *76*, 315–325. [CrossRef] [PubMed]

31. Vanherwegen, A.S.; Gysemans, C.; Mathieu, C. Regulation of immune function by vitamin d and its use in diseases of immunity. *Endocrinol. Metab. Clin. N. Am.* **2017**, *46*, 1061–1094. [CrossRef] [PubMed]
32. Berridge, M.J. Vitamin D deficiency: Infertility and neurodevelopmental diseases (attention deficit hyperactivity disorder, autism, and schizophrenia). *Am. J. Physiol. Cell Physiol.* **2018**, *314*, C135–C151. [CrossRef] [PubMed]
33. Liu, N.Q.; Hewison, M. Vitamin d, the placenta and pregnancy. *Arch. Biochem. Biophys.* **2012**, *523*, 37–47. [CrossRef] [PubMed]
34. Ganguly, A.; Tamblyn, J.A.; Finn-Sell, S.; Chan, S.Y.; Westwood, M.; Gupta, J.; Kilby, M.D.; Gross, S.R.; Hewison, M. Vitamin D, the placenta and early pregnancy: Effects on trophoblast function. *J. Endocrinol.* **2018**, *236*, R93–R103. [CrossRef] [PubMed]
35. Shin, J.S.; Choi, M.Y.; Longtine, M.S.; Nelson, D.M. Vitamin d effects on pregnancy and the placenta. *Placenta* **2010**, *31*, 1027–1034. [CrossRef] [PubMed]
36. Knabl, J.; Vattai, A.; Ye, Y.; Jueckstock, J.; Hutter, S.; Kainer, F.; Mahner, S.; Jeschke, U. Role of placental VDR expression and function in common late pregnancy disorders. *Int. J. Mol. Sci.* **2017**, *18*, 2340. [CrossRef] [PubMed]
37. Lorenzen, M.; Boisen, I.M.; Mortensen, L.J.; Lanske, B.; Juul, A.; Blomberg Jensen, M. Reproductive endocrinology of vitamin D. *Mol. Cell. Endocrinol.* **2017**, *453*, 103–112. [CrossRef] [PubMed]
38. Cui, X.; Gooch, H.; Petty, A.; McGrath, J.J.; Eyles, D. Vitamin D and the brain: Genomic and non-genomic actions. *Mol. Cell. Endocrinol.* **2017**, *453*, 131–143. [CrossRef] [PubMed]
39. Di Somma, C.; Scarano, E.; Barrea, L.; Zhukouskaya, V.V.; Savastano, S.; Mele, C.; Scacchi, M.; Aimaretti, G.; Colao, A.; Marzullo, P. Vitamin D and neurological diseases: An endocrine view. *Int. J. Mol. Sci.* **2017**, *18*, 2482. [CrossRef] [PubMed]
40. Welsh, J. Function of the vitamin D endocrine system in mammary gland and breast cancer. *Mol. Cell. Endocrinol.* **2017**, *453*, 88–95. [CrossRef] [PubMed]
41. Angellotti, E.; Pittas, A.G. The role of vitamin d in the prevention of type 2 diabetes: To D or not to D? *Endocrinology* **2017**, *158*, 2013–2021. [CrossRef] [PubMed]
42. Dimova, R.; Tankova, T.; Chakarova, N. Vitamin d in the spectrum of prediabetes and cardiovascular autonomic dysfunction. *J. Nutr.* **2017**, *147*, 1607–1615. [CrossRef] [PubMed]
43. Berridge, M.J. Vitamin D deficiency and diabetes. *Biochem. J.* **2017**, *474*, 1321–1332. [CrossRef] [PubMed]
44. Kassi, E.; Nasiri-Ansari, N.; Papavassiliou, A.G. Vitamin d affects glucocorticoid action in target cells. *Oncotarget* **2017**, *8*, 7220–7221. [CrossRef] [PubMed]
45. Plum, L.A.; DeLuca, H.F. Vitamin D, disease and therapeutic opportunities. *Nat. Rev. Drug Discov.* **2010**, *9*, 941–955. [CrossRef] [PubMed]
46. Feldman, D.; Krishnan, A.V.; Swami, S.; Giovannucci, E.; Feldman, B.J. The role of vitamin d in reducing cancer risk and progression. *Nat. Rev. Cancer* **2014**, *14*, 342–357. [CrossRef] [PubMed]
47. Fleet, J.C.; DeSmet, M.; Johnson, R.; Li, Y. Vitamin d and cancer: A review of molecular mechanisms. *Biochem. J.* **2012**, *441*, 61–76. [CrossRef] [PubMed]
48. Masuda, S.; Jones, G. Promise of vitamin d analogues in the treatment of hyperproliferative conditions. *Mol. Cancer Ther.* **2006**, *5*, 797–808. [CrossRef] [PubMed]
49. Slominski, A.T.; Brozyna, A.A.; Skobowiat, C.; Zmijewski, M.A.; Kim, T.K.; Janjetovic, Z.; Oak, A.S.; Jozwicki, W.; Jetten, A.M.; Mason, R.S.; et al. On the role of classical and novel forms of vitamin d in melanoma progression and management. *J. Steroid Biochem. Mol. Biol.* **2018**, *177*, 159–170. [CrossRef] [PubMed]
50. Slominski, A.T.; Brozyna, A.A.; Zmijewski, M.A.; Jozwicki, W.; Jetten, A.M.; Mason, R.S.; Tuckey, R.C.; Elmets, C.A. Vitamin D signaling and melanoma: Role of vitamin d and its receptors in melanoma progression and management. *Lab. Investig.* **2017**, *97*, 706–724. [CrossRef] [PubMed]
51. Norman, A.W. Minireview: Vitamin d receptor: New assignments for an already busy receptor. *Endocrinology* **2006**, *147*, 5542–5548. [CrossRef] [PubMed]
52. Mason, R.S.; Reichrath, J. Sunlight vitamin d and skin cancer. *Anticancer Agents Med. Chem.* **2013**, *13*, 83–97. [CrossRef] [PubMed]
53. Bikle, D.D.; Elalieh, H.; Welsh, J.; Oh, D.; Cleaver, J.; Teichert, A. Protective role of vitamin D signaling in skin cancer formation. *J. Steroid Biochem. Mol. Biol.* **2013**, *136*, 271–279. [CrossRef] [PubMed]

54. Neme, A.; Seuter, S.; Carlberg, C. Selective regulation of biological processes by vitamin d based on the spatio-temporal cistrome of its receptor. *Biochim. Biophys. Acta* **2017**, *1860*, 952–961. [CrossRef] [PubMed]
55. Bikle, D.D. Vitamin D receptor, UVR, and skin cancer: A potential protective mechanism. *J. Investig. Dermatol.* **2008**, *128*, 2357–2361. [CrossRef] [PubMed]
56. Elias, P.M. Structure and function of the stratum corneum extracellular matrix. *J. Investig. Dermatol.* **2012**, *132*, 2131–2133. [CrossRef] [PubMed]
57. Dixon, K.M.; Norman, A.W.; Sequeira, V.B.; Mohan, R.; Rybchyn, M.S.; Reeve, V.E.; Halliday, G.M.; Mason, R.S. 1alpha,25(OH)(2)-vitamin D and a nongenomic vitamin d analogue inhibit ultraviolet radiation-induced skin carcinogenesis. *Cancer Prev. Res. (Phila)* **2011**, *4*, 1485–1494. [CrossRef] [PubMed]
58. Makarova, A.; Wang, G.; Dolorito, J.A.; Kc, S.; Libove, E.; Epstein, E.H., Jr. Vitamin D3 produced by skin exposure to UVR inhibits murine basal cell carcinoma carcinogenesis. *J. Investig. Dermatol.* **2017**, *137*, 2613–2619. [CrossRef] [PubMed]
59. Slominski, A.T.; Zmijewski, M.A.; Semak, I.; Zbytek, B.; Pisarchik, A.; Li, W.; Zjawiony, J.; Tuckey, R.C. Cytochromes P450 and skin cancer: Role of local endocrine pathways. *Anticancer Agents Med. Chem.* **2014**, *14*, 77–96. [CrossRef] [PubMed]
60. Slominski, A.T.; Kim, T.K.; Hobrath, J.V.; Oak, A.S.W.; Tang, E.K.Y.; Tieu, E.W.; Li, W.; Tuckey, R.C.; Jetten, A.M. Endogenously produced nonclassical vitamin D hydroxy-metabolites act as "Biased" Agonists on VDR and inverse agonists on RORalpha and RORgamma. *J. Steroid Biochem. Mol. Biol.* **2017**, *173*, 42–56. [CrossRef] [PubMed]
61. Wang, J.; Slominski, A.; Tuckey, R.C.; Janjetovic, Z.; Kulkarni, A.; Chen, J.; Postlethwaite, A.E.; Miller, D.; Li, W. 20-Hydroxyvitamin D(3) inhibits proliferation of cancer cells with high efficacy while being non-toxic. *Anticancer Res.* **2012**, *32*, 739–746. [PubMed]
62. Slominski, A.T.; Janjetovic, Z.; Fuller, B.E.; Zmijewski, M.A.; Tuckey, R.C.; Nguyen, M.N.; Sweatman, T.; Li, W.; Zjawiony, J.; Miller, D.; et al. Products of vitamin D3 or 7-dehydrocholesterol metabolism by cytochrome P450scc show anti-leukemia effects, having low or absent calcemic activity. *PLoS ONE* **2010**, *5*, e9907. [CrossRef] [PubMed]
63. Chen, J.; Wang, J.; Kim, T.K.; Tieu, E.W.; Tang, E.K.; Lin, Z.; Kovacic, D.; Miller, D.D.; Postlethwaite, A.; Tuckey, R.C.; et al. Novel vitamin d analogs as potential therapeutics: Metabolism, toxicity profiling, and antiproliferative activity. *Anticancer Res.* **2014**, *34*, 2153–2163. [PubMed]
64. Tongkao-On, W.; Carter, S.; Reeve, V.E.; Dixon, K.M.; Gordon-Thomson, C.; Halliday, G.M.; Tuckey, R.C.; Mason, R.S. Cyp11a1 in skin: An alternative route to photoprotection by vitamin D compounds. *J. Steroid Biochem. Mol. Biol.* **2015**, *148*, 72–78. [CrossRef] [PubMed]
65. Slominski, A.; Janjetovic, Z.; Tuckey, R.C.; Nguyen, M.N.; Bhattacharya, K.G.; Wang, J.; Li, W.; Jiao, Y.; Gu, W.; Brown, M.; et al. 20s-hydroxyvitamin D3, noncalcemic product of CYP11A1 action on vitamin D3, exhibits potent antifibrogenic activity in vivo. *J. Clin. Endocrinol. Metab.* **2013**, *98*, E298–E303. [CrossRef] [PubMed]
66. Tuckey, R.C.; Li, W.; Shehabi, H.Z.; Janjetovic, Z.; Nguyen, M.N.; Kim, T.K.; Chen, J.; Howell, D.E.; Benson, H.A.; Sweatman, T.; et al. Production of 22-hydroxy metabolites of vitamin D3 by cytochrome P450scc (CYP11A1) and analysis of their biological activities on skin cells. *Drug Metab. Dispos.* **2011**, *39*, 1577–1588. [CrossRef] [PubMed]
67. Zbytek, B.; Janjetovic, Z.; Tuckey, R.C.; Zmijewski, M.A.; Sweatman, T.W.; Jones, E.; Nguyen, M.N.; Slominski, A.T. 20-Hydroxyvitamin D3, a product of vitamin D3 hydroxylation by cytochrome P450scc, stimulates keratinocyte differentiation. *J. Investig. Dermatol.* **2008**, *128*, 2271–2280. [CrossRef] [PubMed]
68. Janjetovic, Z.; Zmijewski, M.A.; Tuckey, R.C.; DeLeon, D.A.; Nguyen, M.N.; Pfeffer, L.M.; Slominski, A.T. 20-Hydroxycholecalciferol, product of vitamin D3 hydroxylation by P450scc, decreases NF-kappaB activity by increasing IkappaB alpha levels in human keratinocytes. *PLoS ONE* **2009**, *4*, e5988. [CrossRef] [PubMed]
69. Janjetovic, Z.; Tuckey, R.C.; Nguyen, M.N.; Thorpe, E.M., Jr.; Slominski, A.T. 20,23-dihydroxyvitamin D3, novel P450scc product, stimulates differentiation and inhibits proliferation and NF-kappaB activity in human keratinocytes. *J. Cell. Physiol.* **2010**, *223*, 36–48. [PubMed]
70. Wasiewicz, T.; Szyszka, P.; Cichorek, M.; Janjetovic, Z.; Tuckey, R.C.; Slominski, A.T.; Zmijewski, M.A. Antitumor effects of vitamin D analogs on hamster and mouse melanoma cell lines in relation to melanin pigmentation. *Int. J. Mol. Sci.* **2015**, *16*, 6645–6667. [CrossRef] [PubMed]

71. Wierzbicka, J.M.; Zmijewski, M.A.; Piotrowska, A.; Nedoszytko, B.; Lange, M.; Tuckey, R.C.; Slominski, A.T. Bioactive forms of vitamin d selectively stimulate the skin analog of the hypothalamus-pituitary-adrenal axis in human epidermal keratinocytes. *Mol. Cell. Endocrinol.* **2016**, *437*, 312–322. [CrossRef] [PubMed]
72. Skobowiat, C.; Oak, A.S.; Kim, T.K.; Yang, C.H.; Pfeffer, L.M.; Tuckey, R.C.; Slominski, A.T. Noncalcemic 20-hydroxyvitamin D3 inhibits human melanoma growth in in vitro and in vivo models. *Oncotarget* **2017**, *8*, 9823–9834. [CrossRef] [PubMed]
73. Janjetovic, Z.; Brozyna, A.A.; Tuckey, R.C.; Kim, T.K.; Nguyen, M.N.; Jozwicki, W.; Pfeffer, S.R.; Pfeffer, L.M.; Slominski, A.T. High basal NF-kappaB activity in nonpigmented melanoma cells is associated with an enhanced sensitivity to vitamin D3 derivatives. *Br. J. Cancer* **2011**, *105*, 1874–1884. [CrossRef] [PubMed]
74. Wierzbicka, J.M.; Binek, A.; Ahrends, T.; Nowacka, J.D.; Szydlowska, A.; Turczyk, L.; Wasiewicz, T.; Wierzbicki, P.M.; Sadej, R.; Tuckey, R.C.; et al. Differential antitumor effects of vitamin d analogues on colorectal carcinoma in culture. *Int. J. Oncol.* **2015**, *47*, 1084–1096. [CrossRef] [PubMed]
75. Piotrowska, A.; Wierzbicka, J.; Slebioda, T.; Wozniak, M.; Tuckey, R.C.; Slominski, A.T.; Zmijewski, M.A. Vitamin D derivatives enhance cytotoxic effects of H_2O_2 or cisplatin on human keratinocytes. *Steroids* **2016**, *110*, 49–61. [CrossRef] [PubMed]
76. Lin, Z.; Marepally, S.R.; Goh, E.S.Y.; Cheng, C.Y.S.; Janjetovic, Z.; Kim, T.K.; Miller, D.D.; Postlethwaite, A.E.; Slominski, A.T.; Tuckey, R.C.; et al. Investigation of 20s-hydroxyvitamin D3 analogs and their 1alpha-OH derivatives as potent vitamin d receptor agonists with anti-inflammatory activities. *Sci. Rep.* **2018**, *8*, 1478. [CrossRef] [PubMed]
77. Lin, Z.; Chen, H.; Belorusova, A.Y.; Bollinger, J.C.; Tang, E.K.Y.; Janjetovic, Z.; Kim, T.K.; Wu, Z.; Miller, D.D.; Slominski, A.T.; et al. 1alpha,20S-dihydroxyvitamin D3 interacts with vitamin D receptor: Crystal structure and route of chemical synthesis. *Sci. Rep.* **2017**, *7*, 10193. [CrossRef] [PubMed]
78. Slominski, A.T.; Kim, T.K.; Takeda, Y.; Janjetovic, Z.; Brozyna, A.A.; Skobowiat, C.; Wang, J.; Postlethwaite, A.; Li, W.; Tuckey, R.C.; et al. RORalpha and ROR gamma are expressed in human skin and serve as receptors for endogenously produced noncalcemic 20-hydroxy- and 20,23-dihydroxyvitamin D. *FASEB J.* **2014**, *28*, 2775–2789. [CrossRef] [PubMed]
79. Le Poole, I.C.; van den Berg, F.M.; van den Wijngaard, R.M.; Galloway, D.A.; van Amstel, P.J.; Buffing, A.A.; Smits, H.L.; Westerhof, W.; Das, P.K. Generation of a human melanocyte cell line by introduction of HPV16 E6 and E7 genes. *In Vitro Cell. Dev. Biol. Anim.* **1997**, *33*, 42–49. [CrossRef] [PubMed]
80. Slominski, A.T.; Kim, T.K.; Li, W.; Yi, A.K.; Postlethwaite, A.; Tuckey, R.C. The role of CYP11A1 in the production of vitamin D metabolites and their role in the regulation of epidermal functions. *J. Steroid Biochem. Mol. Biol.* **2014**, *144PA*, 28–39. [CrossRef] [PubMed]
81. Bikle, D.D.; Oda, Y.; Tu, C.L.; Jiang, Y. Novel mechanisms for the vitamin d receptor (VDR) in the skin and in skin cancer. *J. Steroid Biochem. Mol. Biol.* **2015**, *148*, 47–51. [CrossRef] [PubMed]
82. Carlberg, C. What do we learn from the genome-wide perspective on vitamin D3? *Anticancer Res.* **2015**, *35*, 1143–1151. [PubMed]
83. Kim, T.K.; Wang, J.; Janjetovic, Z.; Chen, J.; Tuckey, R.C.; Nguyen, M.N.; Tang, E.K.; Miller, D.; Li, W.; Slominski, A.T. Correlation between secosteroid-induced vitamin D receptor activity in melanoma cells and computer-modeled receptor binding strength. *Mol. Cell. Endocrinol.* **2012**, *361*, 143–152. [CrossRef] [PubMed]
84. Slominski, A.T.; Janjetovic, Z.; Kim, T.K.; Wright, A.C.; Grese, L.N.; Riney, S.J.; Nguyen, M.N.; Tuckey, R.C. Novel vitamin D hydroxyderivatives inhibit melanoma growth and show differential effects on normal melanocytes. *Anticancer Res.* **2012**, *32*, 3733–3742. [PubMed]
85. Soshilov, A.A.; Denison, M.S. Ligand promiscuity of aryl hydrocarbon receptor agonists and antagonists revealed by site-directed mutagenesis. *Mol. Cell. Biol.* **2014**, *34*, 1707–1719. [CrossRef] [PubMed]
86. Soshilov, A.; Denison, M.S. Ligand displaces heat shock protein 90 from overlapping binding sites within the aryl hydrocarbon receptor ligand-binding domain. *J. Biol. Chem.* **2011**, *286*, 35275–35282. [CrossRef] [PubMed]
87. Tuckey, R.C.; Janjetovic, Z.; Li, W.; Nguyen, M.N.; Zmijewski, M.A.; Zjawiony, J.; Slominski, A. Metabolism of 1alpha-hydroxyvitamin D3 by cytochrome P450scc to biologically active 1alpha,20-dihydroxyvitamin D3. *J. Steroid Biochem. Mol. Biol.* **2008**, *112*, 213–219. [CrossRef] [PubMed]

88. Hiwatashi, A.; Nishii, Y.; Ichikawa, Y. Purification of cytochrome P-450d1 alpha (25-hydroxyvitamin D3-1 alpha-hydroxylase) of bovine kidney mitochondria. *Biochem. Biophys. Res. Commun.* **1982**, *105*, 320–327. [CrossRef]

89. Janjetovic, Z.; Nahmias, Z.P.; Hanna, S.; Jarrett, S.G.; Kim, T.K.; Reiter, R.J.; Slominski, A.T. Melatonin and its metabolites ameliorate ultraviolet b-induced damage in human epidermal keratinocytes. *J. Pineal Res.* **2014**, *57*, 90–102. [CrossRef] [PubMed]

4

Disparities in Head and Neck Cancer: A Case for Chemoprevention with Vitamin D

Mirela Ibrahimovic [1,2], Elizabeth Franzmann [3,4], Alison M. Mondul [1,2], Katherine M. Weh [1,5], Connor Howard [1,5], Jennifer J. Hu [3,6], W. Jarrard Goodwin [3,6] and Laura A. Kresty [1,5,*]

1 The Rogel Cancer Center, University of Michigan, Ann Arbor, MI 48109, USA; imirela@umich.edu (M.I.); amondul@umich.edu (A.M.M.); kweh@med.umich.edu (K.M.W.); conhow@med.umich.edu (C.H.)
2 Department of Epidemiology, School of Public Health, University of Michigan, Ann Arbor, MI 48109, USA
3 Sylvester Comprehensive Cancer Center, University of Miami School of Medicine, Miami, FL 33136, USA; efranzman@med.miami.edu (E.F.); jhu@med.miami.edu (J.J.H.); wgoodwin@med.miami.edu (W.J.G.)
4 Department of Otolaryngology, University of Miami School of Medicine, Miami, FL 33136, USA
5 Department of Surgery, Thoracic Surgery Section, University of Michigan, Ann Arbor, MI 48109, USA
6 Department of Public Health Sciences, University of Miami School of Medicine, Miami, FL 33136, USA
* Correspondence: lkresty@med.umich.edu

Abstract: Blacks experience disproportionate head and neck cancer (HNC) recurrence and mortality compared to Whites. Overall, vitamin D status is inversely associated to HNC pointing to a potential protective linkage. Although hypovitaminosis D in Blacks is well documented it has not been investigated in Black HNC patients. Thus, we conducted a prospective pilot study accessing vitamin D status in newly diagnosed HNC patients stratified by race and conducted in vitro studies to investigate mechanisms associated with potential cancer inhibitory effects of vitamin D. Outcome measures included circulating levels of vitamin D, related nutrients, and risk factor characterization as well as dietary and supplemental estimates. Vitamin D-based in vitro assays utilized proteome and microRNA (miR) profiling. Nineteen patients were enrolled, mean circulating vitamin D levels were significantly reduced in Black compared to White HNC patients, 27.3 and 20.0 ng/mL, respectively. Whites also supplemented vitamin D more frequently than Blacks who had non-significantly higher vitamin D from dietary sources. Vitamin D treatment of HNC cell lines revealed five significantly altered miRs regulating genes targeting multiple pathways in cancer based on enrichment analysis (i.e., negative regulation of cell proliferation, angiogenesis, chemokine, MAPK, and WNT signaling). Vitamin D further altered proteins involved in cancer progression, metastasis and survival supporting a potential role for vitamin D in targeted cancer prevention.

Keywords: head and neck cancer; racial disparities; vitamin D; chemoprevention; UVB; microRNA; proteomic profiling

---

1. Introduction

Head and neck cancer (HNC) is the ninth most commonly diagnosed cancer in the United States and is associated with significant morbidity, mortality, and economic loss [1,2]. Important racial disparities persist for HNC [3]. Historically, HNC was more common in Black Americans than Whites, however, the incidence rate in the latter has increased since the 1990s in parallel with human papillomavirus (HPV)—positive HNC, which is diagnosed more among White males [4]. Black Americans tend to have lower rates of HPV-associated HNC which generally present as oropharyngeal cancers and are associated with better response to treatment and improved five-year survival rates compared to HPV-negative HNC [5,6]. Overall, HNC in Black patients is associated with a much lower five-year survival rate, about 30% compared to 57% in White patients [5,6]. Disparate survival rates have been investigated in recent years, yet consensus regarding the causative factors remains to be fully elucidated. Published reports document that Black HNC patients present with more advanced disease at initial diagnosis, experience greater delays in treatment initiation, and experience more gaps in health insurance coverage compared to Whites [7–9]. Still, our understanding of racial disparities in HNC remains incomplete. Research assessing potential biological mechanisms underlying HNC in racially diverse populations is lacking, as is information on the contribution of modifiable dietary factors to HNC incidence and progression. An inverse association between vitamin D status and cancer incidence, prognosis, and mortality has been reported in several cancer types, HNC included [10–14]. Moreover, it is well documented that Black Americans are at a higher risk for low vitamin D status, yet the link between HNC and vitamin D status has not been evaluated among Black patients [15,16].

Studies investigating vitamin D have identified a multitude of health benefits including improved calcium absorption, improved immune function, and an increase in bone density [17,18]. It has been speculated that vitamin D has potential anticarcinogenic effects through multiple biologic functions; however, clinical interventions and observational studies evaluating vitamin D have yielded mixed results across different cancers [10]. Nonetheless, a recent prospective cohort study targeting HNC in a population without race reported shows that higher vitamin D intake levels are associated with decreased risk of HNC recurrence [13]. Conversely, vitamin D deficiency has been linked to lymphatic metastasis among HNC patients [19].

The goal of this prospective pilot study was to assess vitamin D status in newly diagnosed Black and White HNC patients and to conduct in vitro studies to improve our understanding of mechanisms associated with the potential cancer inhibitory effects of vitamin D in the context of HNC. To our knowledge, there have been no studies evaluating the association between vitamin D levels and HNC in Black patients despite their increased risk of vitamin D deficiency and increased risk of HNC recurrence as well as reduced five-year survival rates compared to White patients. In the present analysis, we examine vitamin D levels and other characteristics in Black and White HNC patients treated for HNC in Miami, Florida. Further, to explore anti-cancer mechanisms of vitamin D microRNA (miR) and proteomic profiling was conducted on human HNC cancer cell lines following vitamin D treatment.

Our research findings support that Black HNC patients present at an earlier age and with reduced levels of circulating vitamin D levels compared to Whites even in sunny South Florida. In addition, none of our Black HNC patients had vitamin D levels greater than or equal to 30 ng/mL, the level associated with optimal regulation of parathyroid hormone (PTH), calcium absorption, and bone health. Parallel in vitro studies revealed that vitamin D treatment of HNC cell lines significantly altered miRs regulating genes involved in many cancer pathways (i.e., steroid biosynthesis, cell proliferation, angiogenesis, chemokine, stem cell pluripotency, MAPK, and WNT signaling). Similarly, proteomic profiling following vitamin D treatment revealed modulation of proteins with roles in HNC cancer progression, metastasis, chemoresistance, and cancer recurrence and further supporting a potential role vitamin D in targeted cancer prevention [20–23].

2. Materials and Methods

2.1. Characteristics of the Head and Neck Cancer Patient Population

Nineteen HNC patients (10 non-Hispanic Whites and 9 Blacks) were recruited from the Sylvester Cancer Center or Jackson Memorial Hospital in Miami, Florida. Patients 18 years of age or older were included if they had a new diagnosis of HNC cancer (including primary lesions of the oral cavity, excluding HPV-linked cancers of the oropharynx); primary lesions of stage I–IV were included. All subjects gave their informed consent for inclusion before they participated in the study. The study was conducted in accordance with the Declaration of Helsinki, and the protocol was approved by the Institutional Review Board and Ethics Committee of the University of Miami (Project ID: 81110). Both male and female patients were enrolled in the study on a rolling basis. If the participant was pregnant, suffered from other illnesses or used chronic medication known to impact vitamin D metabolism they were excluded from the study. Human subject inclusion codes were G1A, M1A, and C3A. Additional information collected included basic demographic and socioeconomic factors (i.e., age, sex, height, weight, residency, annual income, highest education level completed, risk factors, and occupational history).

2.2. Dietary Intake Information and Risk Factor Characterization

Block Dietary Data Systems screeners were used to collect data on the patients' dietary intake including fruit and vegetable consumption as well as calcium and vitamin D intake. In addition to this, physical activity and sun exposure data were collected. Smoking status and alcohol consumption data were acquired by utilizing Tobacco Product Assessment Consortium (TobPRAC) tools.

2.3. Blood Measures

Blood levels of both the circulating metabolite (25-hydroxyvitamin D) and active metabolite (1,25-dihydroxyvitamin D) of vitamin D were measured from serum. Plasma was utilized to determine calcium and PTH levels. Levels of 25-hydroxyvitamin D and 1,25-dihydroxyvitamin D were determined using a two-step process involving rapid extraction and purification and (radioimmunoassay) RIA with specific antibodies (DiaSorin, Stillwater, MN, USA). PTH levels were determined utilizing the Immulite Immunometric assay (Diagnostic Products Corp., Los Angeles, CA, USA). Quest Diagnostics (San Juan Capistrano, CA, USA and Miramar, FL, USA) analyzed the samples utilizing well validated methods as previously reported [24]. Patients were categorized on the basis of four serum concentrations informed by the literature. 25-hydroxyvitamin D: <10.0 ng/mL, 10.0–19.9 ng/mL, 20.0–29.9 ng/mL, and >30.0 ng/mL. The first cut point is the classic definition of vitamin D deficiency and the second the level at which blood PTH homeostasis is achieved, the third a level proposed to classify an insufficient state and the fourth a level postulated for optimal regulation of PTH, calcium absorption and bone density [25]. The other two blood-based markers were assessed on a continuous scale. Students T-test were used to determine if there were statistically significant differences in blood or nutrient levels between Black and White patients. Chi-Square test was utilized to determine differences between racial groups by level and a p-value of 0.05 was considered statistically significant.

2.4. Head and Neck Cancer Cell Lines

SCC-25 (CR-1628™) and CAL-27 (CRL-2095™) cell lines were both obtained from American Type Culture Collection (ATCC). SCC-25 cells were isolated from a 70 year old White male who had squamous cell carcinoma of the tongue at T2N1 [26]. Likewise, CAL-27 cells were isolated from squamous cell carcinoma of the tongue in a White male who was 56 years old [27]. The two cell lines were plated at 3.5E06 and 1E06, respectively, and allowed to adhere for 30 h in T-75 flasks with DMEM:F12 complete medium, 10% FBS. Cells were then treated with either 2 μM of vitamin D in the form of cholecalciferol (vitamin D3, Sigma, St Louis, MO, USA) or vehicle (dilute EtOH) and harvested 24 h post-treatment utilizing a cell scraper. Cells were placed in D-PBS (without calcium or magnesium) and centrifuged at low speed (500× g) to pellet. The pellets were snap frozen in liquid nitrogen and stored at −80 °C until they were processed for RNA isolation, proteomic profiling, or evaluation of individual vitamin D linked proteins. The concentration of Vitamin D3 utilized for the HNSCC cell line studies were based on our preliminary viability investigations as shown (Figure S1) which show the LD50 in the range or 0.5 to 2uM as well as consideration of the published literature, both in preclinical and clinical studies [28–33]. As discussed above, circulating levels of vitamin D in humans have been targeted at >30 ng/mL (75 nmol/L or 0.075uM) [33] for optimal health. However, precise dose extrapolation from cell lines to physiological relevant human concentrations of vitamin D is complicated by the fact that levels may not accurately reflect tissue or intracellular concentrations [34]. Furthermore, human intervention studies or supplementation in free-living populations frequently involve daily vitamin D intake or in some intervention studies multiple times a day, whereas the in vitro studies herein are based on a single dose of vitamin D. Considering these factors a concentration of 2 μM was chosen for all cell-based assays.

2.5. RNA Isolation and microRNA Assay

RNA was isolated utilizing standard phenol-chloroform extraction procedures as previously described [35]. RNA quality was determined by Nanodrop using the 8000 Spectrophotometer (Thermo Scientific, Wilmington, NC, USA) and RNA integrity and presence of the small RNA fraction was determined using the Bioanalyzer 2100 capillary electrophoresis system (Agilent, Santa Clara, CA, USA). Sixty nanograms of total RNA was reverse transcribed using the human Megaplex Primer Pools A and B and the TaqMan miR reverse transcription kit (Applied Biosystems, Foster City, CA, USA) [35]. Each sample was pre-amplified for 12 cycles using human pool A and B Taqman® Megaplex™ PreAmp Primers and PreAmp Master Mix (Applied Biosystems) and the preamplification reactions diluted, combined with TaqMan ® Gene-Expression Master Mix (Applied Biosystems) divided into eight aliquots and each aliquot was added to one of the eight sample ports of the TaqMan® Array A or B (v2.0), respectively. The TaqMan® Array Human miR Card Set v2.0 (Thermo Fisher Scientific, Waltham, MA, USA) enables detection of 667 human miRs, 3 miR endogenous reference controls, and 1 miR assay not related to human as a negative control. Table S1 includes relevant miR platform and sequence information. The real-time PCR reactions were run according to the manufacturer's instructions. RealTime Statminer Software (Integromics, Philadelphia, PA, USA) was used to analyze the data. The global geometric mean of all expressed miR assays was used to normalize the data. Significantly altered miRs were determined based on the most stringent criteria with a *p*-value cutoff of 1E-05 was used to determine statistically significant miRs.

2.6. MiR Gene Targets and Enrichment Analysis

Validated gene targets from miRs significantly altered by vitamin D treatment were determined using miRTarBase (The Chinese University of Hongkong, Shenzhen, China) [36]. The miRTarBase software and database enables users to search for validated gene targets based on the miR ID. This database was chosen as it is relatively stable and miRTarBase has been shown to be broader and more comprehensive when compared to other miR target validation databases [37]. Database for Annotation, Visualization, and Integrated Discovery (DAVID, v6.8, Frederick National Laboratory for Cancer Research, Frederick, MD, USA) was utilized to analyze the validated gene targets regulated by up or down-regulated miRs. Additionally, MetaCore software (Clarviate Analytics, Philadelphia, PA, USA) was used to further explore functional analysis of common gene targets for CAL-27 and SCC-25. *p*-values are calculated for the terms in each ontology after enrichment; the terms are then tested as separate hypotheses. The resultant *q*-value illustrates the corrected-values accounting for the total terms in the ontology including the rank of each term. This provides an estimate of the Benjamini False Discovery Rate (FDR).

2.7. Proteomic Profiling

Protein resuspension was achieved in 2-D cell lysis buffer (30 mM Tris-HCl, pH 8.8, containing 7 M urea, 2 M thiourea, and 4% CHAPS). This mixture was then sonicated at 4 °C followed by shaking for 30 min at room temperature, centrifugation at 4 °C (14,000 rpm) for 30 min and supernatant collection. Bio-Rads protein assay was used to measure protein concentration. The protein lysate was further processed for global proteome profiling including CyDye labeling, running of SDS gels, gel imaging, resolving protein spots, spot digestion, and MALDI-TOF MS and TOF/TOF tandem MS/MS methods were conducted in collaboration with Applied Biomics (Hayward, CA, USA).

2.8. Lysate Collection and Western Blot Analysis of HNC Cancer Cells Following Vitamin D

CAL-27 (7E5) and SCC-25 (7E5) cells were seeded in T-25 flasks (Corning, Thermofisher Scientific, Waltham, MA, USA) and adhered overnight prior to treatment with 2 μM vitamin D (Sigma Aldrich, Saint Louis, MO, USA) or vehicle (dilute ethanol) dissolved in phenol red free complete RPMI medium (Thermo Fisher Scientific, Scientific, Waltham, MA, USA). Cell lysates were harvested at 24 and 48 h post-treatment using RPPA lysis buffer (1% Triton X-100, 50 mM HEPES, pH 7.4, 150 mM NaCl, 1.5 mM $MgCl_2$, 1 mM EGTA, 100 mM NaF, 10 mM sodium pyrophosphate, 1 mM sodium orthovanadate, and 10% glycerol) with complete EDTA-free protease and PhosSTOP phosphatase inhibitors (Sigma Aldrich, Saint Louis, MO, USA). Protein was quantified using the DC protein assay (Bio-Rad, Hercules, CA, USA). Approximately 15 μg of protein was loaded in precast 4–20% Criterion TGX gels (Bio-Rad, Hercules, CA, USA), ran for 1 h, transferred to a PVDF membrane with the Trans-Blot® Turbo™ system (Bio-Rad, Hercules, CA, USA) for 30 min, blocked for 1 h at room temperature, incubated overnight with primary antibodies and incubated with the secondary antibody for 1 h. Images were captured via the ChemiDoc Molecular Imager and band quantification with ImageLab analysis software (both Bio-Rad, Hercules, CA, USA). Expression values were determined by chemiluminescent immunodetection and normalized to appropriate loading controls. Immunoblotting was performed using commercially available antibodies from Abcam (Cambridge, MA USA): DAB2 (#ab33441; 1:500), Cell Signaling Technology (Danvers, MA USA): GAPDH (#2118; 1:25,000), LsBio (Seattle, WA USA): LRP2 (#LS-c667890; 1:250), Santa Cruz Biotechnology (Dallas, TX USA): Vitamin D receptor (#sc-13133; 1:100), GAPDH (#sc-32233; 1:40,000), and Thermo Fisher Scientific, Scientific, Waltham, MA, USA): Vitamin D binding protein (#PA5-29082; 1:500).

3. Results

3.1. Patient Characteristics

Patient demographics, tobacco and alcohol use, and nutrient levels are summarized in Table 1. A total of nineteen HNC patients enrolled, 9 Black and 10 White. Black patients were significantly younger (53.6 years ± 9.4) upon HNC diagnosis compared to White patients (64.3 years ± 14.4) (p-value = 0.036). One hundred percent of the participants reported alcohol use. Compared to White patients, Black patients were both more likely to have a history of smoking and reported higher current smoking status. Ever smoking was reported by 66.7% of Black patients versus 30% of Whites. Among patients who smoked the average years of smoking was 24.6 years among Blacks and 34.7 years among White patients, in alignment with Whites being diagnosed at a later age. Black patients had non-significantly elevated mean body mass index (BMI) compared to Whites. All patients reported low fruit and vegetable consumption, two servings per day. Whites reported significantly higher rates of sun protection via sunscreen or protective clothing when sun exposure was ≥2 h/daily (p-value = 0.003, Chi-square). All Blacks reporting protecting from the sun did so by clothing or hats, not sunscreen use, whereas Whites protected with both sunscreen and apparel. Both groups reported similar sun exposure in terms of intense sun exposure, weekly sun exposure, and exposure during summer and winter months. Blacks and Whites did not differ significantly based on months living in Florida. Blacks averaged 11.0 months and Whites 10.4 months in Florida, with one Black and 3 White patients reporting living outside of Florida for at least three months. Black and White HNC patients differed significantly in terms of education, with Whites reporting significantly higher rates of college graduation as well as completing graduate or professional degrees. In contrast the highest level of education for Blacks was high school graduation, 55.6% vs. 10% among White patients. Reported annual income levels were significantly lower among Black compared to White HNC patients. Physical activity levels were low for both Black and White patients with over 70% reporting rarely or never exercising.

Table 1. Characteristics of newly diagnosed head and neck cancer patients.

Characteristics	Race	
	Black	White
Average Age (years, ±SD)	53.6 (±9.4)	64.3 (±14.4) #
Ratio of Men:Women (*n*)	5:4	8:2
Alcohol Use	100%	100%
Current Smoker	33.3%	20%
Ever Smoker	66.7%	30%
Body Mass Index (mean kg/m^2)	27.1	24.2
Fruit & Vegetable Servings/Daily	2.0	2.1
Sun Protection, Never or Seldom	89.9%	20.0%
Sun Protection, Always or Mostly	11.1%	80.0% #
Middle School or Some High School (*n*)	22.2% (2)	0%
High School Graduate (*n*)	55.6% (5)	10% (1)
Some College (*n*)	11.1% (1)	30.0% (3)
College Graduate or Professional Degree (*n*)	11.1% (1)	60.0% (6) #

Education is reported as highest level achieved; Sun protection use refers to using clothing or sunscreen for periods of sun exposer ≥2 h a day; and # Statistically significantly different based on Students *T*-Test or the Chi-Square test statistic for population differences across categories (*p*-value < 0.05).

3.2. Blood Levels of Vitamin D, Parathyroid, and Calcium Among Head and Neck Cancer Patients

Table 2 reports serum and plasma measurements by patient racial group. Generally, the circulating metabolite, 25-Hydroxyvitamin D (25-OH) vitamin D is considered the most valid indicator of vitamin D status as it reflects the last 15 days; compared to the active metabolite which reflects approximately the last 15 h. The mean level of 25-Hydroxyvitamin D among Blacks diagnosed with HNC (20 ng/mL) was significantly lower than the mean among Whites (27.30 ng/mL, *p*-value = 0.04). In addition, to mean 25-Hydroxyvitamin D levels being lower in Blacks, no Black HNC patients had vitamin D levels greater than or equal to 30 ng/mL, the level associated with optimal regulation of PTH, calcium absorption and bone density. In contrast, 30% of White patients had 25-Hydroxyvitamin D levels over 30 ng/mL. About 50% of Blacks presented with 25-Hydroxyvitamin D levels in the 10–19.9 ng/mL range compared to only 10% of Whites further supporting that even in sunny South Florida vitamin D levels are lower in Blacks HNC patients compared to White HNC patients. There were no differences noted in 1,25-Dihydroxyvitamin D, which has relatively short half-life and is not considered an indicator of true vitamin D status, but rather a marker modulated only in cases of severe deficiency. Similarly, there were no differences in circulating PTH or calcium levels between the two patient populations.

Table 2. Blood levels of vitamin D, parathyroid, and calcium among head and neck cancer patients.

Measurement	Race		*p*-Value
	Black	White	
25-Hydroxyvitamin D (ng/mL)	20.00 (±5.98)	27.30 (±9.86)	0.04
1,25-Dihydroxyvitamin D (pg/mL)	43.86 (±20.80)	36.80 (±14.33)	0.21
Patients with Low Vitamin D (<19.9 ng/mL)	50%	10%	
Patients with Intermediate Vitamin D (20.0–29.9 ng/mL)	50%	60%	
Patients with Sufficient Vitamin D (≥30 ng/mL)	0%	30%	0.06
Parathyroid (pg/mL)	35.50 (±23.95)	35.89 (±14.93)	0.48
Calcium (pg/mL)	9.34 (0.58)	9.09 (±0.68)	0.21

p-value based on Students *T*-test for nutrient levels and Chi-square test statistic for vitamin D differences by concentrations in the populations (<0.05 considered statistically significant).

3.3. Nutrient Levels of Vitamin D and Calcium Based on Dietary Screeners

Block Vitamin D and Calcium Screeners were utilized to gain insight into how dietary and supplement sources of vitamin D may impact circulating levels with the results summarized in Table 3.

Black HNC patients reported (non-significantly) lower total vitamin D intake compared to Whites. Interestingly, compared to Whites, Black patients reported marginally higher intake of vitamin D from dietary sources (p-value = 0.07), whereas White patients reported non-significantly higher supplemental intake of both vitamin D and also calcium; 50% of Whites reported use of supplemental vitamin D compared to 22.2% of Black HNC patients.

Table 3. Nutrient levels of vitamin D and calcium based on dietary screeners.

Measurement	Race		*p*-Value
	Black	White	
Total Vitamin D (IU)	174.70 (±154.37)	276.93 (±206.03)	0.23
Dietary Vitamin D (IU)	121.24 (±113.77)	62.92 (±40.10)	0.07
Supplemental Vitamin D (IU)	88.89 (±176.38)	200.00 (±210.82)	0.12
Patients Supplementing Vitamin D	22.2%	50.0%	0.21
Total Calcium (mg)	678.40 (±450.42)	542.93 (±280.74)	0.22
Dietary Calcium (mg)	535.16 (±317.30)	447.87 (±286.89)	0.27
Supplemental Calcium (mean, mg)	25.28 (±56.10)	83.69 (±82.94)	0.31
Patients Supplementing Calcium	44.4%	60.0%	0.34

p-Value based on Students T-test or Chi-square test for population measures (<0.05 considered statistically significant).

3.4. *Top miRs Dysregulated in HNC Cell Lines by Vitamin D*

A total of 5 miRs were highly significantly dysregulated (p < 5.00E-04) in either CAL-27 or SCC-25 cell lines following vitamin D treatment as shown in Figure 1. In CAL-27 cells, hsa-miR-7-1-3p and hsa-miR-632 were significantly dysregulated by vitamin D as compared to a vehicle treated cells (p-value = 2.36E-05, −26.459 Fold-change and p-value = 9.56E-05 and 47.487 Fold-change, respectively) (Figure 1A). Vitamin D treatment of the SCC-25 cells resulted in significantly altered hsa-miR-331-5p (p-value = 3.82E-05, −45.008 Fold Change), hsa-miR-335 (p-value = 3.83E-05, −63.611 Fold Change), and hsa-miR-616 (p-value = 6.73E-05, 66.355 Fold Change), respectively (Figure 1A).

Figure 1C,D illustrate the total gene targets for all significantly down and up-regulated miRs, respectively, and overlapping gene targets of miRs altered in the same direction by vitamin D treatment (detailed in Table S4). The total 157 validated genes stem from the three up-regulated miRs which contrasts to 3082 genes regulated by the two down-regulated miRs. In Figure 1C, down-regulated miR-335 contributes the majority of presumably up-regulated gene targets compared to miR-7-1-3p. The two down-regulated miRs share 32 validated gene targets (Table S4) with diverse cancer-associated functions. Figure 1D illustrates the lack of overlapping genes among up-regulated miRs. There is only one common gene target, POLD3, that is shared between miR-632 and miR-331-5p, but not miR-616-3p. Overall, there is a considerably reduced number of validated gene targets for the up-regulated miRs compared to the down-regulated; still, a number of resultant genes have documented roles in cell proliferation, DNA damage response, cancer stemness, extracellular matrix organization, and genome stability (Table S5). In contrast with the down-regulated miRs, all three of the up-regulated miRs have similar numbers of validated gene targets.

Next, validated gene targets regulated by the vitamin D altered miRNAs were determined using miRTarBase. The number of validated gene targets associated with significantly altered miRs in each cell line are depicted in Figure 1B. In SCC-25 and CAL-27 cells a total of 3014 and 225 validated gene targets were identified, respectively (Figure 1B). Specifically, 63 validated gene targets were identified for hsa-miR-331-5p, 2898 for hsa-miR-335, and 53 for hsa-miR-616 in SCC-25 cells, respectively. In CAL-27 cells, 184 validated gene targets were stemmed from hsa-miR-7-1 and 41 from hsa-miR-632. Figure 1B shows the total number of validated gene targets regulated by vitamin D altered miRs stratified by cell line, including 45 common or overlapping genes. A comprehensive list of validated gene targets and their respective miRs is available in Table S2, with Table S3 (n = 45) and Table S4 (n = 32), showing the identity of overlapping genes depicted in Figure 1B–D, respectively.

A Dysregulated miRs following Vitamin D Treatment of Head and Neck Cancer Cell Lines.

Cell line	MicroRNA	Direction of Change	Fold-Change	*p*-Value	Validated Gene Targets
Cal 27	miR-632	Up regulated	47.49	9.56 E-05	41
	miR-7-1-3p	Down regulated	26.46	2.36 E-05	184
SCC-25	miR-331-5p	Up regulated	45.01	3.82 E-05	63
	miR-616-3p	Up regulated	66.36	6.73 E-05	53
	miR-335	Down regulated	63.61	3.83 E-05	2898

B Dysregulated miRs and Regulated Gene Targets (n)

C Down-Regulated miRs and Regulated Gene Targets (n)

D Up-Regulated miRs and Regulated Gene Targets (n)

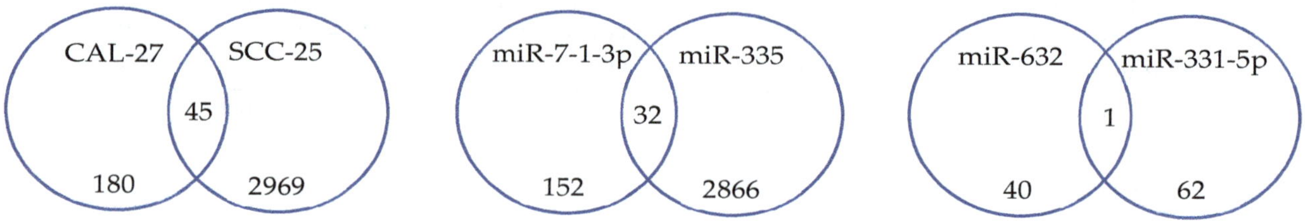

Figure 1. Summary of Significantly Dysregulated miRs following Vitamin D Treatment of Head and Neck Cancer Cell Lines. (**A**) Vitamin D altered miRs in CAL-27 and SCC-25 cells, the direction of change, and the number of validated gene targets regulated by each miR with 45 overlapping genes. (**B**) Validated gene targets regulated by Vitamin D modulated miRs in CAL-27 and SCC-25 cells and overlapping gene targets. (**C**) Specific miRs down regulated by Vitamin D in CAL-27 and SCC-25 cells, with overlapping genes identified (n = 32). (**D**) Up-regulated miRs showing individual results and overlapping gene targets (n = 1).

3.5. DAVID Enrichment Analysis

Two approaches of enrichment analysis were applied. The first based on the direction of miR change and resultant genes (157 and 3082) regulated by those miRs altered by vitamin D and the second based on all miRs and resultant common genes altered in both cell lines by vitamin D treatment (n = 45). The genes regulated by vitamin D driven miR dysregulation were analyzed for their respective Kyoto Encyclopedia of Genes and Genomes (KEGG) pathways, biological processes, molecular function, and disease linkages. Table 4 summarizes the top most significantly altered functional terms based on all up or down-regulated miRs and subsequent validated gene targets (n = 157 and 3082). The top KEGG pathway for the up-regulated miRs, presumably down-regulated gene targets, is Pathways in cancer (p-value = 0.01, FDR = 0.90) with nine genes contributing *(CKD4, DVL3, ETS1, MSH6, XIAP, RHOA, SMAD4, CCDC6,* and *LPAR2*). Expanded results, beyond the top changes, are detailed in Table S5. Stemming from vitamin D down-regulated miRs, the most significant identified KEGG pathway (Table 4) is Steroid biosynthesis (p-value = 7.72E-06, FDR = 2.2E-03, 13 genes), followed by MAPK signaling pathway (p-value = 3.89E-05, FDR = 5.52E-03, 65 genes), and Signaling pathways regulating pluripotency of stem cells (p-value = 6.80E-05, FDR = 6.43E-03, 41 genes). Additional significantly altered pathways linked to down-regulated miRs include Estrogen, PI3K-AKT, RAS, and Chemokine signaling (Table S5).

Table 4. Top pathways, biological processes, and molecular functions and diseases for altered MiR. Target Genes following vitamin D Treatment of CAL-27 and SCC-25 head and neck cell lines.

Functional Parameter	MiR Alteration	Term (*n*)	*p*-Value	Benjamini-Hochberg FDR
KEGG Pathway	Up-regulated	Pathways in Cancer (9)	0.01	0.90
	Down-regulated	Steroid Biosynthesis (13)	7.72E-06	2.2E-03
Biological Process	Up-regulated	Positive regulation of transcription from RNA polymerase II promoter (18)	3.31E-03	0.97
	Down-regulated	Negative regulation of cell proliferation (95)	5.27E-06	0.03
Molecular Function	Up-regulated	Protein binding (96)	1.50E-04	0.04
	Down-regulated	Transcription factor activity, sequence-specific DNA binding (194)	1.47E-05	0.03
Diseases	Up-regulated	Cancer (95)	4.30 E-04	7.71E-03
	Down-regulated	Chemodependency (736)	2.91E-12	5.53E-11

FDR: False Discovery Rate.

Nine biological processes were significantly altered by vitamin D based on genes linked to down-regulated miRs including Negative regulation of cell proliferation (*p*-value = 5.27E-06, FDR = 0.03, 95 genes), Angiogenesis (*p*-value = 1.03E-05, FDR = 0.03, 60 genes), and Canonical WNT signaling (*p*-value = 2.26E-05, FDR = 0.03, 29 genes) as well as Extracellular matrix and Cell adhesion. Genes stemming from up-regulated miRs resulted in Positive regulation of transcription from RNA polymerase II promoter as the top process, but it was not significant once FDR corrected.

In terms of molecular function, vitamin D linked up-regulated miRs and subsequent genes identified only Protein binding (*p*-value = 1.50E-04, FDR = 0.04, 96 genes) as a significant function.

Down-regulated miRs and related genes revealed only Transcription factor activity, sequence-specific DNA binding (*p*-value = 1.47E-05, FDR = 0.03, 194 genes). Finally, top diseases identified based on miRs up and down-regulated by vitamin D include Cancer and Chemodependency, respectively.

In addition, enrichment analysis was conducted based on the 45 validated gene targets shared in both vitamin D treated HNC cell lines (as illustrated in Figure 1A and detailed in Table S3) revealing Focal adhesion as the only significant pathway (*p*-value = 3.20E-04, FDR = 2.90E-02, 6 genes) following vitamin D treatment. Genes included *COL4A1*, *EGFR*, *IGF1R*, *ITGA1*, *PAK3*, and *VEGFA*, many with relevance to HNC. Similar to the results stemming from up or down-regulated miR driven genes (Figure 1C,D), Protein binding was the top molecular function identified based on the 45 shared genes in CAL-27 and SCC-25 cells.

3.6. Protein Level Changes in HNC Cells Following Vitamin D Treatment

Western blot results implicate response differences to vitamin D treatment between CAL-27 cells and SCC-25 cells (Figure 2). Western results show that levels of LRP2 and DAB2 proteins are constitutively lower in CAL-27 cells as compared to SCC-25 cells. The vitamin D receptor is expressed more strongly in SCC-25 as well. However, vitamin D binding protein is expressed more strongly in CAL-27 cells. Vitamin D treatment increased levels of the vitamin D receptor in both HNC cell lines, with strongest effects noted in SCC-25 cells. Vitamin D treatment modestly increased DAB2 levels only in CAL-27 cells. Vitamin D driven LRP2 increases were only observed in SCC-25 cells supporting differential responses between the cell lines. Findings may reflect that HNC cells increase their ability to endocytose vitamin D and bind vitamin D at the nuclear receptor in response to vitamin D treatment. The observed differences between cell lines may be due to molecular differences between them, raising the possibility that there may also be different molecular profiles in patient populations; expression of these proteins should be examined in patient samples. These findings may have relevance to the relative importance of free versus bound vitamin D in HNC and to the metabolism and processing of vitamin D in vivo [38,39].

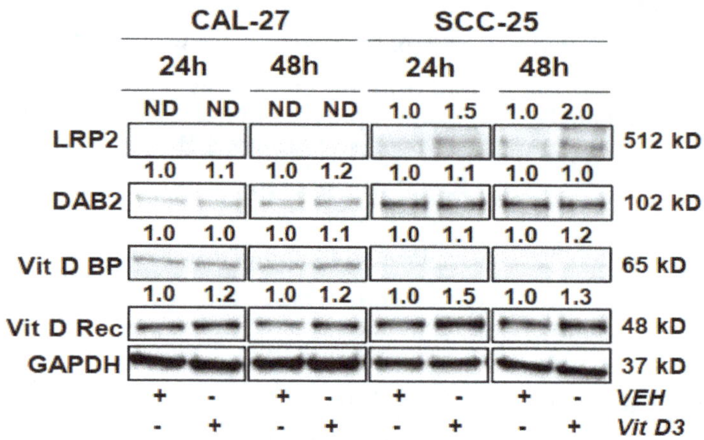

Figure 2. Modulation of vitamin D related proteins. Western blot results for CAL-27 and SCC-25 HNC cell lines following 2 μM vitamin D treatment. ND indicates no detection. Quantitation was normalized to GAPDH as a loading control and fold-change from vehicle reported.

Proteomic profiling was also employed as an untargeted approach to determine additional proteins modified by vitamin D utilizing of SCC-25 and CAL-27 human HNC cell lines with results summarized in Table 5. A total of six proteins were identified as highly dysregulated by vitamin D. Nucleophosmin, Lactoylglutathione lyase, Heat shock protein beta-1, and Ras-related protein Rap-2b were markedly downregulated in SCC-25 cells. In CAL-27 cells, Peroxiredoxin-1 and Histone H2A type 1-J were down and up-regulated, respectively (Table 5).

Table 5. Proteins modified by vitamin D treatment of head and neck cancer cell lines.

Cells	Spot	Protein	Symbol	Fold-Change	Uniprot No.
SCC-25	15/16 *	Nucleophosmin	NPM_HUMAN	−2.36	P06748
	28	Lactoylglutathione lyase	LGUL_HUMAN	−2.73	Q04760
	31	Heat shock protein beta-1	HSPB1_HUMAN	−2.57	P04792
	51	Ras-related protein Rap-2b	RAP2B_HUMAN	−3.39	P61225
CAL-27	30	Peroxiredoxin-1	PRDX1_HUMAN	−2.60	Q06830
	31	Histone H2A type 1-J	H2A1J_HUMAN	+2.48	Q99878

* The fold-change for Nucleophosmin is an average of the two detected spots 15 and 16 following treatment with vitamin D.

4. Discussion

Many studies have investigated the underlying factors that contribute to racial disparities in HNC patients pointing to a complex and multifactorial etiology. Black HNC patients have a 20–30% reduction in five-year relative survival compared to Whites [40,41]. In turn, Black Americans have higher age-adjusted HNC mortality rates compared to Whites [42]. The literature supports that Black patients are more likely to be diagnosed with higher stage disease and distant metastases, and experience increased mortality following a diagnosis of HNC [9,43,44]. Black HNC patients are also significantly less likely to undergo surgical treatment, even among patients with similar health insurance status [9,45,46]. Sociodemographic factors are frequently cited as dominate causes to cancer disparities, including HNC [47–50]. However, a recent meta-analysis including ten studies with greater than 100,000 patients reported poorer survival among Black HNC patients after controlling for socioeconomic factors as well as tumor stage and treatment variables supporting that additional factors contribute to the observed racial differences [51]. Thus, the objective of this prospective pilot study was to assess vitamin D status in newly diagnosed HNC patients stratified by race and to gain potential mechanistic insight by performing in vitro studies utilizing human HNC cell lines. Among Whites vitamin D status is inversely associated with HNC, low vitamin D levels in White HNC patients is also linked to cancer progression, increased recurrence, and metastatic disease [13,14,19]. Despite well documented hypovitaminosis D in Blacks, vitamin D status has not been assessed in HNC patients stratified by race.

Our pilot study results showed significantly lower levels of circulating vitamin D (25-hydroxyvitamin D) in newly diagnosed Black HNC patients (20.0 ng/mL) compared to the White patients (27.3 ng/mL). Although this is the first such report in Blacks with HNC, it does align with earlier research in Blacks without cancer which also reported reduced vitamin D levels in the range of 18.0–25.1 ng/mL [15,16,52–55]. Higher levels of melanin pigmentation in darker skin is known to be a contributory cause of lower levels of vitamin D among Blacks. In addition, an inverse association between BMI and vitamin D level has been noted previously, including during interventional studies [56–58]. Although the mean BMI was higher among Black HNC patients and more Blacks were overweight based on BMI, the differences were not statistically significant. Sun exposure is also known to impact vitamin D levels and to interact with obesity [59]. All HNC patients reported similar levels of sun exposure, but Whites reported more frequent use of sunscreen compared to Blacks. Overall, both groups of HNC patients had low levels of vitamin D, with none of the Black patients and only 30% of the White patients having levels ≥30 ng/mL, which is required for optimal PTH regulation, calcium absorption, and bone density [25]. Moreover, 50% of Black HNC patients had deficient vitamin D levels, below 20 ng/mL. Interestingly, dietary and supplement intake measures also indicated that Black HNC patients had lower total vitamin D, but they received more from dietary sources, whereas White patients supplemented more frequently. Two previous studies have also reported lower supplemental vitamin D intake in Blacks compared to Whites [60,61]. Although randomized clinical trials and interventional studies with vitamin D have had mixed results, targeting deficient populations may prove beneficial, especially in the context of racial disparities [10,62,63].

Similar to previous larger studies and published metanalysis focused on racial disparities in HNC [8,9,64,65], our pilot study results support that Black and White HNC patients differ significantly in terms of highest educational obtainment and annual income level. Exposure to other known HNC risk factors appeared similar between Whites and Blacks, including alcohol use and current smoking status. Blacks HNC patients did have non-significantly increased rates of ever smoking compared to Whites, and they were diagnosed about ten years earlier than Whites with HNC for reasons that remain unclear. In addition, Blacks who smoked, did so on average for 10 fewer years compared to Whites when diagnosed with HNC, raising the possibility that other, less well characterized factors may indeed be contributing to HNC progression and disparate survival among Blacks.

Tobacco, alcohol, and HPV are considered among the major modifiable risk factors for HNC [5]. Tobacco use has declined in the United States reducing tobacco linked HNC and in turn reducing age adjusted HNC incidence rates among Blacks [8,66]; yet, Blacks still have elevated age adjusted mortality rates for HNC compared to Whites [3,8,42,67]. In addition, HPV-positive HNC has markedly increased in recent years, but is generally more common among White males and has more favorable treatment outcomes [68–71]; thus, neither tobacco use or HPV prevalence patterns appear to fully explain the racial disparity in HNC outcomes. Although this is a small pilot study, we report differences in vitamin D levels among newly diagnosed Black and White HNC patients which may contribute to disparities in HNC outcomes. The topic merits further investigation in a larger cohort study incorporating additional relevant clinical variables such as cancer stage, grade, subsite analysis, treatment choice and survival outcomes.

In vitro studies were undertaken to explore potential mechanisms of vitamin D activity in two human HNC cell lines, CAL-27 and SCC-25, both of squamous cell origin. Vitamin D treatment significantly altered five miRs, each regulating between 41 to 2898 genes. Of the miRs modulated by vitamin D, Hsa-miR-7-1 and hsa-miR-335 were significantly down-regulated; whereas, hsa-miR-331-5p, hsa-miR-616, and hsa-miR-632 were significantly up-regulated. Enrichment analysis via DAVID was conducted based on the genes regulated by each miR within a cell line, and also separately based on genes regulated by vitamin D induced up or down-regulated miRs revealing effects on multiple cancer relevant pathways and processes. There is evidence that both down-regulated miRs have oncogenic activity in HNC or precursors lesions [72–85]. Analysis of genes regulated by down-regulated miRs revealed modulation of multiple pathways relevant to HNC including MAPK, PI3K, RAS, and Chemokine signaling. Additionally, the top biological processes altered based on genes regulated by down-regulated miRs was Negative regulation of cellular proliferation followed by Angiogenesis; Canonical WNT signaling and Cell adhesion were also among the significant processes. Two previous studies investigating the role of miR-7 in lung cancer, which shares risk factors with HNC, reported that miR-7 is induced by EGFR/Ras/ERK/Myc signaling leading to aberrant cell proliferation and migration [75,86]. Together these results support a cancer inhibitory role for vitamin D through impacting key drivers identified in HNC [87]. Considering that HPV-positive HNC are documented to have double the PI3-kinase activating mutations (50% as compared to HPV-negative ones, which have about 25%) future studies should expand evaluations to include HPV-positive models or tissues [88].

Vitamin D treatment of HNC cell lines up-regulated hsa- miR-331-5p, hsa-miR-616-3p, and hsa-miR-632. Combined, these miRs presumably down-regulate 157 gene targets, many with well documented roles in cell proliferation, signal transduction, DNA damage response, cancer stemness, adhesion, extracellular matrix (EMT) organization, and genome stability (i.e., *MDM4, CDK4, MSH6, XIAP, ETS1, RHOA, SMAD4, POLD3, COL3A1, FGF2, FOXF2,* and *SOX5*). Notably, *MDM4* plays a role in regulating p53 and has been linked to cancer recurrence and poor outcomes in HNC patients [89–91]. As another example, the transcription of *CDK4* is linked to tobacco mediated oral carcinogenesis and acts as a potent cyclin dependent Kinase 4 Regulatory Factor (KRF) and a potential cancer target [92]. In terms of specific miRs, vitamin D treatment increased miR-331-5p. Reports support that miR-331-5p, as well as the 3p strand, differ in patients with laryngeal squamous cell carcinoma [80,82,93]. Moreover, overexpression of miR-331-3p inhibits cell proliferation and invasion while promoting apoptosis via reduced expression of elF4B and subsequent inhibition of the phosphorylation of PI3K/AKT signaling molecules [94]. Similarly, in lung cancer, increased expression of miR-331 has cancer inhibitory effects through down-regulation of MAPK, suppression of EMT as well as inhibition of metastatic ability of cancer cells in vitro and in vivo [95,96]. Results for miR-632 in the context of HNC appear mixed. One study reported that under-expression of miR-632 in saliva from oral squamous cell carcinoma patients compared to healthy controls suggesting increasing levels by vitamin D may prove favorable [97]. Similarly, Lu et al. suggested miR-632 to be a tumor suppressor in laryngeal cancers where it is down-regulated potentially via CCR6 and p38 dependent mechanisms [98]. Conversely, another study reported that increased expression of miR-632 in laryngeal tissues and cell lines accelerates cell proliferation, migration, and invasion supporting a more oncogenic function [99]. Contradictory finding may be due to heterogeneity of cell lines and even patient samples. It is well documented that miRs can act in a cancer specific manner, but there is less research documenting site specific effects within a target or evaluating additional sources of heterogeneity. To our knowledge miR-616-3p has not been reported as dysregulated in HNC. Our data supports that vitamin D modulates a select panel of miRs in HNC cell lines, which ultimately interferes with many cancer hallmarks. Additional research has evaluated vitamin D modulation of miRs in lung, cervical, and breast cancers [66]. However, the miRs identified in previously published studies do not overlap with those identified as significantly modulated by vitamin D in HNC cell lines.

Proteomic profiling was conducted to assess whether vitamin D held potential to impact or correct known defects in protein machinery associated with HNC. In total, vitamin D markedly increased one protein and down-regulated five proteins, all with documented roles in cancer [22,100–104]. Nucleophosmin (NPM), is associated with evasion of apoptosis, increased cancer cell viability, growth, and cell proliferation [105], and was down-regulated following vitamin D treatment of SCC-25 cells.

In a recent study increased expression of NPM was reported in 82% of laryngeal cancer tissues and NPM knockdown inhibited laryngeal cancer cell survival [23]. The full results revealed an oncogenic role for NPM in laryngeal cancer through its effects on apoptosis and cellular growth. Overexpression of NPM has been documented in oral squamous cell carcinoma (OSCC); immunohistochemistry and immunofluorescent staining showed significantly elevated expression levels in OSCC patient samples compared to control [106]. Another OSCC focused study reported NPM silencing induced genes involved in apoptosis and downregulated of procarcinogenesis genes [107]. The down-regulation of NPM following vitamin D treatment is consistent with our enrichment analysis results given NPM has a role in the Myc-ARF-p53 pathway and the molecule functions as a histone chaperone [108,109]. The latter may also explain the reduction noted in Histone H2A type 1-j (H2A1J) following vitamin D. Similarly, lactoylglutathione lyase (GLO1), was down-regulated in HNC cell lines after vitamin D treatment and is documented to be significantly overexpressed in OSCC tissues [110]. Importantly, there is recent evidence that GLO1 plays a critical role in invasion and metastasis of oropharyngeal tumors, in addition to initiation and maintenance of tumor growth. It has been reported that patients with high GLO1 expression have significantly shorter disease-specific survival [110]. GLO1 has only been characterized in a small number of HNC studies as cited; however, it is shown to have multiple roles in promoting cancer cell survival, proliferation, and is a likely target for chemotherapy based on the broader literature [111].

Vitamin D down-regulated Heat shock protein beta-1 (HSP27), a multi-functional protein with well documented roles in HNC inflammation, proliferation, cancer progression, stemness, EMT, and more recently radio-sensitization and therapeutic resistance [21,112–117]. Moreover, in SCC of the tongue HSP27 inhibition represses apoptosis and enhances sensitivity to chemotherapies [21] supporting a role for agents that reduce or impair HSP27. HSP27 is also a downstream target of the PI3K/AKT signaling pathway [112] which links our proteomic results to our enrichment analysis based on vitamin D induced miR alterations. Finally, expression levels of a number of RAB family members segregate metastatic versus non-metastatic oral cancers, including *RAB2B* [118]. In addition, the latter study reported knock-down of *RAB5, RAB7*, and *RAB11* in SCC-25 cells inhibits cancer cell migration and invasion supporting that agents downregulating RAB family members may impart cancer inhibitory potential.

Two additional proteins were altered by vitamin D treatment specifically in CAL-27 HNC cells. H2A1-J was up-regulated by vitamin D but has not been reported on in HNC. However, H2A1 depletion is linked to induction of cancer cell stemness in hepatocellular carcinoma [119] which aligns with gene enrichment analysis conducted based on miRs dysregulated by vitamin D in our study. Additionally, modulated by vitamin D in CAL-27 cells was Peroxiredoxin-1 (PRX-1). It was down-regulated, further supporting a role for vitamin D in suppressing HNC associated pathways. An evaluation of Prx-1 in human OSCC tissues showed elevated expression in OSCC samples compared to controls; interestingly investigators also saw a dose-dependent elevation in Prx-1 such that expression was highest in smokers with OSCC and lowest in control tissues [120]. Additional research has shown silencing of Prx-1 in CAL-27 and SCC-15 blocks promotion of proliferation and migration and Prx-1 has the ability to promote EMT processes via NFκB linked activity, as has been reported for NPM and HSP27 [120,121]. Thus, vitamin D treatment of HNC cell lines results in potent down-regulation of proteins implicated in multiple aspects of cancer, from inflammation, to aberrant proliferation, to migration, altered EMT, adhesion, and therapeutic resistance. Interestingly, a number of the vitamin D inhibited proteins are known to converge on a common transcription factor, NFkB which has also been proposed as a potential target for increased therapeutic efficacy in HNC [122].

5. Conclusions

Limitations of our research include a relatively small sample size, but this was intended to be a first assessment for determining whether a larger study was warranted. In addition, our small sample size of 19 HNC patients precludes making any linkages to sex, stage, grade, site-specific effects, or survival. Finally, to our knowledge there are no HNC cell lines available for research which are derived from Black patients; thus, our in vitro work was limited to HNC cell lines derived from White HNC patients.

Still, our data shows for the first time that circulating vitamin D levels are significantly depressed in newly diagnosed Black HNC patients compared to Whites. Furthermore, in vitro studies targeting mechanisms by which vitamin D may inhibit HNC revealed activity targeting early to late cancer related events; spanning from inflammation and chemokine changes to alterations in EMT, drivers of recurrence, and therapeutic resistance. Despite mixed results from vitamin D trials in other targets, our results support that vitamin D modulates a number of cancer pathways, biological processes, genes, and proteins with well documented roles in HNC development, response to therapy and disease recurrence which remains a significant issue. Study results support conducting future research to evaluate vitamin D in larger cohorts stratified by race and with sufficient power to interpret key clinical correlates and survival outcomes. Our results also revealed new vitamin D induced miR alterations which paralleled changes in many HNC relevant proteins paving the way for future genetic studies to interrogate miR dysregulation relative protein function. Ultimately, our results may inform and guide future in vitro, in vivo, and clinical chemoprevention studies assessing the efficacy of vitamin D as an intervention strategy for vulnerable or high risk populations, whether it be based on race or other variables imparting increased risk for HNC.

Supplementary Materials:
Figure S1: Vitamin D3 inhibits HNC cell viability, Table S1: MicroRNA platform and sequence information, Table S2: Comprehensive list of vitamin D altered miRs stratified by direction of change and individual validated gene targets, Table S3: Validated gene targets altered in both CAL-27 and SCC-25 HNC cell lines by vitamin D (n = 45), Table S4: Overlapping target genes of miRs altered in the same direction by vitamin D (n = 32), Table S5: Top pathways, biological processes, molecular functions and diseases for vitamin D altered miRs and validated gene targets in HNC cell Lines.

Author Contributions: Conceptualization, L.A.K., W.J.G., J.J.H., and E.F.; methodology, L.A.K., E.F., J.J.H., W.J.G., and A.M.M.; validation, K.M.W., M.I., and C.H.; formal analysis, M.I., C.H., and L.A.K.; investigation, W.J.G., E.F., K.M.W., and L.A.K.; resources, L.A.K. and W.J.G.; data curation, L.A.K., M.I., C.H., and K.M.W.; writing—original draft preparation, L.A.K. and M.I.; writing—review and editing, M.I., A.M.M., K.M.W., J.J.H., C.H., and L.A.K.; visualization, L.A.K., and M.I.; supervision, W.J.G. and L.A.K.; project administration, L.A.K.; and funding acquisition, W.J.G. and L.A.K. All authors have read and agreed to the published version of the manuscript.

Acknowledgments: We thank the patients who participated in the research and clinical and technical support staff.

References

1. Rettig, E.M.; D'Souza, G. Epidemiology of Head and Neck Cancer. *Surg. Oncol. Clin. N. Am.* **2015**, *24*, 379–396. [CrossRef] [PubMed]
2. Wissinger, E.; Griebsch, I.; Lungershausen, J.; Foster, T.; Pashos, C.L. The Economic Burden of Head and Neck Cancer: A Systematic Literature Review. *Pharmacoeconomics* **2014**, *32*, 865–882. [CrossRef] [PubMed]
3. Daraei, P.; Moore, C.E. Racial Disparity among the Head and Neck Cancer Population. *J. Cancer Educ.* **2015**, *30*, 546–551. [CrossRef] [PubMed]
4. Chaturvedi, A.K.; Engels, E.A.; Pfeiffer, R.M.; Hernandez, B.Y.; Xiao, W.; Kim, E.; Jiang, B.; Goodman, M.T.; Sibug-Saber, M.; Cozen, W.; et al. Human Papillomavirus and Rising Oropharyngeal Cancer Incidence in the United States. *J. Clin. Oncol.* **2011**, *29*, 4294–4301. [CrossRef] [PubMed]
5. Benson, E.; Li, R.; Eisele, D.; Fakhry, C. The Clinical Impact of HPV Tumor Status upon Head and Neck Squamous Cell Carcinomas. *Oral Oncol.* **2014**, *50*, 565–574. [CrossRef]
6. O'Rorke, M.A.; Ellison, M.V.; Murray, L.J.; Moran, M.; James, J.; Anderson, L.A. Human Papillomavirus Related Head and Neck Cancer Survival: A Systematic Review and Meta-Analysis. *Oral Oncol.* **2012**, *48*, 1191–1201. [CrossRef]

7. Al-Othman, M.O.F.; Morris, C.G.; Logan, H.L.; Hinerman, R.W.; Amdur, R.J.; Mendenhall, W.M. Impact of Race on Outcome after Definitive Radiotherapy for Squamous Cell Carcinoma of the Head and Neck. *Cancer* **2003**, *98*, 2467–2472. [CrossRef]
8. Goodwin, W.J.; Thomas, G.R.; Parker, D.F.; Joseph, D.; Levis, S.; Franzmann, E.; Anello, C.; Hu, J.J. Unequal Burden of Head and Neck Cancer in the United States. *Head Neck* **2008**, *30*, 358–371. [CrossRef]
9. Kompelli, A.; Cartmell, K.B.; Sterba, K.R.; Alberg, A.J.; Xiao, C.C.; Sood, A.J.; Garrett-Mayer, E.; White-Gilbertson, S.J.; Rosenzweig, S.A.; Day, T.A. An Assessment of Racial Differences in Epidemiological, Clinical and Psychosocial Factors among Head and Neck Cancer Patients at the Time of Surgery. *World J. Otorhinolaryngol. Head Neck Surg.* **2020**, *6*, 41–48. [CrossRef]
10. Mondul, A.M.; Weinstein, S.J.; Layne, T.M.; Albanes, D. Vitamin D and Cancer Risk and Mortality: State of the Science, Gaps, and Challenges. *Epidemiol. Rev.* **2017**, *39*, 28–48. [CrossRef]
11. Zhao, Y.; Chen, C.; Pan, W.; Gao, M.; He, W.; Mao, R.; Lin, T.; Huang, J. Comparative Efficacy of Vitamin D Status in Reducing the Risk of Bladder Cancer: A Systematic Review and Network Meta-Analysis. *Nutrition* **2016**, *32*, 515–523. [CrossRef] [PubMed]
12. Xu, Y.; Shao, X.; Yao, Y.; Xu, L.; Chang, L.; Jiang, Z.; Lin, Z. Positive Association between Circulating 25-Hydroxyvitamin D Levels and Prostate Cancer Risk: New Findings from an Updated Meta-Analysis. *J. Cancer Res. Clin. Oncol.* **2014**, *140*, 1465–1477. [CrossRef] [PubMed]
13. Yokosawa, E.B.; Arthur, A.E.; Rentschler, K.M.; Wolf, G.T.; Rozek, L.S.; Mondul, A.M. Vitamin D Intake and Survival and Recurrence in Head and Neck Cancer Patients. *Laryngoscope* **2018**, *128*, E371–E376. [CrossRef] [PubMed]
14. Vaughan-Shaw, P.G.; O'Sullivan, F.; Farrington, S.M.; Theodoratou, E.; Campbell, H.; Dunlop, M.G.; Zgaga, L. The Impact of Vitamin D Pathway Genetic Variation and Circulating 25-HydroxyVitamin D on Cancer Outcome: Systematic Review and Meta-Analysis. *Br. J. Cancer* **2017**, *116*, 1092–1110. [CrossRef]
15. Chan, J.; Jaceldo-Siegl, K.; Fraser, G.E. Determinants of Serum 25 Hydroxyvitamin D Levels in a Nationwide Cohort of Blacks and Non-Hispanic Whites. *Cancer Causes Control* **2010**, *21*, 501–511. [CrossRef]
16. Freedman, D.M.; Cahoon, E.K.; Rajaraman, P.; Major, J.M.; Doody, M.M.; Alexander, B.H.; Hoffbeck, R.W.; Kimlin, M.G.; Graubard, B.I.; Linet, M.S. Sunlight and Other Determinants of Circulating 25-Hydroxyvitamin D Levels in Black and White Participants in a Nationwide US Study. *Am. J. Epidemiol.* **2013**, *177*, 180–192. [CrossRef]
17. Aranow, C. Vitamin D and the Immune System. *J. Investig. Med.* **2011**, *59*, 881–886. [CrossRef]
18. Dawson-Hughes, B.; Harris, S.S.; Krall, E.A.; Dallal, G.E. Effect of Calcium and Vitamin D Supplementation on Bone Density in Men and Women 65 Years of Age or Older. *N. Engl. J. Med.* **1997**, *337*, 670–676. [CrossRef]
19. Bochen, F.; Balensiefer, B.; Körner, S.; Bittenbring, J.T.; Neumann, F.; Koch, A.; Bumm, K.; Marx, A.; Wemmert, S.; Papaspyrou, G.; et al. Vitamin D Deficiency in Head and Neck Cancer Patients–Prevalence, Prognostic Value and Impact on Immune Function. *Oncoimmunology* **2018**, *7*. [CrossRef]
20. Coutinho-Camillo, C.M.; Lourenço, S.V.; Nishimoto, I.N.; Kowalski, L.P.; Soares, F.A. Nucleophosmin, P53, and Ki-67 Expression Patterns on an Oral Squamous Cell Carcinoma Tissue Microarray. *Hum. Pathol.* **2010**, *41*, 1079–1086. [CrossRef]
21. Zheng, G.; Zhang, Z.; Liu, H.; Xiong, Y.; Luo, L.; Jia, X.; Peng, C.; Zhang, Q.; Li, N.; Gu, Y.; et al. Hsp27-Mediated Extracellular and Intracellular Signaling Pathways Synergistically Confer Chemoresistance in Squamous Cell Carcinoma of Tongue. *Clin. Cancer Res.* **2018**, *24*, 1163–1175. [CrossRef] [PubMed]
22. Yanagawa, T.; Omura, K.; Harada, H.; Ishii, T.; Uwayama, J.; Nakaso, K.; Iwasa, S.; Koyama, Y.; Onizawa, K.; Yusa, H.; et al. Peroxiredoxin I Expression in Tongue Squamous Cell Carcinomas as Involved in Tumor Recurrence. *Int. J. Oral Maxillofac. Surg.* **2005**, *34*, 915–920. [CrossRef]
23. Wang, H.T.; Tong, X.; Zhang, Z.X.; Sun, Y.Y.; Yan, W.; Xu, Z.M.; Fu, W.N. MYCT1 Represses Apoptosis of Laryngeal Cancerous Cells through the MAX/MiR-181a/NPM1 Pathway. *FEBS J.* **2019**, *286*, 3892–3908. [CrossRef] [PubMed]
24. QuestAssureD TM 25-Hydroxy and 1,25-Dihydroxyvitamin D. Test Detail. Quest Diagnostics. Available online: https://testdirectory.questdiagnostics.com/test/test-detail/16761/questassured-25-hydroxy-and-125-dihydroxyvitamin-d?p=r&q=25-hydroxyvitaminD&cc=MASTER (accessed on 23 April 2020).
25. Holick, M.F.; Binkley, N.C.; Bischoff-Ferrari, H.A.; Gordon, C.M.; Hanley, D.A.; Heaney, R.P.; Murad, M.H.; Weaver, C.M. Evaluation, Treatment, and Prevention of Vitamin D Deficiency: An Endocrine Society Clinical Practice Guideline. *J. Clin. Endocrinol. Metab.* **2011**, *96*, 1911–1930. [CrossRef] [PubMed]

26. Rheinwald, J.G.; Beckett, M.A. Tumorigenic Keratinocyte Lines Requiring Anchorage and Fibroblast Support Cultured from Human Squamous Cell Carcinomas1. *Cancer Res.* **1981**, *41*, 1657–1663.
27. Gioanni, J.; Samson, M.; Zanghellini, E.; Mazeau, C.; Ettore, F.; Demard, F.; Chauvel, P.; Duplay, H.; Schneider, M.; Laurent, J.-C.; et al. Characterization of a New Surface Epitope Specific for Human Epithelial Cells Defined by a Monoclonal Antibody and Application to Tumor Diagnosis. *Cancer Res.* **1987**, *47*, 4417–4424.
28. Bhoora, S.; Pather, Y.; Marais, S.; Punchoo, R. Cholecalciferol Inhibits Cell Growth and Induces Apoptosis in the CaSki Cell Line. *Med. Sci. (Basel)* **2020**, *8*. [CrossRef]
29. Shruthi, N.; Prashanthkumar, M.; Venugopalreddy, B.; Suma, M.; Subba Rao, V. Analysis of the Cytotoxic Effects of Vitamin D3 on Colorectal, Breast and Cervical Carcinoma Cell Lines. *Biochem. Anal. Biochem.* **2017**, *6*. [CrossRef]
30. Baek, S.; Lee, Y.S.; Shim, H.E.; Yoon, S.; Baek, S.Y.; Kim, B.S.; Oh, S.O. Vitamin D3 regulates cell viability in gastric cancer and cholangiocarcinoma. *Anat. Cell Biol.* **2011**, *44*, 204–209. [CrossRef]
31. Bennett, R.G.; Wakeley, S.E.; Hamel, F.G.; High, R.R.; Korch, C.; Goldner, W.S. Gene expression of vitamin D metabolic enzymes at baseline and in response to vitamin D treatment in thyroid cancer cell lines. *Oncology* **2012**, *83*, 264–272. [CrossRef]
32. Santos, J.M.; Khan, Z.S.; Munir, M.T.; Tarafdar, K.; Rahman, S.M.; Hussain, F. Vitamin D3 decreases glycolysis and invasiveness, and increases cellular stiffness in breast cancer cells. *J. Nutr. Biochem.* **2018**, *53*, 111–120. [CrossRef] [PubMed]
33. Charoenngam, N.; Holick, M.F. Immunologic Effects of Vitamin D on Human Health and Disease. *Nutrients* **2020**, *12*. [CrossRef] [PubMed]
34. Berlin, J.L.; Shantha, G.P.; Yeager, H.; Thomas-Hemak, L. Serum vitamin D levels may not reflect tissue-level vitamin D in sarcoidosis. *BMJ Case Rep.* **2014**, *2014*. [CrossRef] [PubMed]
35. Kresty, L.; Clarke, J.; Ezell, K.; Exum, A.; Howell, A.; Guettouche, T. MicroRNA Alterations in Barrett's Esophagus, Esophageal Adenocarcinoma, and Esophageal Adenocarcinoma Cell Lines Following Cranberry Extract Treatment: Insights for Chemoprevention. *J. Carcinog.* **2011**, *10*. [CrossRef]
36. Chou, C.H.; Shrestha, S.; Yang, C.D.; Chang, N.W.; Lin, Y.L.; Liao, K.W.; Huang, W.C.; Sun, T.H.; Tu, S.J.; Lee, W.H.; et al. MiRTarBase Update 2018: A Resource for Experimentally Validated MicroRNA-Target Interactions. *Nucleic Acids Res.* **2018**, *46*, D296–D302. [CrossRef]
37. Lee, Y.J.; Kim, V.; Muth, D.C.; Witwer, K.W. Validated MicroRNA Target Databases: An Evaluation. *Drug Dev. Res.* **2015**, *76*, 389–396. [CrossRef]
38. Tsuprykov, O.; Chen, X.; Hocher, C.F.; Skoblo, R.; Yin, L.; Hocher, B. Why Should We Measure Free 25(OH) Vitamin D? *J. Steroid Biochem. Mol. Biol.* **2018**, *180*, 87–104. [CrossRef]
39. Nagai, J.; Christensen, E.I.; Morris, S.M.; Willnow, T.E.; Cooper, J.A.; Nielsen, R. Mutually Dependent Localization of Megalin and Dab2 in the Renal Proximal Tubule. *Am. J. Physiol. Ren. Physiol.* **2005**, *289*. [CrossRef]
40. Rose, B.S.; Jeong, J.H.; Nath, S.K.; Lu, S.M.; Mell, L.K. Population-Based Study of Competing Mortality in Head and Neck Cancer. *J. Clin. Oncol.* **2011**, *29*, 3503–3509. [CrossRef]
41. American Cancer Society. *Cancer Facts & Figures 2020*; American Cancer Society: Atlanta, GA, USA, 2020.
42. American Cancer Society. *Cancer Facts and Figures for African Americans 2019–2021*; American Cancer Society: Atlanta, GA, USA, 2019.
43. Mahal, B.A.; Inverso, G.; Aizer, A.A.; Bruce Donoff, R.; Chuang, S.K. Impact of African-American Race on Presentation, Treatment, and Survival of Head and Neck Cancer. *Oral Oncol.* **2014**, *50*, 1177–1181. [CrossRef]
44. Zakeri, K.; Macewan, I.; Vazirnia, A.; Cohen, E.E.W.; Spiotto, M.T.; Haraf, D.J.; Vokes, E.E.; Weichselbaum, R.R.; Mell, L.K. Race and Competing Mortality in Advanced Head and Neck Cancer. *Oral Oncol.* **2014**, *50*, 40–44. [CrossRef] [PubMed]
45. Subramanian, S.; Chen, A. Treatment Patterns and Survival among Low-Income Medicaid Patients with Head and Neck Cancer. *JAMA Otolaryngol. Head Neck Surg.* **2013**, *139*, 489–495. [CrossRef] [PubMed]
46. Du, X.L.; Liu, C.C. Racial/Ethnic Disparities in Socioeconomic Status, Diagnosis, Treatment and Survival among Medicare-Insured Men and Women with Head and Neck Cancer. *J. Health Care Poor Underserved* **2010**, *21*, 913–930. [CrossRef] [PubMed]

47. Molina, M.A.; Cheung, M.C.; Perez, E.A.; Byrne, M.M.; Franceschi, D.; Moffat, F.L.; Livingstone, A.S.; Goodwin, W.J.; Gutierrez, J.C.; Koniaris, L.G. African American and Poor Patients Have a Dramatically Worse Prognosis for Head and Neck Cancer: An Examination of 20,915 Patients. *Cancer* **2008**, *113*, 2797–2806. [CrossRef]
48. Arbes, S.J. Factors Contributing to the Poorer Survival of Black Americans Diagnosed with Oral Cancer (United States). *Cancer Causes Control* **1999**, *10*, 513–523. [CrossRef]
49. Ellis, L.; Canchola, A.J.; Spiegel, D.; Ladabaum, U.; Haile, R.; Gomez, S.L. Racial and Ethnic Disparities in Cancer Survival: The Contribution of Tumor, Sociodemographic, Institutional, and Neighborhood Characteristics. *J. Clin. Oncol.* **2018**, *36*, 25–33. [CrossRef]
50. Saini, A.T.; Genden, E.M.; Megwalu, U.C. Sociodemographic Disparities in Choice of Therapy and Survival in Advanced Laryngeal Cancer. *Am. J. Otolaryngol. Head Neck Med. Surg.* **2016**, *37*, 65–69. [CrossRef]
51. Russo, D.P.; Tham, T.; Bardash, Y.; Kraus, D. The Effect of Race in Head and Neck Cancer: A Meta-Analysis Controlling for Socioeconomic Status. *Am. J. Otolaryngol.* **2020**, *41*, 102624. [CrossRef]
52. Yetley, E.A. Assessing the Vitamin D Status of the US Population. *Am. J. Clin. Nutr.* **2008**, *88*, 558–564. [CrossRef]
53. Harris, S.S.; Soteriades, E.; Coolidge, J.A.S.; Mudgal, S.; Dawson-Hughes, B. Vitamin D Insufficiency and Hyperparathyroidism in a Low Income, Multiracial, Elderly Population. *J. Clin. Endocrinol. Metab.* **2000**, *85*, 4125–4130. [CrossRef]
54. Jacobs, E.T.; Alberts, D.S.; Foote, J.A.; Green, S.B.; Hollis, B.W.; Yu, Z.; Martínez, M.E. Vitamin D Insufficiency in Southern Arizona. *Am. J. Clin. Nutr.* **2008**, *87*, 608–613. [CrossRef] [PubMed]
55. Shea, M.K.; Houston, D.K.; Tooze, J.A.; Davis, C.C.; Johnson, M.A.; Hausman, D.B.; Cauley, J.A.; Bauer, D.C.; Tylavsky, F.; Harris, T.B.; et al. Correlates and Prevalence of Insufficient 25-Hydroxyvitamin D Status in Black and White Older Adults: The Health, Aging and Body Composition Study. *J. Am. Geriatr. Soc.* **2011**, *59*, 1165–1174. [CrossRef] [PubMed]
56. Camozzi, V.; Frigo, A.C.; Zaninotto, M.; Sanguin, F.; Plebani, M.; Boscaro, M.; Schiavon, L.; Luisetto, G. 25-Hydroxycholecalciferol Response to Single Oral Cholecalciferol Loading in the Normal Weight, Overweight, and Obese. *Osteoporos. Int.* **2016**, *27*, 2593–2602. [CrossRef]
57. Gallagher, J.C.; Yalamanchili, V.; Smith, L.M. The Effect of Vitamin D Supplementation on Serum 25OHD in Thin and Obese Women. *J. Steroid Biochem. Mol. Biol.* **2013**, 195–200. [CrossRef]
58. Blum, M.; Dawson-Hughes, B.; Dallal, G.E. Body Size and Serum 25 Hydroxy Vitamin D Response to Oral Supplements in Healthy Older Adults. *J. Am. Coll. Nutr.* **2008**, *27*, 274–279. [CrossRef] [PubMed]
59. Savastano, S.; Barrea, L.; Savanelli, M.C.; Nappi, F.; Di Somma, C.; Orio, F.; Colao, A. Low Vitamin D Status and Obesity: Role of Nutritionist. *Rev. Endocr. Metab. Disord.* **2017**, *18*, 215–225. [CrossRef] [PubMed]
60. Rock, C.L. Multivitamin-Multimineral Supplements: Who Uses Them? *Am. J. Clin. Nutr.* **2007**, *85*, 277–279. [CrossRef]
61. Radimer, K.; Bindewald, B.; Hughes, J.; Ervin, B.; Swanson, C.; Picciano, M.F. Dietary Supplement Use by US Adults: Data from the National Health and Nutrition Examination Survey, 1999–2000. *Am. J. Epidemiol.* **2004**, *160*, 339–349. [CrossRef]
62. Giammanco, M.; Di Majo, D.; La Guardia, M.; Aiello, S.; Crescimannno, M.; Flandina, C.; Tumminello, F.M.; Leto, G. Vitamin D in Cancer Chemoprevention. *Pharm. Biol.* **2015**, *53*, 1399–1434. [CrossRef]
63. Kennel, K.A.; Drake, M.T. Vitamin D in the Cancer Patient. *Curr. Opin. Support. Palliat. Care* **2013**, *7*, 272–277. [CrossRef]
64. Lenze, N.R.; Farquhar, D.R.; Mazul, A.L.; Masood, M.M.; Zevallos, J.P. Racial Disparities and Human Papillomavirus Status in Oropharyngeal Cancer: A Systematic Review and Meta-Analysis. *Head Neck* **2019**, *41*, 256–261. [CrossRef] [PubMed]
65. Peterson, C.E.; Khosla, S.; Chen, L.F.; Joslin, C.E.; Davis, F.G.; Fitzgibbon, M.L.; Freels, S.; Hoskins, K. Racial Differences in Head and Neck Squamous Cell Carcinomas among Non-Hispanic Black and White Males Identified through the National Cancer Database (1998–2012). *J. Cancer Res. Clin. Oncol.* **2016**, *142*, 1715–1726. [CrossRef] [PubMed]
66. Sturgis, E.M.; Cinciripini, P.M. Trends in Head and Neck Cancer Incidence in Relation to Smoking Prevalence: An Emerging Epidemic of Human Papillomavirus-Associated Cancers? *Cancer* **2007**, *110*, 1429–1435. [CrossRef] [PubMed]

67. Morse, D.E.; Kerr, A.R. Disparities in Oral and Pharyngeal Cancer Incidence, Mortality and Survival among Black and White Americans. *J. Am. Dent. Assoc.* **2006**, *137*, 203–212. [CrossRef]
68. Gillison, M.L.; D'Souza, G.; Westra, W.; Sugar, E.; Xiao, W.; Begum, S.; Viscidi, R. Distinct Risk Factor Profiles for Human Papillomavirus Type 16-Positive and Human Papillomavirus Type 16-Negative Head and Neck Cancers. *J. Natl. Cancer Inst.* **2008**, *100*, 407–420. [CrossRef]
69. Schwartz, S.R.; Yueh, B.; McDougall, J.K.; Daling, J.R.; Schwartz, S.M. Human Papillomavirus Infection and Survival in Oral Squamous Cell Cancer: A Population-Based Study. *Otolaryngol. Head Neck Surg.* **2001**, *125*, 1–9. [CrossRef]
70. Dayyani, F.; Etzel, C.J.; Liu, M.; Ho, C.H.; Lippman, S.M.; Tsao, A.S. Meta-Analysis of the Impact of Human Papillomavirus (HPV) on Cancer Risk and Overall Survival in Head and Neck Squamous Cell Carcinomas (HNSCC). *Head Neck Oncol.* **2010**, *2*. [CrossRef]
71. Fakhry, C.; Westra, W.H.; Li, S.; Cmelak, A.; Ridge, J.A.; Pinto, H.; Forastiere, A.; Gillison, M.L. Improved Survival of Patients with Human Papillomavirus-Positive Head and Neck Squamous Cell Carcinoma in a Prospective Clinical Trial. *J. Natl. Cancer Inst.* **2008**, *100*, 261–269. [CrossRef]
72. Huang, Q.; Yang, J.; Zheng, J.; Hsueh, C.; Guo, Y.; Zhou, L. Characterization of Selective Exosomal MicroRNA Expression Profile Derived from Laryngeal Squamous Cell Carcinoma Detected by next Generation Sequencing. *Oncol. Rep.* **2018**, *40*, 2584–2594. [CrossRef]
73. Zeljic, K.; Supic, G.; Magic, Z. New Insights into Vitamin D Anticancer Properties: Focus on MiRNA Modulation. *Mol. Genet. Genom.* **2017**, *292*, 511–524. [CrossRef]
74. Kalinowski, F.C.; Giles, K.M.; Candy, P.A.; Ali, A.; Ganda, C.; Epis, M.R.; Webster, R.J.; Leedman, P.J. Regulation of Epidermal Growth Factor Receptor Signaling and Erlotinib Sensitivity in Head and Neck Cancer Cells by MiR-7. *PLoS ONE* **2012**, *7*. [CrossRef] [PubMed]
75. Horsham, J.; Kalinowski, F.; Epis, M.; Ganda, C.; Brown, R.; Leedman, P. Clinical Potential of MicroRNA-7 in Cancer. *J. Clin. Med.* **2015**, *4*, 1668–1687. [CrossRef]
76. Yang, J.H.; Lin, L.K.; Zhang, S. Epigenetic Silencing of MicroRNA-335 Contributes to Nasopharyngeal Carcinoma Metastasis. *Am. J. Otolaryngol. Head Neck Med. Surg.* **2020**, *41*. [CrossRef] [PubMed]
77. Ou, D.; Wu, Y.; Liu, J.; Lao, X.; Zhang, S.; Liao, G. MiRNA-335 and MiRNA-182 Affect the Occurrence of Tongue Squamous Cell Carcinoma by Targeting Survivin. *Oncol. Lett.* **2016**, *12*, 2531–2537. [CrossRef] [PubMed]
78. Cheng, A.M.; Byrom, M.W.; Shelton, J.; Ford, L.P. Antisense Inhibition of Human MiRNAs and Indications for an Involvement of MiRNA in Cell Growth and Apoptosis. *Nucleic Acids Res.* **2005**, *33*, 1290–1297. [CrossRef] [PubMed]
79. Sethi, N.; Wright, A.; Wood, H.; Rabbitts, P. MicroRNAs and Head and Neck Cancer: Reviewing the First Decade of Research. *Eur. J. Cancer* **2014**, 2619–2635. [CrossRef] [PubMed]
80. Ayaz, L.; Görür, A.; Yaroğlu, H.Y.; Özcan, C.; Tamer, L. Differential Expression of MicroRNAs in Plasma of Patients with Laryngeal Squamous Cell Carcinoma: Potential Early-Detection Markers for Laryngeal Squamous Cell Carcinoma. *J. Cancer Res. Clin. Oncol.* **2013**, *139*, 1499–1506. [CrossRef]
81. MacLellan, S.A.; Lawson, J.; Baik, J.; Guillaud, M.; Poh, C.F.Y.; Garnis, C. Differential Expression of MiRNAs in the Serum of Patients with High-Risk Oral Lesions. *Cancer Med.* **2012**, *1*, 268–274. [CrossRef]
82. Yang, Y.; Li, Y.X.; Yang, X.; Jiang, L.; Zhou, Z.J.; Zhu, Y.Q. Progress Risk Assessment of Oral Premalignant Lesions with Saliva MiRNA Analysis. *BMC Cancer* **2013**, *13*. [CrossRef]
83. Hsu, C.M.; Lin, P.M.; Wang, Y.M.; Chen, Z.J.; Lin, S.F.; Yang, M.Y. Circulating MiRNA Is a Novel Marker for Head and Neck Squamous Cell Carcinoma. *Tumour Biol.* **2012**, *33*, 1933–1942. [CrossRef]
84. Ramdas, L.; Giri, U.; Ashorn, C.L.; Coombes, K.R.; El-Naggar, A.; Ang, K.K.; Story, M.D. MiRNA Expression Profiles in Head and Neck Squamous Cell Carcinoma and Adjacent Normal Tissue. *Head Neck* **2009**, *31*, 642–654. [CrossRef] [PubMed]
85. Rentoft, M.; Fahlén, J.; Coates, P.J.; Laurell, G.; Sjöström, B.; Rydén, P.; Nylander, K. MiRNA Analysis of Formalin-Fixed Squamous Cell Carcinomas of the Tongue Is Affected by Age of the Samples. *Int. J. Oncol.* **2011**, *38*, 61–69. [CrossRef]
86. Chou, Y.T.; Lin, H.H.; Lien, Y.C.; Wang, Y.H.; Hong, C.F.; Kao, Y.R.; Lin, S.C.; Chang, Y.C.; Lin, S.Y.; Chen, S.J.; et al. EGFR Promotes Lung Tumorigenesis by Activating MiR-7 through a Ras/ERK/Myc Pathway That Targets the Ets2 Transcriptional Repressor ERF. *Cancer Res.* **2010**, *70*, 8822–8831. [CrossRef] [PubMed]

87. Alsahafi, E.; Begg, K.; Amelio, I.; Raulf, N.; Lucarelli, P.; Sauter, T.; Tavassoli, M. Clinical Update on Head and Neck Cancer: Molecular Biology and Ongoing Challenges. *Cell Death Dis.* **2019**. [CrossRef]
88. Lechner, M.; Frampton, G.M.; Fenton, T.; Feber, A.; Palmer, G.; Jay, A.; Pillay, N.; Forster, M.; Cronin, M.T.; Lipson, D.; et al. Targeted Next-Generation Sequencing of Head and Neck Squamous Cell Carcinoma Identifies Novel Genetic Alterations in HPV+ and HPV- Tumors. *Genome Med.* **2013**, *5*, 49. [CrossRef]
89. Jackson-Weaver, O.; Ungvijanpunya, N.; Yuan, Y.; Qian, J.; Gou, Y.; Wu, J.; Shen, H.; Chen, Y.; Li, M.; Richard, S.; et al. PRMT1-P53 Pathway Controls Epicardial EMT and Invasion. *Cell Rep.* **2020**, *31*. [CrossRef] [PubMed]
90. Lu, Z.; Sturgis, E.M.; Zhu, L.; Zhang, H.; Tao, Y.; Wei, P.; Wei, Q.; Li, G. Mouse Double Minute 4 Variants Modify Susceptibility to Risk of Recurrence in Patients with Squamous Cell Carcinoma of the Oropharynx. *Mol. Carcinog.* **2018**, *57*, 361–369. [CrossRef]
91. Ach, T.; Schwarz-Furlan, S.; Ach, S.; Agaimy, A.; Gerken, M.; Rohrmeier, C.; Zenk, J.; Iro, H.; Brockhoff, G.; Ettl, T. Genomic Aberrations of MDM2, MDM4, FGFR1 and FGFR3 Are Associated with Poor Outcome in Patients with Salivary Gland Cancer. *J. Oral Pathol. Med.* **2016**, *45*, 500–509. [CrossRef]
92. Mishra, R.; Ranjan Das, B. Early Overexpression of Cdk4 and Possible Role of KRF and C-Myc in Chewing Tobacco Mediated Oral Cancer Development. *Mol. Biol. Rep.* **2003**, *30*, 207–213. [CrossRef]
93. Yu, C.; Xing, F.; Zhang, J.; Xu, J.; Li, Y. A Combination of MRNA Expression Profile and MiRNA Expression Profile Identifies Detection Biomarkers in Different Tumor Stages of Laryngeal Squamous Cell Carcinoma. *Eur. Rev. Med. Pharmacol. Sci.* **2018**, *22*, 7296–7304.
94. Xuefang, Z.; Ruinian, Z.; Liji, J.; Chun, Z.; Qiaolan, Z.; Jun, J.; Yuming, C.; Junrong, H. MiR-331-3p Inhibits Proliferation and Promotes Apoptosis of Nasopharyngeal Carcinoma Cells by Targeting Elf4B-PI3K-AKT Pathway. *Technol. Cancer Res. Treat.* **2020**, *19*, 153303381989225. [CrossRef]
95. Li, X.; Zhu, J.; Liu, Y.; Duan, C.; Chang, R.; Zhang, C. MicroRNA-331-3p Inhibits Epithelial-mesenchymal Transition by Targeting ErbB2 and VAV2 through the Rac1/PAK1/B-catenin Axis in Non-small-cell Lung Cancer. *Cancer Sci.* **2019**, *110*, cas.14014. [CrossRef]
96. Zhan, J.; Jiao, D.; Wang, Y.; Song, J.; Wu, J.; Wu, L.; Chen, Q.; Ma, S. Integrated MicroRNA and Gene Expression Profiling Reveals the Crucial MiRNAs in Curcumin Anti-Lung Cancer Cell Invasion. *Thorac. Cancer* **2017**, *8*, 461–470. [CrossRef] [PubMed]
97. Momen-Heravi, F.; Trachtenberg, A.J.; Kuo, W.P.; Cheng, Y.S. Genomewide Study of Salivary MicroRNAs for Detection of Oral Cancer. *J. Dent. Res.* **2014**, *93*, 86S–93S. [CrossRef]
98. Lu, E.; Su, J.; Zhou, Y.; Zhang, C.; Wang, Y. CCL20/CCR6 Promotes Cell Proliferation and Metastasis in Laryngeal Cancer by Activating P38 Pathway. *Biomed. Pharmacother.* **2017**, *85*, 486–492. [CrossRef]
99. Zhou, Z.X.; Zhang, Z.P.; Tao, Z.Z.; Tan, T.Z. MiR-632 Promotes Laryngeal Carcinoma Cell Proliferation, Migration, and Invasion through Negative Regulation of GSK3β. *Oncol. Res.* **2020**, *28*, 21–31. [CrossRef]
100. Grisendi, S.; Mecucci, C.; Falini, B.; Pandolfi, P.P. Nucleophosmin and Cancer. *Nat. Rev. Cancer* **2006**, 493–505. [CrossRef] [PubMed]
101. Saini, J.; Sharma, P.K. Clinical, Prognostic and Therapeutic Significance of Heat Shock Proteins in Cancer. *Curr. Drug Targets* **2018**, *19*, 1478–1490. [CrossRef] [PubMed]
102. Rabbani, N.; Xue, M.; Weickert, M.O.; Thornalley, P.J. Multiple Roles of Glyoxalase 1-Mediated Suppression of Methylglyoxal Glycation in Cancer Biology—Involvement in Tumour Suppression, Tumour Growth, Multidrug Resistance and Target for Chemotherapy. *Semin. Cancer Biol.* **2018**, 83–93. [CrossRef]
103. Kumar, N.; Prasad, P.; Jash, E.; Saini, M.; Husain, A.; Goldman, A.; Sehrawat, S. Insights into Exchange Factor Directly Activated by CAMP (EPAC) as Potential Target for Cancer Treatment. *Mol. Cell. Biochem.* **2018**, *447*, 77–92. [CrossRef]
104. Monteiro, F.L.; Baptista, T.; Amado, F.; Vitorino, R.; Jerónimo, C.; Helguero, L.A. Expression and Functionality of Histone H2A Variants in Cancer. *Oncotarget* **2014**, *5*, 3428–3443. [CrossRef]
105. Dhar, S.K.; St. Clair, D.K. Nucleophosmin Blocks Mitochondrial Localization of P53 and Apoptosis. *J. Biol. Chem.* **2009**, *284*, 16409–16418. [CrossRef]
106. Jeon, Y.J.; Cho, J.H.; Lee, S.Y.; Choi, Y.H.; Park, H.; Jung, S.; Shim, J.H.; Chae, J.I. Esculetin Induces Apoptosis Through EGFR/PI3K/Akt Signaling Pathway and Nucleophosmin Relocalization. *J. Cell. Biochem.* **2016**, *117*, 1210–1221. [CrossRef] [PubMed]
107. Shandilya, J.; Swaminathan, V.; Gadad, S.S.; Choudhari, R.; Kodaganur, G.S.; Kundu, T.K. Acetylated NPM1 Localizes in the Nucleoplasm and Regulates Transcriptional Activation of Genes Implicated in Oral Cancer Manifestation. *Mol. Cell. Biol.* **2009**, *29*, 5115–5127. [CrossRef] [PubMed]

108. Onikubo, T.; Nicklay, J.J.; Xing, L.; Warren, C.; Anson, B.; Wang, W.L.; Burgos, E.S.; Ruff, S.E.; Shabanowitz, J.; Cheng, R.H.; et al. Developmentally Regulated Post-Translational Modification of Nucleoplasmin Controls Histone Sequestration and Deposition. *Cell Rep.* **2015**, *10*, 1735–1748. [CrossRef]
109. Lindström, M.S. NPM1/B23: A Multifunctional Chaperone in Ribosome Biogenesis and Chromatin Remodeling. *Biochem. Res. Int.* **2011**, *2011*. [CrossRef] [PubMed]
110. Kreycy, N.; Gotzian, C.; Fleming, T.; Flechtenmacher, C.; Grabe, N.; Plinkert, P.; Hess, J.; Zaoui, K. Glyoxalase 1 Expression Is Associated with an Unfavorable Prognosis of Oropharyngeal Squamous Cell Carcinoma. *BMC Cancer* **2017**, *17*. [CrossRef] [PubMed]
111. Geng, X.; Ma, J.; Zhang, F.; Xu, C. Glyoxalase i in Tumor Cell Proliferation and Survival and as a Potential Target for Anticancer Therapy. *Oncol. Res. Treat.* **2014**, *37*, 570–574. [CrossRef] [PubMed]
112. Ernst, B.P.; Wiesmann, N.; Gieringer, R.; Eckrich, J.; Brieger, J. HSP27 Regulates Viability and Migration of Cancer Cell Lines Following Irradiation. *J. Proteom.* **2020**, *226*, 103886. [CrossRef]
113. Guttmann, D.M.; Hart, L.; Du, K.; Seletsky, A.; Koumenis, C. Inhibition of Hsp27 Radiosensitizes Head-and-Neck Cancer by Modulating Deoxyribonucleic Acid Repair. *Int. J. Radiat. Oncol. Biol. Phys.* **2013**, *87*, 168–175. [CrossRef]
114. Zhu, Z.K.; Wang, Y.S.; Xu, X. Biology Behavior of Head and Neck Squamous Cell Cancer Cells Changes after Knocking down Heat Shock Protein 27. *Hua Xi Kou Qiang Yi Xue Za Zhi* **2020**, *38*, 139–144. [CrossRef] [PubMed]
115. Berggren, K.L.; Restrepo Cruz, S.; Hixon, M.D.; Cowan, A.T.; Keysar, S.B.; Craig, S.; James, J.; Barry, M.; Ozbun, M.A.; Jimeno, A.; et al. MAPKAPK2 (MK2) Inhibition Mediates Radiation-Induced Inflammatory Cytokine Production and Tumor Growth in Head and Neck Squamous Cell Carcinoma. *Oncogene* **2019**, *38*, 7329–7341. [CrossRef] [PubMed]
116. Chen, W.; Ren, X.; Wu, J.; Gao, X.; Cen, X.; Wang, S.; Sheng, S.; Chen, Q.; Tang, Y.J.; Liang, X.H.; et al. HSP27 Associates with Epithelial–Mesenchymal Transition, Stemness and Radioresistance of Salivary Adenoid Cystic Carcinoma. *J. Cell. Mol. Med.* **2018**, *22*, 2283–2298. [CrossRef] [PubMed]
117. Kim, J.; Lim, H.; Kim, S.; Cho, H.; Kim, Y.; Li, X.; Choi, H.; Kim, O. Effects of HSP27 Downregulation on PDT Resistance through PDT-Induced Autophagy in Head and Neck Cancer Cells. *Oncol. Rep.* **2016**, *35*, 2237–2245. [CrossRef]
118. da Silva, S.D.; Marchi, F.A.; Xu, B.; Bijian, K.; Alobaid, F.; Mlynarek, A.; Rogatto, S.R.; Hier, M.; Kowalski, L.P.; Alaoui-Jamali, M.A. Predominant Rab-GTPase Amplicons Contributing to Oral Squamous Cell Carcinoma Progression to Metastasis. *Oncotarget* **2015**, *6*, 21950–21963. [CrossRef]
119. Lo Re, O.; Fusilli, C.; Rappa, F.; Van Haele, M.; Douet, J.; Pindjakova, J.; Rocha, S.W.; Pata, I.; Valčíková, B.; Uldrijan, S.; et al. Induction of Cancer Cell Stemness by Depletion of Macrohistone H2A1 in Hepatocellular Carcinoma. *Hepatology* **2018**, *67*, 636–650. [CrossRef]
120. Niu, W.; Zhang, M.; Chen, H.; Wang, C.; Shi, N.; Jing, X.; Ge, L.; Chen, T.; Tang, X. Peroxiredoxin 1 Promotes Invasion and Migration by Regulating Epithelial-to-Mesenchymal Transition during Oral Carcinogenesis. *Oncotarget* **2016**, *7*, 47042–47051. [CrossRef]
121. Jiang, Y.; Cao, W.; Wu, K.; Qin, X.; Wang, X.; Li, Y.; Yu, B.; Zhang, Z.; Wang, X.; Yan, M.; et al. LncRNA LINC00460 Promotes EMT in Head and Neck Squamous Cell Carcinoma by Facilitating Peroxiredoxin-1 into the Nucleus. *J. Exp. Clin. Cancer Res.* **2019**, *38*, 1–19. [CrossRef]
122. Monisha, J.; Kishor Roy, N.; Bordoloi, D.; Kumar, A.; Golla, R.; Kotoky, J.; Padmavathi, G.; B. Kunnumakkara, A. Nuclear Factor Kappa B: A Potential Target to Persecute Head and Neck Cancer. *Curr. Drug Targets* **2016**, *18*, 232–253. [CrossRef]

5

The Effect of Vitamin D Supplementation on its Metabolism and the Vitamin D Metabolite Ratio

Vito Francic [1,†], Stan R. Ursem [2,†], Niek F. Dirks [2], Martin H. Keppel [3], Verena Theiler-Schwetz [1], Christian Trummer [1], Marlene Pandis [1], Valentin Borzan [1], Martin R. Grübler [1], Nicolas D. Verheyen [4], Winfried März [5], Andreas Tomaschitz [6], Stefan Pilz [1], Annemieke C. Heijboer [2] and Barbara Obermayer-Pietsch [1,*]

1 Division of Endocrinology and Diabetology, Endocrinology Lab Platform, Department of Internal Medicine, Medical University of Graz, 8036 Graz, Austria; vito.francic@medunigraz.at (V.F.); verena.schwetz@medunigraz.at (V.T.-S.); christian.trummer@medunigraz.at (C.T.); marlene.pandis@medunigraz.at (M.P.); valentin.borzan@medunigraz.at (V.B.); martin.gruebler@gmx.net (M.R.G.); stefan.pilz@chello.at (S.P.)

2 Department of Clinical Chemistry, Endocrine Laboratory, Amsterdam Gastroenterology & Metabolism, Vrije Universiteit Amsterdam and University of Amsterdam, Amsterdam UMC, 1105 Amsterdam, The Netherlands; s.ursem@amsterdamumc.nl (S.R.U.); n.dirks@amsterdamumc.nl (N.F.D.); a.heijboer@amsterdamumc.nl (A.C.H.)

3 Department of Laboratory Medicine, Paracelsus Medical University Salzburg, 5020 Salzburg, Austria; keppel.martin@gmail.com

4 Division of Cardiology, Department of Internal Medicine, Medical University of Graz, 8036 Graz, Austria; nicolas.verheyen@medunigraz.at

5 Synlab Academy, Synlab Holding Germany GmbH, 68163 Mannheim, Germany; Winfried.Maerz@synlab.com

6 Health Center Trofaiach-Gössgrabenstrasse, 8739 Trofaiach, Austria; andreas.tomaschitz@gmx.at

* Correspondence: barbara.obermayer@medunigraz.at

† These authors contributed equally to this work.

Abstract: 25-hydroxyvitamin D (25(OH)D) is commonly measured to assess vitamin D status. Other vitamin D metabolites such as 24,25-dihydroxyvitamin D (24,25$(OH)_2$D) provide additional insights into vitamin D status or metabolism. Earlier studies suggested that the vitamin D metabolite ratio (VMR), calculated as 24,25$(OH)_2$D/25(OH)D, could predict the 25(OH)D increase after vitamin D supplementation. However, the evidence for this additional value is inconclusive. Therefore, our aim was to assess whether the increase in 25(OH)D after supplementation was predicted by the VMR better than baseline 25(OH)D. Plasma samples of 106 individuals (25(OH)D < 75 nmol/L) with hypertension who completed the Styrian Vitamin D Hypertension Trial (NC.T.02136771) were analyzed. Participants received vitamin D (2800 IU daily) or placebo for 8 weeks. The treatment effect (ANCOVA) for 25(OH)D_3, 24,25$(OH)_2D_3$ and the VMR was 32 nmol/L, 3.3 nmol/L and 0.015 (all $p < 0.001$), respectively. Baseline 25(OH)D_3 and 24,25$(OH)_2D_3$ predicted the change in 25(OH)D_3 with comparable strength and magnitude. Correlation and regression analysis showed that the VMR did not predict the change in 25(OH)D_3. Therefore, our data do not support routine measurement of 24,25$(OH)_2D_3$ in order to individually optimize the dosage of vitamin D supplementation. Our data also suggest that activity of 24-hydroxylase increases after vitamin D supplementation.

Keywords: vitamin D metabolites; vitamin D supplementation; vitamin D metabolite ratio; randomized controlled trial; 24,25-dihydroxy vitamin D

1. Introduction

Vitamin D plays an essential role in calcium and phosphate homeostasis [1]. Vitamin D status is most commonly assessed by determining the 25-hydroxyvitamin D (25(OH)D) concentration in serum or plasma. However, several other vitamin D-related metabolites can be measured to provide a better understanding of individual vitamin D status and metabolism. Among them, 24,25(OH)$_2$D has emerged as a metabolite with potentially high utility [2].

In the kidneys, 25(OH)D is converted by 1-alpha-hydroxylase (CYP27B1) into 1,25-dihydroxyvitamin D (1,25(OH)$_2$D; also called active vitamin D or calcitriol) (Figure 1). 1,25(OH)$_2$D can bind to the vitamin D receptor (VDR) with high affinity. The subsequent signaling results in an increase in serum calcium and phosphate concentrations, mainly mediated by an increased intestinal uptake. In addition, 1,25(OH)$_2$D has effects on the parathyroid gland, kidneys and bones, all resulting in an increase in serum calcium and phosphate concentrations [1]. Furthermore, 1,25(OH)2D has major effects on modulating the immune system, which might be relevant for the treatment of autoimmune diseases, infections, cancer and cardiovascular diseases [3]. An excess of both 1,25(OH)$_2$D and/or 25(OH)D lead to their catabolism by the enzyme 24-hydroxylase (CYP24A1). This results in the formation of metabolites 1,24,25(OH)$_2$D and 24,25(OH)$_2$D, respectively [4]. It is still unclear whether 24,25(OH)$_2$D has a physiological role in humans [5].

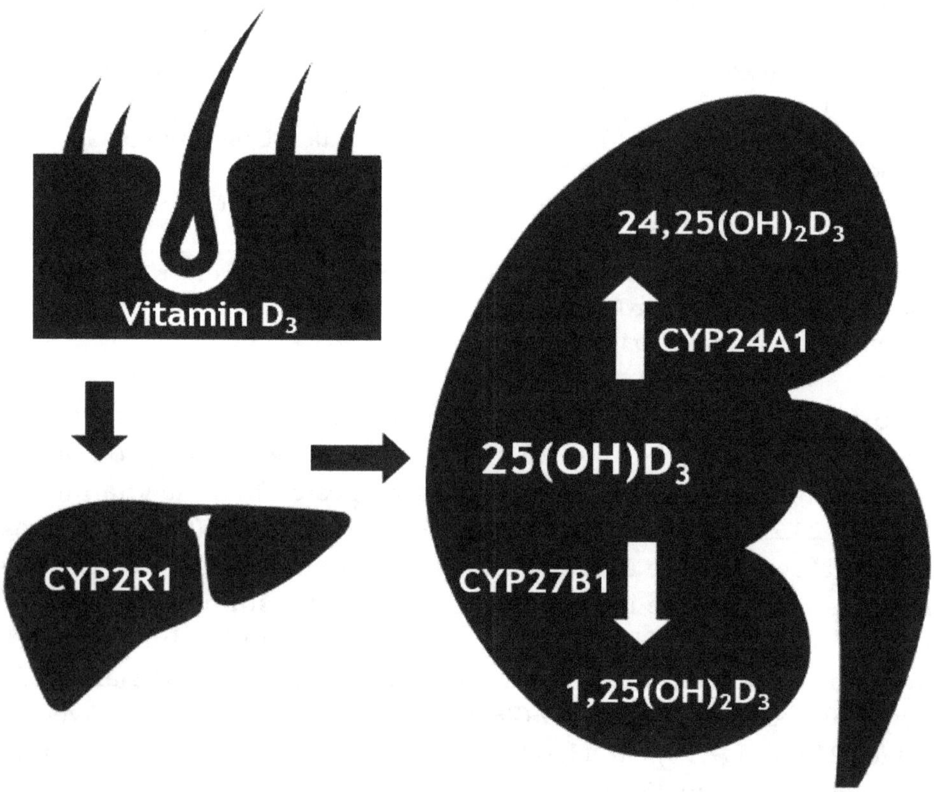

Figure 1. Metabolism of vitamin D. Vitamin D$_3$ (cholecalciferol) is produced in the skin when exposed to sunlight. The hepatic enzyme CYP2R1 then converts this into 25(OH)D$_3$ (calcifediol). In the kidneys, 25(OH)D$_3$ can be converted into the active form, 1,25(OH)$_2$D$_3$ (calcitriol), by CYP27B1 (1-α-hydroxylase). In the kidneys, CYP24A1 (24-hydroxylase) can catabolize the 25(OH)D$_3$ into 24,25(OH)$_2$D$_3$.

Using an LC-MS/MS method, 25(OH)D and 24,25(OH)$_2$D can be measured simultaneously, which allows for determination of the 24,25(OH)$_2$D/25(OH)D ratio, also known as the vitamin D metabolite ratio (VMR) [2]. The VMR is an indicator of CYP24A1 activity and thereby of vitamin D catabolism. It is currently used for diagnosing idiopathic infantile hypercalcemia, a rare genetic disorder in which a mutation in CYP24A1 results in severe hypercalcemia and suppressed parathyroid hormone (PTH) levels [5]. The VMR may also reflect vitamin D receptor (VDR) activity since CYP24A1 expression is upregulated in response to 1,25$(OH)_2$D [2].

In recent years, there has been an increasing interest in the use of the VMR when assessing vitamin D status. For example, it has been postulated to better reflect vitamin D deficiency [6]. In addition, it has been speculated that the ratio could provide useful information regarding bone health [7]. Interestingly, several studies show that the VMR can predict the change seen in 25(OH)D after vitamin D supplementation, although results are inconclusive [6,8–11]. The CYP24A1 activity could be partially responsible for the individual differences seen in the effect of vitamin D supplementation on serum levels of 25(OH)D. Theoretically, if CYP24A1 activity is a major predictor of the effect of vitamin D supplementation, the VMR could be used to personalize the treatment dosage. At present, 25(OH)D concentrations at the start of supplementation, as well as BMI, age, ethnicity and genetic background have been most commonly studied in regard to predicting the response to vitamin D supplementation, and studies involving 1,25$(OH)_2$D, 24,25$(OH)_2$D, free and bioavailable 25(OH)D and the VMR are scarce [12].

Therefore, we set out to determine whether baseline VMR measurements can predict changes in vitamin D-related metabolite levels after vitamin D supplementation. To that extent, we measured 25$(OH)D_3$, 1,25$(OH)_2$D and 24,25$(OH)_2D_3$ in a randomized clinical trial of patients (25(OH)D < 75 nmol/L) receiving vitamin D supplementation [13]. We hypothesized that measurements of baseline VMR would be advantageous over baseline 25(OH)D measurements for the prediction of the change in 25(OH)D upon supplementation.

2. Materials and Methods

2.1. Study Cohort

The present post-hoc analysis was conducted in adults (>18 years old) with 25(OH)D levels <75 nmol/L and hypertension, who completed the randomized, placebo-controlled Styrian Vitamin D Hypertension Trial (NC.T.02136771). The participants of this trial were treated with either placebo or 2800 IU daily of vitamin D_3 (Oleovit D_3, Fresenius Kabi, Graz, Austria) for 8 weeks. A total of 188 study participants completed the original study and sufficient material for analysis from both study visits was available for 106 of these subjects. The details regarding the study, including inclusion and exclusion criteria, can be found in the publication of the original study by Pilz et al. [13].

Study participants provided written informed consent. The study complied with the Declaration of Helsinki and was approved by the ethics committee of the Medical University of Graz, Austria.

2.2. Measurements

For the original study by Pilz et al, the 25(OH)D levels were determined with the ChemiLuminescence assay (IDS-iSYS 25-hydroxyvitamin D assay; Immunodiagnostic Systems Ltd., Boldon, UK) on an IDS-iSYS multidiscipline automated analyser [13]. The intra- and inter-assay CVs were 6.2% and 11.6%, respectively.

In the present study, 25$(OH)D_3$ and 24,25$(OH)_2D_3$ were measured in plasma samples by isotope dilution liquid chromatography-tandem mass spectrometry at the Endocrine Laboratory of the Amsterdam UMC, as described previously [14]. For 25$(OH)D_3$, the lower limit of quantitation (LLOQ) was 1.2 nmol/L and the inter- and intra-assay coefficients of variation (CV) were 6% and 3%, respectively. For 24,25$(OH)_2D_3$, the LLOQ was 0.1 nmol/L and the inter- and intra-assay coefficients of variation (CV) were 9% and 5%, respectively. 25$(OH)D_2$ was also measured, but as the concentrations were all very low (<7.9 nmol/L) and supplementation was given as vitamin D_3, these data were not taken into account in this paper. In order to calculate the VMR and as it is the golden standard, the LC/MS-MS method was used for the current study. Using this method, 7 subjects had 25(OH)D levels >75 nmol/L at baseline. Measurements of other study parameters have been described previously [13].

To calculate free and biologically available 25$(OH)D_3$ we used the equations from Powe et al. [15].

2.3. *Statistical Analysis*

Continuous data following a normal distribution are reported as means with standard deviations (SD). Variables with a skewed distribution are shown as medians with interquartile ranges. Categorical variables are shown as percentages of observations. Groups at baseline were compared using the unpaired Students t-test, the Mann–Whitney U test or the chi-squared test. Skewed variables were log transformed before being used in parametric analyses.

The changes from baseline for 25(OH)D_3, 1,25(OH)$_2$D and 24,25(OH)$_2D_3$ in the vitamin-D-treated group were calculated as the difference between the value at the final study visit and the value at baseline. They are depicted as Δ25(OH)D_3, Δ1,25(OH)$_2$D and Δ24,25(OH)$_2D_3$. The VMR was calculated as the ratio between 24,25(OH)$_2D_3$ and 25(OH)D_3.

Analysis of covariance (ANCOVA) was used to calculate the treatment effects with adjustment for baseline values. Pearson correlation analysis was used to determine the strength of associations between vitamin-D-related parameters and Δ25(OH)D_3, Δ1,25(OH)$_2$D, as well as Δ24,25(OH)$_2D_3$. Bonferroni correction was applied to account for multiple testing. Univariate linear regression analysis was used to determine the relation between Δ25(OH)D_3 and baseline 25(OH)D_3, 24,25(OH)$_2D_3$ and VMR.

Using the LC/MS-MS method, 7 subjects had 25(OH)D levels >75 nmol/L at baseline. Therefore, we explored whether inclusion of these subjects had an effect on the analyses. In addition, we also investigated whether the inclusion of only subjects with 25(OH)D levels <50 nmol/L at baseline would affect the analyses.

If outliers were detected in the analyses by the software, defined as cases with standardized residuals greater than 3 standard deviations for ANCOVA analyses or as cases with values higher or lower than 1.5*IQR (interquartile range) for correlation analyses, they were removed and the analysis repeated to determine their potential effect on the analysis. In the case of Pearson correlation analyses, one extreme outlier was removed (25(OH)D > 4xSD at baseline) because of its significant effect on all of the analyses. This is marked in the results section. If the outliers had no significant effect on the analysis, the results including the outliers are reported. A p-value < 0.05 was considered statistically significant. All analyses were performed using S.P.SS version 25 (S.P.SS, Chicago, IL, USA).

3. Results

The baseline characteristics of study participants can be found in Table 1. There were no differences between the placebo and vitamin-D-treated groups in any of the parameters at baseline.

Table 1. Baseline characteristics.

Parameter	All (n = 106)	Placebo (n = 54)	Vitamin D (n = 52)	p-value
Age (years)	62.0 (51.3–68.7)	64.8 (50.8–70.2)	59.6 (52.4–66.6)	0.318
Body mass index (kg/m^2)	30.0 ± 5.4	29.7 ± 5.9	30.3 ± 4.9	0.562
Gender (% female)	57	57	56	0.865
24,25(OH)$_2D_3$ (nmol/L)	3.5 ± 1.6	3.4 ± 1.5	3.6 ± 1.5	0.419
25(OH)D_3 (nmol/L)	48 ± 18	46 ± 19	49 ± 18	0.401
VMR ((nmol/L)/(nmol/L))	0.073 ± 0.017	0.072 ± 0.018	0.073 ± 0.017	0.768
PTH (pmol/L)	5.5 (4.1–6.7)	5.5 (4.0–6.7)	5.3 (4.1–6.7)	0.779
1,25(OH)$_2$D (pmol/L)	126 ± 53	118 ± 52	133 ± 52	0.142
Serum phosphate (mmol/L)	0.94 ± 0.17	0.96 ± 0.17	0.92 ± 0.16	0.282
Serum calcium (mmol/L)	2.26 (2.21–2.33)	2.26 (2.21–2.34)	2.26 (2.20–2.33)	0.773
eGFR (mL/min/1.73m^2)	72 ± 17	69 ± 16	74 ± 18	0.152
24h urinary calcium excretion (mmol/24h)	3.30 (1.90–5.00)	2.95 (1.83–4.78)	3.70 (2.10–6.30)	0.222
Calculated free 25(OH)D_3 (pmol/L)	15 (9–21)	12 (8–21)	17 (11–20)	0.153
Vitamin D binding protein (µg/mL)	247.1 ± 109.5	254.8 ± 110.6	239.3 ± 109.0	0.772
Calculated bioavailable 25(OH)D_3 (nmol/L)	5.9 (3.9–8.2)	5.2 (3.2–8.5)	6.6 (4.1–8.0)	0.149
1,25(OH)$_2$D /25(OH)D_3 ((nmol/L)/(nmol/L))	0.0023 (0.0019–0.0036)	0.0027 (0.0018–0.0039)	0.0028 (0.0021–0.0035)	0.753
1,25(OH)$_2$D /24,25(OH)$_2D_3$ ((nmol/L)/(nmol/L))	0.036 (0.025–0.05)	0.036 (0.024–0.051)	0.035 (0.026–0.050)	0.893

The calculated treatment effects after vitamin D supplementation are depicted in Table 2. We observed significant treatment effects for all included vitamin-D-related parameters. For 25(OH)D_3, the treatment effect was 32 nmol/L (95% CI: 26 to 39; p < 0.001), for 1,25(OH)$_2$D 26 pmol/L (9 to 42; p = 0.003), for 24,25(OH)$_2D_3$ 3.3 nmol/L (2.7 to 3.9; p < 0.001), for the VMR 0.015 (nmol/L)/(nmol/L)

(0.010–0.019; $p < 0.001$), for calculated free 25(OH)D_3 12 pmol/L (6 to 18; $p < 0.001$), for calculated bioavailable 25(OH)D_3 4.66 nmol/L (2.63 to 6.68; $p < 0.001$), for the 1,25(OH)$_2$D/25(OH)D_3 ratio −0.0010 (nmol/L)/(nmol/L) (−0.0013 to −0.0006; $p < 0.001$) and for the 1,25(OH)$_2$D/24,25(OH)$_2D_3$ ratio −0.020 (nmol/L)/(nmol/L) (−0.026 to −0.015; $p < 0.001$). In the subgroup of subjects with 25(OH)D_3 levels below 50 nmol/L, the treatment effects and *p*-values were comparable for all parameters.

Table 2. Analysis of covariance (ANCOVA) analysis for the effect of vitamin D or placebo treatment on vitamin-D-related parameters.

Parameter	Group	Baseline	Follow-up	Treatment Effect (95% CI)	*p*-value
25(OH)D_3 (nmol/L)	Placebo, n=54 Vitamin D, n=52	46 ± 19 49 ± 18	45 ± 20 79 ± 19	32 (26 to 39)	<0.001
1,25(OH)$_2$D (pmol/L)	Placebo, n=52 Vitamin D, n=52	118 ± 52 133 ± 52	114 ± 39 150 ± 63	26 (9 to 42)	0.003
24,25(OH)$_2D_3$ (nmol/L)	Placebo, n=54 Vitamin D, n=52	3.4 ± 1.5 3.6 ± 1.6	3.3 ± 1.8 6.8 ± 1.7	3.3 (2.7 to 3.9)	<0.001
VMR	Placebo, n=54 Vitamin D, n=52	0.072 ± 0.018 0.073 ± 0.017	0.071 ± 0.017 0.087 ± 0.018	0.015 (0.010 to 0.020)	<0.001
Calculated free 25(OH)D_3 (pmol/L)*	Placebo, n=53 Vitamin D, n=51	12 (8–21) 17 (11–20)	12 (8–18) 21 (17–31)	12 (6 to 18)	<0.001
Calculated bioavailable 25(OH)D_3 (nmol/L) *	Placebo, n=53 Vitamin D, n=51	5.22 (3.15–8.51) 6.60 (4.10–8.02)	4.99 (2.95–6.83) 8.69 (6.58–12.51)	4.66 (2.63 to 6.68)	<0.001
1,25(OH)$_2$D/ 25(OH)D_3 *	Placebo, n=52 Vitamin D, n=52	0.0027 (0.0018–0.0039) 0.0028 (0.0021–0.0035)	0.0026 (0.0019–0.0036) 0.0019 (0.0014–0.0026)	−0.0010 (−0.0013 to −0.0006)	<0.001
1,25(OH)$_2$D /24,25(OH)$_2D_3$ *	Placebo, n=52 Vitamin D, n=52	0.036 (0.024–0.051) 0.035 (0.026–0.050)	0.037 (0.026–0.052) 0.022 (0.016–0.028)	−0.020 (−0.026 to −-0.015)	<0.001

* Log-transformed parameters.

The overall correlation between 25(OH)D_3 and 24,25(OH)$_2D_3$ at baseline was r = 0.815, $p < 0.001$. Results of the regression analyses of the Δ25(OH)D_3 in the vitamin-D-supplemented group are shown in Figure 2. The slope of the linear regression, *p*-values and R^2 values are highly similar for baseline 25(OH)D_3 and 24,25(OH)$_2D_3$. The VMR, however, could not predict the increase in 25(OH)D_3 concentration. The results of the correlation analyses in the vitamin-D-treated group are summarized in Table 3. None of the vitamin-D-related parameters correlated significantly with Δ25(OH)D_3 or Δ1,25(OH)$_2$D after Bonferroni correction. Also, in the subgroup of subjects with 25(OH)D levels below 50 nmol/L, none of the parameters correlated significantly with Δ25(OH)D_3 or Δ1,25(OH)$_2$D after Bonferroni correction. For Δ25(OH)D_3, a trend was seen for baseline 25(OH)D_3 and baseline 24,25(OH)$_2D_3$ (r = −0.388, $p = 0.056$ and r = −0.374, $p = 0.056$). This trend with Δ25(OH)D_3 was also observed for calculated free 25(OH)D_3 and calculated bioavailable 25(OH)D_3 (r = −0.373, $p = 0.056$ and r = −0.375, $p = 0.056$). Δ24,25(OH)$_2D_3$ was significantly associated with baseline 25(OH)D_3, 24,25(OH)$_2D_3$, calculated free 25(OH)D_3 and calculated bioavailable 25(OH)D_3 (r = −0.562, $p < 0.001$; r = −0.476, $p = 0.003$; r = −0.382, $p = 0.048$ and r = −0.393, $p = 0.032$, respectively), but not with other parameters. In the subgroup of subjects with 25(OH)D_3 levels below 50 nmol/L, none of the parameters correlated significantly with Δ24,25(OH)$_2D_3$ after Bonferroni correction.

Correlation analyses after adjustment for gender, age, BMI, PTH, eGFR, serum phosphate and serum calcium showed that none of the vitamin-D-related parameters were significantly associated with Δ25(OH)D_3 or Δ1,25(OH)$_2$D after Bonferroni correction (Table A1). However, when corrected for the above-mentioned parameters, only baseline 25(OH)D_3 was still significantly associated with Δ24,25(OH)$_2D_3$ (r = −0.657, $p = 0.008$). In the subgroup of subjects with 25(OH)D_3 levels below 50 nmol/L, none of the parameters correlated significantly with Δ25(OH)D_3, Δ1,25(OH)$_2$D or Δ24,25(OH)$_2D_3$ after Bonferroni correction.

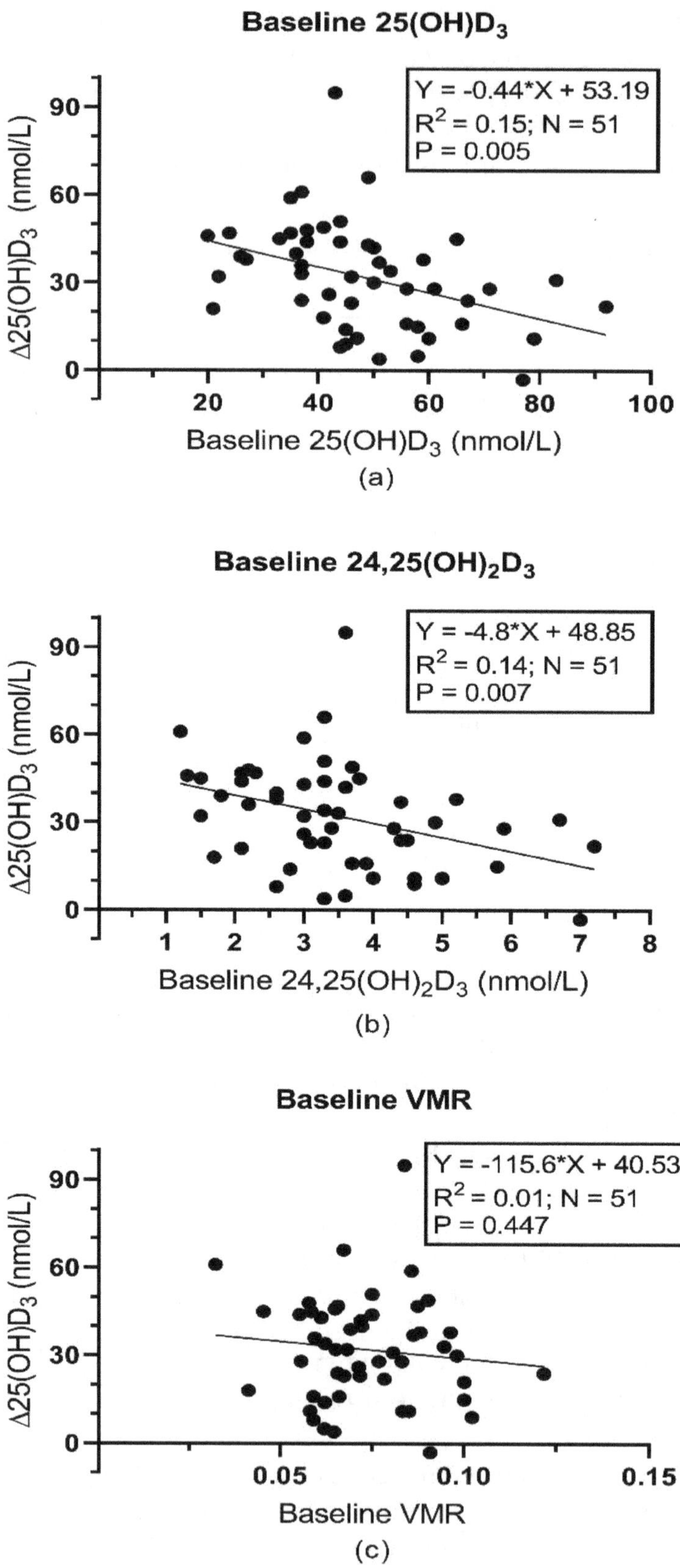

Figure 2. Univariate linear regression analysis for the change in 25(OH)D_3 concentration in the vitamin D intervention group and (**a**) baseline 25(OH)D_3, (**b**) baseline 24,25$(OH)_2D_3$ and (**c**) baseline VMR (Vitamin D Metabolite Ratio).

Table 3. Pearson correlations with unadjusted p-values and Bonferroni adjusted p-values of baseline vitamin-D-related parameters with the changes from baseline of $25(OH)D_3$, $1,25(OH)_2D$ and $24,25(OH)_2D_3$ after vitamin D supplementation.

Baseline Parameters		$\Delta 25(OH)D_3$	$\Delta 1,25(OH)_2D$	$\Delta 24,25(OH)_2D_3$
$25(OH)D_3$	r	−0.388	−0.142	−0.562
	p-value	0.005	0.322	<0.001
	Adjusted p-value	0.056	1.000	<0.001
$1,25(OH)_2D$	r	−0.287	−0.260	−0.272
	p-value	0.041	0.065	0.053
	Adjusted p-value	0.328	0.520	0.424
$24,25(OH)_2D_3$	r	−0.374	−0.122	−0.476
	p-value	0.007	0.392	<0.001
	Adjusted p-value	0.056	1.000	0.003
VMR	r	−0.109	−0.027	−0.015
	p-value	0.448	0.850	0.916
	Adjusted p-value	1.000	1.000	1.000
Calculated free $25(OH)D_3$ *	r	−0.373	−0.281	−0.382
	p-value	0.007	0.046	0.006
	Adjusted p-value	0.056	0.368	0.048
Calculated bioavailable $25(OH)D_3$ *	r	−0.375	−0.280	−0.393
	p-value	0.007	0.047	0.004
	Adjusted p-value	0.056	0.376	0.032
$1,25(OH)_2D/25(OH)D_3$ *	r	−0.004	−0.058	0.176
	p-value	0.980	0.687	0.216
	Adjusted p-value	1.000	1.000	1.000
$1,25(OH)_2D/24,25(OH)_2D_3$ *	r	0.053	−0.028	0.181
	p-value	0.711	0.843	0.204
	Adjusted p-value	1.000	1.000	1.000

* Log-transformed parameters.

4. Discussion

The goal of our study was to assess whether vitamin D metabolites can predict the increase of 25(OH)D after vitamin D supplementation. As elaborated above, CYP24A1 activity (24-hydroxylase) is reflected by the ratio of $24,25(OH)_2D$ over 25(OH)D, i.e. the VMR. In addition, the ratio between $1,25(OH)_2D$ and $24,25(OH)_2D_3$ was recently proposed as part of a three-dimensional model for assessing vitamin D metabolic pathways [16]. It was previously suggested that vitamin D metabolites and their ratios could provide additional information for predicting vitamin D treatment response [8,9]. The findings in this vitamin D RC.T. in patients with 25(OH)D levels <75 nmol/L and hypertension do not support this hypothesis.

In our study, the VMR did not predict $\Delta 25(OH)D_3$ in the treatment arm of the RC.T.. In a regression model, baseline $24,25(OH)_2D_3$ and baseline $25(OH)D_3$ did, with comparable strength and magnitude, predict the increase in $25(OH)D_3$ upon treatment. When adjusting for multiple testing in correlation analyses, no correlations of any of the included parameters with $\Delta 25(OH)D_3$ retained significance. Yet, we did observe trends for $\Delta 25(OH)D_3$ with baseline $25(OH)D_3$, $24,25(OH)_2D_3$, free $25(OH)D_3$ and bioavailable $25(OH)D_3$. Notwithstanding their borderline significance, the strength of the correlations is highly similar between these parameters and they do not seem to be superior to baseline 25(OH)D. According to these data, we can infer that CYP24A1 activity, measured by the VMR, does not predict the individual differences in the increase in 25(OH)D after vitamin D supplementation.

Concerning the VMR, the results of this study are in accordance with several other published reports. Saleh et al. performed an RC.T. of 4 weeks with 107 participants receiving a single 100,000 IU dose of vitamin D or placebo [11]. The VMR could not predict the increase of 25(OH)D after 4 weeks, whereas 25(OH)D did predict this increase with a similar R^2-value to our data. However, their data indicated that $24,25(OH)_2D_3$ could not predict the $\Delta 25(OH)D_3$, whereas in our study it did. Aloia et al.

reported on the predictive properties of the VMR in four different small samples (between 14 and 16 participants per group) of placebo or 800, 2000 or 4000 IU vitamin D daily for 10 weeks [6]. They did not show an advantage of the VMR as a predictor, compared to baseline 25(OH)D, 24,25$(OH)_2D_3$ or free 25(OH)D. Binkley et al. investigated the effect of 1800IU of vitamin D in 62 postmenopausal women after 4 months and measured vitamin D metabolites [10]. They observed that neither VMR, 25(OH)D, 24,25$(OH)_2D_3$ nor free 25(OH)D was related to the observed increase in 25(OH)D.

On the contrary, other published studies did suggest a predictive role for the VMR. The study by Wagner et al. included young adults with a mean age of around 27 years that received 28,000 IU (equivalent to 4000 IU per day) of vitamin D once per week for 8 weeks in the form of a supplement or fortified cheese. Wagner et al. showed that the VMR predicted the increase in vitamin-D-receiving subjects ($R^2 = -0.38$, $p = 0.004$, $n = 60$) [8]. Also, Cashman et al. reported a significant correlation between the VMR and the change after vitamin D supplementation ($R^2 = 0.15$, $p < 0.01$) in a study including subjects above 50 years of age that were treated for 15 weeks by 20 μg vitamin D (800 IU) per day [9]. Of note, both studies did not report the R^2-value of baseline 25(OH)D with its increase after supplementation. Therefore, it is not possible to conclude whether the VMR was superior to 25(OH)D in this aspect.

Changes in other vitamin-D-related parameters after vitamin D treatment were also studied. To that end, we assessed if Δ1,25$(OH)_2D$ and Δ24,25$(OH)_2D_3$ could be predicted by baseline parameters included in the study. We found no correlation between any tested baseline parameter and Δ1,25$(OH)_2D$. 1,25$(OH)_2D$ levels are mainly regulated by calcium levels, which could explain this observation [12]. On the other hand, baseline 25$(OH)D_3$, 24,25$(OH)_2D_3$, calculated free 25$(OH)D_3$ and calculated bioavailable 25$(OH)D_3$ all showed a significant correlation with Δ24,25$(OH)_2D_3$. The clinical relevance of this observation is, in our opinion, unclear and should be further studied.

In our study, we observed an increase in the VMR upon vitamin D treatment. This suggests an increase in CYP24A1 activity and catabolism of 25(OH)D upon supplementation. A concurrent decrease in the 1,25$(OH)_2D$/25$(OH)D_3$ ratio implies a reduced conversion of 25(OH)D to 1,25$(OH)_2D$. Indeed, this suggests the physiological shift from anabolic to catabolic pathways when an excess of vitamin D exists. This is also supported by the significant decrease in the 1,25$(OH)_2D$/24,25$(OH)_2D_3$ ratio. In the present study, and all aforementioned studies, the correlation coefficients between baseline 25(OH)D and Δ25$(OH)D_3$ after supplementation were negative, which implies that the change in 25$(OH)D_3$ after vitamin D treatment is smaller in individuals with higher baseline 25$(OH)D_3$ levels [8–10].

We acknowledge that this study has several limitations. First, the results are derived from post-hoc analyses. Second, the study population consisted of hypertensive subjects with 25(OH)D levels <75 nmol/L; therefore, the findings might not be readily extrapolated to the general population. Furthermore, for the vitamin D level inclusion criterion, the 25(OH)D concentrations were measured at study baseline using a chemiluminescence assay, while mass-spectrometry-based methods are currently the gold standard [2]. However, for the current study, 25(OH)D and 24,25$(OH)_2D$ were re-measured using a dedicated LC-MS/MS method. In addition, the intervention period of 8 weeks was relatively short and only a small number of subjects were severely vitamin D deficient. Vitamin D deficiency was defined as a 25(OH)D of <75 nmol/L in the original study by Pilz et al. [13]. There is still an ongoing debate as to whether the cut-off levels should be set at <50 nmol/L or <75 nmol/L [17,18]. In addition, vitamin D sufficiency was defined by measurements of baseline 25$(OH)D_3$, which is currently the critical measurement for defining vitamin D status [19]. Some studies suggest that free 25$(OH)D_3$ could be a better marker for assessing vitamin D status [20]. In our study, calculated free 25$(OH)D_3$ did not predict Δ25(OH)D3 after supplementation better than baseline 25$(OH)D_3$. The RC.T. design and the successful vitamin D intervention are strengths of this study. Also, a high number of parameters were measured with gold-standard methods. In contrast to the majority of exploratory studies on the VMR, p-values of the correlations were adjusted for multiple testing.

In summary, we show that 25$(OH)D_3$, 24,25$(OH)_2D_3$ and the VMR increase after vitamin D treatment. However, 24,25$(OH)_2D_3$ and the VMR could not predict 25$(OH)D_3$ levels after vitamin

D treatment in this cohort better than baseline 25(OH)D_3. As this has been corroborated by other studies, it implicates the routine measurement of 24,25$(OH)_2D_3$ will probably be of no added value when personalizing the treatment dosage of vitamin D.

Author Contributions: Conceptualization, V.F., S.R.U., B.O.P., A.C.H.; methodology, N.F.D.; software, V.F., S.R.U., S.P., A.C.H., B.O.P., W.M., A.T.; validation, A.C.H., B.O.P.; formal analysis, V.F. and S.R.U..; investigation, M.H.K., V.T., C.T., M.P., V.B., M.R.G., N.D.V.; resources, S.P., A.C.H., B.O.P.; data curation, S.P., A.C.H., B.O.P.; writing—original draft preparation, V.F., S.R.U..; writing—review and editing, V.F., S.R.U., S.P., B.O.P., A.C.H., N.F.D.; visualization, V.F., S.R.U.; supervision, S.P., B.O.P., A.C.H.; project administration, S.P., A.C.H., B.O.P.; funding acquisition, n.a.

Acknowledgments: The authors thank all study participants and also Fresenius Kabi for providing the study medication.

Appendix A

Table A1. Pearson correlations of baseline vitamin-D-related parameters adjusted for gender, age, BMI, PTH, eGFR, serum phosphate and serum calcium, with the changes from baseline of 25(OH)D, 1,25$(OH)_2$D and 24,25$(OH)_2$D after vitamin D supplementation. *p*-values without and with Bonferroni adjustment are shown.

Baseline Parameters		Δ25(OH)D_3	Δ1,25$(OH)_2$D	Δ24,25$(OH)_2D_3$
25(OH)D_3	r	−0.508	−0.277	−0.657
	p-value	0.013	0.201	0.001
	Adjusted *p*-value	0.104	1.000	0.008
1,25$(OH)_2$D	r	−0.350	−0.171	−0.430
	p-value	0.102	0.435	0.040
	Adjusted *p*-value	0.816	1.000	0.320
24,25$(OH)_2D_3$	r	−0.490	−0.129	−0.597
	p-value	0.018	0.559	0.003
	Adjusted *p*-value	0.440	1.000	0.096
VMR	r	−0.064	0.137	−0.516
	p-value	0.773	0.534	0.012
	Adjusted *p*-value	1.000	1.000	0.096
Calculated free 25(OH)D_3 *	r	−0.451	−0.363	−0.399
	p-value	0.031	0.089	0.059
	Adjusted *p*-value	0.248	0.712	0.472
Calculated bioavailable 25(OH)D_3 *	r	−0.451	−0.363	−0.404
	p-value	0.031	0.089	0.056
	Adjusted *p*-value	0.248	0.712	0.448
1,25$(OH)_2$D/25(OH)D_3 *	r	0.122	0.272	0.218
	p-value	0.578	0.209	0.318
	Adjusted *p*-value	1.000	1.000	1.000
1,25$(OH)_2$D /24,25$(OH)_2D_3$ *	r	0.126	0.136	0.211
	p-value	0.565	0.536	0.333
	Adjusted *p*-value	1.000	1.000	1.000

* Log-transformed parameters.

References

1. Bergwitz, C.; Jüppner, H. Regulation of Phosphate Homeostasis by PTH, Vitamin D, and FGF23. *Annu. Rev. Med.* **2010**, *61*, 91–104. [CrossRef] [PubMed]
2. Tuckey, R.C.; Cheng, C.Y.S.; Slominski, A.T. The Serum Vitamin D Metabolome: What We Know and What is Still to Discover. *J. Steroid Biochem. Mol. Biol.* **2019**, *186*, 4–21. [CrossRef] [PubMed]
3. Prietl, B.; Treiber, G.; Pieber, T.R.; Amrein, K. Vitamin D and immune function. *Nutrients* **2013**, *5*, 2502–2521. [CrossRef] [PubMed]

4. Jones, G.; Strugnell, S.A.; DeLuca, H.F. Current Understanding of the Molecular Actions of Vitamin D. *Physiol. Rev.* **1998**, *78*, 1193–1231. [CrossRef] [PubMed]
5. Dirks, N.; Ackermans, M.; Lips, P.; de Jongh, R.; Vervloet, M.; de Jonge, R.; Heijboer, A. The When, What & How of Measuring Vitamin D Metabolism in Clinical Medicine. *Nutrients* **2018**, *10*, 482.
6. Aloia, J.; Fazzari, M.; Shieh, A.; Dhaliwal, R.; Mikhail, M.; Hoofnagle, A.N.; Ragolia, L. The vitamin D metabolite ratio (VMR) as a predictor of functional biomarkers of bone health. *Clin. Endocrinol. (Oxf.)* **2017**, *86*, 674–679. [CrossRef] [PubMed]
7. Ginsberg, C.; Katz, R.; de Boer, I.H.; Kestenbaum, B.R.; Chonchol, M.; Shlipak, M.G.; Sarnak, M.J.; Hoofnagle, A.N.; Rifkin, D.E.; Garimella, P.S.; et al. The 24,25 to 25-hydroxyvitamin D Ratio and Fracture Risk in Older Adults: The Cardiovascular Health Study. *Bone* **2018**, *107*, 124–130. [CrossRef] [PubMed]
8. Wagner, D.; Hanwell, H.E.; Schnabl, K.; Yazdanpanah, M.; Kimball, S.; Fu, L.; Sidhom, G.; Rousseau, D.; Cole, D.E.C.; Vieth, R. The Ratio of Serum 24,25-dihydroxyvitamin D3 to 25-hydroxyvitamin D3 is Predictive of 25-hydroxyvitamin D3 Response to Vitamin D3 Supplementation. *J. Steroid Biochem. Mol. Biol.* **2011**, *126*, 72–77. [CrossRef] [PubMed]
9. Cashman, K.D.; Hayes, A.; Galvin, K.; Merkel, J.; Jones, G.; Kaufmann, M.; Hoofnagle, A.N.; Carter, G.D.; Durazo-Arvizu, R.A.; Sempos, C.T. Significance of Serum 24,25-Dihydroxyvitamin D in the Assessment of Vitamin D Status: A Double-edged Sword? *Clin. Chem.* **2015**, *61*, 636–645. [CrossRef] [PubMed]
10. Binkley, N.; Borchardt, G.; Siglinsky, E.; Krueger, D. Does Vitamin D Metabolite Measurement Help Predict 25(OH)D Change Following Vitamin D Supplementation? *Endocr. Pract.* **2017**, *23*, 432–441. [CrossRef] [PubMed]
11. Saleh, L.; Tang, J.; Gawinecka, J.; Boesch, L.; Fraser, W.D.; von Eckardstein, A.; Nowak, A. Impact of a Single Oral Dose of 100,000 IU Vitamin D3 on Profiles of Serum 25(OH)D3 and its Metabolites 24,25(OH)2D3, 3-epi-25(OH)D3, and 1,25(OH)2D3 in Adults with Vitamin D Insufficiency. *Clin. Chem. Lab. Med.* **2017**, *55*, 1912–1921. [CrossRef] [PubMed]
12. Mazahery, H.; von Hurst, P. Factors Affecting 25-Hydroxyvitamin D Concentration in Response to Vitamin D Supplementation. *Nutrients* **2015**, *7*, 5111–5142. [CrossRef] [PubMed]
13. Pilz, S.; Gaksch, M.; Kienreich, K.; Grübler, M.; Verheyen, N.; Fahrleitner-Pammer, A.; Treiber, G.; Drechsler, C.; Hartaigh, B.Ó.; Obermayer-Pietsch, B.; et al. Effects of Vitamin D on Blood Pressure and Cardiovascular Risk Factors. *Hypertension* **2015**, *65*, 1195–1201. [CrossRef] [PubMed]
14. Dirks, N.F.; Ackermans, M.T.; de Jonge, R.; Heijboer, A.C. Reference Values for 24,25-dihydroxyvitamin D and the 25-hydroxyvitamin D/24,25-dihydroxyvitamin D Ratio. *Clin. Chem. Lab. Med.* **2019**, *25*, 24–26. [CrossRef] [PubMed]
15. Powe, C.E.; Ricciardi, C.; Berg, A.H.; Erdenesanaa, D.; Collerone, G.; Ankers, E.; Wenger, J.; Karumanchi, S.A.; Thadhani, R.; Bhan, I. Vitamin D-binding protein modifies the vitamin D-bone mineral density relationship. *J. Bone Miner. Res.* **2011**, *26*, 1609–1616. [CrossRef] [PubMed]
16. Tang, J.C.Y.; Jackson, S.; Walsh, N.P.; Greeves, J.; Fraser, W.D. Bioanalytical Facility team The Dynamic Relationships Between the Active and Catabolic Vitamin D Metabolites, their ratios, and Associations with PTH. *Sci. Rep.* **2019**, *9*, 6974. [CrossRef] [PubMed]
17. Pilz, S.; Zittermann, A.; Trummer, C.; Theiler-Schwetz, V.; Lerchbaum, E.; Keppel, M.H.; Grübler, M.R.; März, W.; Pandis, M. Vitamin D testing and treatment: A narrative review of current evidence. *Endocr. Connect.* **2019**, *8*, R27–R43. [CrossRef] [PubMed]
18. Holick, M.F. Vitamin D Deficiency. *N. Engl. J. Med.* **2007**, *357*, 266–281. [CrossRef] [PubMed]
19. Sempos, C.T.; Heijboer, A.C.; Bikle, D.D.; Bollerslev, J.; Bouillon, R.; Brannon, P.M.; DeLuca, H.F.; Jones, G.; Munns, C.F.; Bilezikian, J.P.; et al. Vitamin D assays and the definition of hypovitaminosis D: Results from the First International Conference on Controversies in Vitamin D. *Br. J. Clin. Pharmacol.* **2018**, *84*, 2194–2207. [CrossRef] [PubMed]
20. Tsuprykov, O.; Chen, X.; Hocher, C.-F.; Skoblo, R.; Yin, L.; Hocher, B. Why should we measure free 25(OH) vitamin D? *J. Steroid Biochem. Mol. Biol.* **2018**, *180*, 87–104. [CrossRef] [PubMed]

6

Correlation between Fecal Calprotectin Levels in Meconium and Vitamin D Levels in Cord Blood: Association with Intestinal Distress

Jae Hoon Jung [1,2] and Sook Hyun Park [1,2,*]

1 Department of Pediatrics, School of Medicine, Kyunpook National University, Daegu 41404, Korea; wogns7602@gmail.com
2 Division of Neonatology, Kyunpook National University Chilgok Hospital, Daegu 41404, Korea
* Correspondence: park_sh@knu.ac.kr

Abstract: We aimed to investigate the correlation between vitamin D status in cord blood and fecal calprotectin concentrations in meconium, and also find their association with intestinal distress symptoms during the first two weeks of life. Two hundred and twenty-eight newborns were enrolled in the study who were delivered at Kyungpook National University Children's Hospital between July 2016 and August 2017. The first passed meconium samples were collected for fecal calprotectin analysis. Intestinal distress involved infants with necrotizing enterocolitis (NEC) and other feeding interruption signs. The median gestational age of the population was 37.0 (34.3–38.4) weeks, and the median birth weight was 2635 (2100–3268) g. The median fecal calprotectin levels in meconium were 134.1 (55.6–403.2) μg/g (range: 11.5–2000 μg/g) and the median 25-hydroxyvitamin D (25-OHD) concentrations in cord blood were 21.0 (15.5–28.8) ng/mL. Sixty infants (26.3%) had intestinal distress, including four patients (1.8%) diagnosed as having NEC. Higher fecal calprotectin concentrations (398.2 (131.8–900.2) μg/g vs. 105.6 (39.4–248.5) μg/g, $p < 0.001$) and lower 25-OHD levels (17.9 (12.8–22.1) ng/mL vs. 23.2 (17.2–33.0) ng/mL, $p < 0.001$) were found in infants with intestinal distress compared to infants without intestinal distress. The cut-off value was set at 359.8 μg/g with a sensitivity of 0.53 and a specificity of 0.82 for the development of intestinal distress in the first two weeks of life. Serum 25-OHD levels in cord blood were inversely correlated with fecal calprotectin concentrations in meconium.

Keywords: vitamin D; calprotectin; necrotizing enterocolitis

---

1. Introduction

Vitamin D is a major regulator of immune function and inflammation and has modulatory effects on the cells of the adaptive and innate immune system. Vitamin D provided biological effects through vitamin D receptors expressed in the kidney, colonic mucosa, and immune cells [1–3]. Vitamin D modulates innate immunity by regulating antimicrobial peptides, which have functions including microbiocidal activity and chemotaxis of inflammatory immune cells [4,5]. Consequently, vitamin D deficiency can result in a pro-inflammatory state and increase susceptibility to intestinal infections [6]. Vitamin D deficiency in the gastrointestinal tract has been presumed to decrease colonic bacterial clearance and lead to expressions of tight junctions in the intestinal epithelium and elevated Th1-mediated inflammation [7–9]. Vitamin D levels have been reported to be associated with severity and the activity of inflammatory bowel disease in adolescents and adults [10]. In infants, maternal 25-hydroxyvitamin D (25-OHD) levels have been associated with necrotizing enterocolitis (NEC) development [11].

Fecal calprotectin is derived mainly from activated neutrophils that have migrated through the gastrointestinal mucosa [12,13]. Migration and accumulation in transepithelial neutrophil at the mucosal surface and within the intestinal lumen are a hallmark of digestive inflammatory pathology [14]. Studies have reported that increased fecal calprotectin levels are correlated with an increased turnover of leukocytes in the intestinal epithelial cells and granulocyte migration toward intestinal lumen [12,15]. It has been previously investigated as a biomarker of mucosal inflammation in various conditions such as NEC, inflammatory bowel disease, and intestinal ischemia-reperfusion [16–21]. Recently, fecal calprotectin levels have been reported to predict cow's milk protein allergy and atopic disease [22,23]. Increased calprotectin levels have also been observed in cases of intolerance to enteral feeding [24].

Under the hypothesis that fecal calprotectin in meconium may reflect the inflammatory status in fetal intestines, the present study aimed to investigate the correlation between vitamin D levels in cord blood and fecal calprotectin concentrations in meconium and also explore its association and intestinal distress symptoms during the first two weeks of life.

2. Materials and Methods

2.1. Study Population and Ethics

The study group enrolled 228 infants who were delivered at Kyungpook National University Children's Hospital between July 2016 and August 2017. Only patients who had results of 25-hydroxyvitamin D (25-OHD) levels through cord blood or at birth were included. The first stool after birth was collected for fecal calprotectin analysis in the meconium. The study excluded patients with any chromosomal or major congenital anomalies. The current study was approved by the Institutional Review Board of Kyungpook National University Chilgok Hospital and was given a waiver of informed consent (2017-03-023).

2.2. Maternal and Neonatal Demographic Data

Maternal and neonatal demographic data were collected through medical record reviews. The maternal demographic features that were recorded included maternal age, premature rupture of membranes (PROM), diabetes, and pregnancy-induced hypertension (PIH). They also included maternal use of antibiotics and steroids for one week before delivery. Neonatal clinical data included gestational age, birth weight, sex, delivery mode, Apgar score at 1 min and 5 min, and small-for-gestational age (SGA) which was defined as under the 10-percentile range for gestational age using the 2013 Fenton growth calculator for preterm infants [25].

2.3. Measurement of Fecal Calprotectin and 25-OHD in Cord Blood

All fecal samples were frozen and stored at −20 °C immediately after collection. Analysis took an average of two to three days. Fecal samples were measured for calprotectin concentration using the supernatant of a centrifuged solution from 0.2 g of stool that was used to evaluate the calprotectin level by ImmunoCap (Phadia 250, Phadia AB (Thermo Scientific), Uppsala, Sweden) after using a Fluorescence Enzyme Immunoassay (FEIA). The detected range of fecal calprotectin concentrations was 11.5–2000 µg/g. The serum 25-OHD levels were measured using radioimmunoassay (DIAsource 25OH-Vit.D3-Ria-CT kit, DIAsource Immuno-Assays S.A., Louvain-la-Neuve, Belgium).

2.4. Definition of Intestinal Distress

In the present study, intestinal distress involved NEC and other feeding interruption signs during the first two weeks of postnatal age. NEC was classified according to the modified Bell's classification [26]. Other feeding interruption signs included infants with one or more episodes of increased gastric residuals (>50%) of previous feeding volume, vomiting, bloody stool, diarrhea, abdominal distension (increased abdominal circumstance > 2 cm), and visible bowel loops on physical examination. Intestinal distress was determined by one neonatologist or two pediatric residents.

2.5. *Statistical Analysis*

Statistical analysis was performed using IBM SPSS Statistics 26.0 software (IBM Corp., Armonk, NY, USA). The Shapiro–Wilk test was applied to check normal distribution between two groups, and the skewness and kurtosis of each variable were studied to test normal distribution. Fecal calprotectin by demographic and clinical factors was compared using the Mann–Whitney test or the chi-square test according to continuous or categorical variables. The Spearman's rank correlation coefficient was used to analyze the correlation between fecal calprotectin concentrations and 25-OHD levels. The analysis of potential confounding factors affecting intestinal distress were performed using logistic regression. The cut-off value for fecal calprotectin in the prediction of intestinal distress was determined using the receiver operating characteristics curve analysis. Statistical significance was defined as p value < 0.05.

3. Results

3.1. *Demographic and Clinical Features of the Study Population*

Demographic and clinical characteristics of patients are shown in Table 1. The median gestational age of the population was 37.0 (34.3–38.4) weeks, and the median birth weight was 2635 (2100–3268) g. The median fecal calprotectin levels in meconium were 134.1 (55.6–403.15) µg/g (range: 11.5–2000 µg/g) and the median 25-OHD concentrations in cord blood were 21.0 (15.5–28.8) ng/mL. Sixty infants (26.3%) had intestinal distress, including four patients (1.8%) who were diagnosed as having NEC. The number of infants with maternal medical history of antibiotics and steroid use was 40 (17.5%), and 31 (13.6%), respectively.

Table 1. Demographic and clinical characteristics of the population.

Variable	Median (IQR) or n (%)
Male sex	118 (51.8)
Gestational age (wks)	37.0 (34.3–38.4)
Birth weight (g)	2635 (2100–3268)
SGA	22 (9.6)
Delivery mode	
Vaginal delivery	68 (29.8)
Cesarean section	160 (70.2)
Maternal features	
Age	33.0 (30.0–36.0)
PROM	35 (14.8)
PIH or Preeclampsia	24 (10.5)
Diabetes	24 (10.5)
Antibiotics	40 (17.5)
Steroid	31 (13.6)
Neonatal features	
Apgar score at 1 min	7.0 (7.0–8.0)
Apgar score at 5 min	9.0 (8.0–9.0)
Intestinal distress	60 (26.3)
NEC	4 (1.8)
25-OHD (ng/mL)	21.0 (15.5–28.8)
Calprotectin (µg/g)	134.1 (55.6–403.2)

Data reported as frequency n (%) or median (IQR). Abbreviations: SGA, small-for-gestational age; PROM, premature rupture of membranes; PIH, pregnancy-induced hypertension; NEC, necrotizing enterocolitis, 25-OHD, 25-hydroxyvitamin D.

3.2. *Fecal Calprotectin Concentrations by Maternal and Neonatal Factors*

Table 2 shows the comparison of fecal calprotectin concentrations by maternal factors. The median fecal calprotectin of infants with maternal PROM (148.1 (62.1–416.6) µg/g) was higher than that of infants without maternal PROM (86.0 (24.9–170.3)) µg/g, $p = 0.039$). There were no statistical differences of fecal calprotectin by maternal PIH or preeclampsia, diabetes, and maternal use of antibiotics and steroid. There were also no significant differences in the median value of fecal calprotectin by sex, prematurity, SGA, or delivery mode (Table 3).

Table 2. Differences of fecal calprotectin concentrations in meconium by maternal factors.

Factors		*n*	FC (μg/g)	*p*-Value
Diabetes	Yes	24	248.6 (84.0–524.0)	0.125
	No	204	126.8 (53.0–403.2)	
PROM	Yes	35	148.1 (62.1–416.6)	0.039
	No	193	86.0 (24.9–170.3)	
PIH or preeclampsia	Yes	24	177.8 (62.3–356.5)	0.739
	No	204	131.7 (55.6–414.3)	
Use of antibiotics	Yes	40	105.8 (49.4–458.3)	0.634
	No	188	134.1 (56.7–369.6)	
Use of steroid	Yes	31	105.8 (68.9–318.9)	0.975
	No	197	136.3 (53.1–416.6)	

Data reported as frequency median (IQR). Abbreviations: FC, fecal calprotectin; PROM, premature rupture of membranes; PIH, pregnancy induced hypertension.

Table 3. Differences of fecal calprotectin concentrations in meconium by neonatal factors.

Factors	*n*	FC (μg/g)	*p*-Value
Sex			
Female	110	122.4 (53.3–364.5)	0.455
Male	118	148.1 (61.5–420.8)	
Gestational age			
Preterm	111	134.4 (61.8–437.2)	0.639
Full-term	117	133.8 (52.8–301.5)	
Fetal growth			
SGA	22	92.3 (22.5–191.3)	0.086
AGA	206	137.2 (61.5–415.8)	
Delivery mode			
Vaginal delivery	68	141.4 (77.6–397.4)	0.420
Cesarean section	160	123.7 (52.9–403.2)	

Data reported as frequency median (IQR). Abbreviations: FC, fecal calprotectin; SGA, small-for-gestational age; AGA, appropriate-for-gestational age.

3.3. *Correlation between Fecal Calprotectin Concentrations and 25-OHD Levels*

Fecal calprotectin levels in meconium were not correlated with gestational age ($\rho = -0.080$, $p = 0.232$) and birth weight ($\rho = -0.020$, $p = 0.769$). Apgar scores at 1 min ($\rho = 0.096$, $p = 0.161$) and 5 min ($\rho = 0.116$, $p = 0.090$) were not correlated with fecal calprotectin levels in meconium. Results also indicate that fecal calprotectin concentrations were significantly correlated with 25-OHD levels ($\rho = -0.352$, $p < 0.001$, Figure 1).

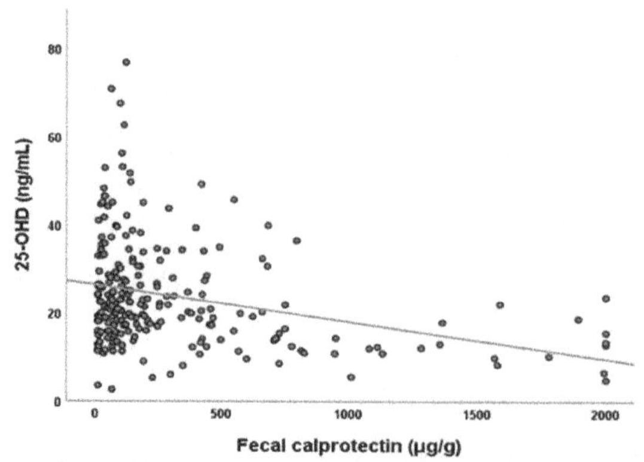

Figure 1. Correlation between 25-hydroxyvitamin D (25-OHD) levels in cord blood and fecal calprotectin concentration of meconium.

3.4. *Association between Intestinal Distress and Fecal Calprotectin Concentrations*

Infants with intestinal distress had lower gestational age and lower birth weight, and older maternal age (Table 4). Higher fecal calprotectin concentrations (398.2 (131.8–900.2) μg/g vs. 105.6 (39.4–248.5) μg/g, $p < 0.001$) and lower 25-OHD levels (17.9 (12.8–22.1) ng/mL vs. 23.2 (17.2–33.0) ng/mL, $p < 0.001$) were found in infants with intestinal distress compared to infants without intestinal distress. The fecal calprotectin concentrations of the two infants diagnosed as having NEC stage III were 32.3 μg/g and 86.0 μg/g, respectively, and the two infants with NEC stage IIb were 180.3 μg/g and 169.5 μg/g, respectively. The 25-OHD levels of the two infants diagnosed as having NEC stage III were 13.77 ng/mL and 13.37 ng/mL, respectively, and the two infants with NEC stage IIb were 21.85 ng/mL and 30.63 ng/mL, respectively.

Table 4. Demographic and clinical characteristics of patients with intestinal distress.

Variable	ID (n = 60)	Non-ID (n = 168)	p-Value
Male sex	32 (53.3)	86 (51.2)	0.880
Gestational age (weeks)	34.5 (32.1–37.1)	37.4 (35.1–38.7)	<0.001
Birth weight (g)	2185 (1663–2683)	2805 (2238–3373)	<0.001
SGA	4 (6.7)	18 (10.7)	0.452
Cesarean section	46 (76.7)	114 (67.9)	0.250
Maternal features			
Age	34.0 (30.0–37.0)	32.0 (29.0–35.0)	0.034
PROM	11 (18.3)	24 (14.3)	0.531
PIH or preeclampsia	8 (13.3)	16 (9.5)	0.463
Diabetes	9 (15.0)	15 (8.9)	0.221
Antibiotics	16 (26.6)	24 (14.3)	0.263
Steroid	12 (20.0)	19 (11.3)	0.123
Neonatal features			
Apgar score at 1 min	7.0 (6.0–8.0)	7.0 (7.0–8.0)	0.327
Apgar score at 5 min	9.0 (8.0–9.0)	9.0 (8.0–9.0)	0.663
25-OHD (ng/mL)	17.9 (12.8–22.1)	23.2 (17.2–33.0)	<0.001
Calprotectin (μg/g)	398.2 (131.8–900.2)	105.6 (39.4–248.5)	<0.001

Data reported as frequency n (%) or median (IQR). Abbreviations: ID, intestinal distress; SGA, small-for-gestational age; PROM, premature rupture of membranes; PIH, pregnancy induced hypertension; NEC, necrotizing enterocolitis; 25-OHD, 25-hydroxyvitamin D.

After adjusting confounding factors, intestinal distress was associated with lower gestational age, older maternal age, maternal PIH, and lower Apgar score (Table 5). Lower 25-OHD levels (odds ratio (OR), 0.943; 95% confidence interval (CI), 0.897–0.991, p = 0.021) and higher calprotectin concentrations (OR, 1.003; 95% CI, 1.002–1.004, $p < 0.001$) were associated with an increased risk of intestinal distress.

Table 5. Logistic regression analysis of associated factors with intestinal distress.

Factors	Adjusted		
	Odds Ratio	95% CI	p-Value
Male sex	0.673	0.278–1.630	0.380
Gestational age (weeks)	0.675	0.471–0.968	0.032
Birth weight (g)	0.999	0.998–1.001	0.448
SGA	1.828	0.274–12.217	0.533
Cesarean section	0.558	0.199–1.565	0.267
Maternal features			
Age	1.164	1.049–1.292	0.004
PROM	1.541	0.389–6.097	0.538
PIH or preeclampsia	5.240	1.204–22.803	0.027
Diabetes	1.801	0.471–6.882	0.390
Antibiotics	3.649	0.577–23.098	0.169
Steroid	1.515	0.388–5.910	0.550

Table 5. *Cont.*

Factors	Adjusted		
	Odds Ratio	95% CI	*p*-Value
Neonatal features			
Apgar score at 1 min	0.517	0.271–0.986	0.045
Apgar score at 5 min	0.344	0.125–0.951	0.040
25-OHD (ng/mL)	0.943	0.897–0.991	0.021
Calprotectin (μg/g)	1.003	1.002–1.004	<0.001

Abbreviations: CI, Confidence interval; ID, intestinal distress; SGA, small-for-gestational age; PROM, premature rupture of membranes; PIH, pregnancy induced hypertension; NEC, necrotizing enterocolitis; 25-OHD, 25-hydroxyvitamin D.

The cut-off value was set at 359.8 μg/g with a sensitivity of 0.53 and a specificity of 0.82 for the development of intestinal distress in the first two weeks of life. The area under the curve value was 0.738 ($p < 0.001$, 95% CI: 0.661–0.815) (Figure 2).

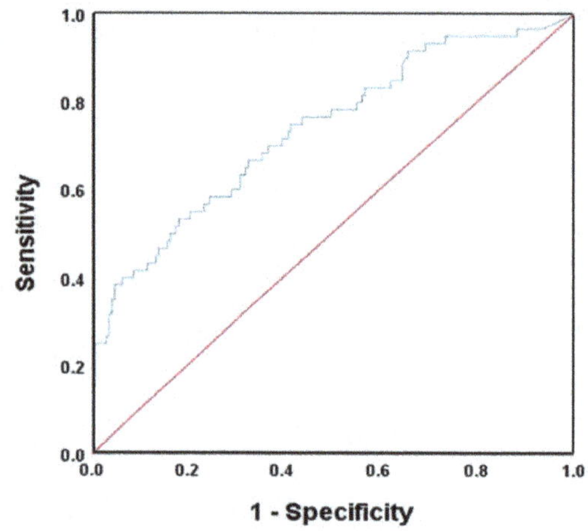

Figure 2. Receiver operating characteristics curves identifying infants with intestinal distress.

4. Discussion

In the present study, median fecal calprotectin levels in meconium were 134.1 (55.6–403.2) μg/g. Fecal calprotectin concentrations in meconium were inversely correlated with 25-OHD levels of cord blood. After adjusting for confounding factors, it was found that intestinal distress was associated with lower gestational age, older maternal age, maternal preeclampsia, lower Apgar score, lower 25-OHD levels, and higher fecal calprotectin levels.

In a previous study, it was shown that fecal calprotectin concentrations in meconium were significantly correlated with birth weight, gestational age, and Apgar score at 5 min [27]. It is thought that prematurity could be associated with immature intestinal mucosa that could induce the transepithelial migration of neutrophil granulocytes or macrophages into the lumen [27]. However, another study similar to the present study showed no statistically significant correlation between fecal calprotectin levels and birth weight, gestational age, or intrauterine growth [28]. This suggests that there might be other factors, aside from prematurity, that may be involved, such as ischemic condition and inflammation determining fecal calprotectin concentrations.

Maternal factors associated with placenta-related oxidative stress can induce endothelial cell injury; this is aggravated in the case of infants having increased mucosal inflammation [29]. It results in a high level of calprotectin in infants with maternal preeclampsia [21]. Under conditions of perinatal asphyxia, high levels of calprotectin in meconium were also found and indicate that ischemic damage to the intestinal mucosa may facilitate the passage of neutrophils [27]. In the present study, Apgar scores at 1 min and 5 min were not correlated with fecal calprotectin levels in meconium, but they were with intestinal distress. Infants with maternal inflammatory conditions, including maternal PROM, had higher fecal calprotectin levels compared to infants without maternal PROM. However, maternal preeclampsia was not correlated with fecal calprotectin levels but, rather, it was associated with intestinal distress.

Vitamin D promotes synthesis of the anti-inflammatory cytokines and inhibits the synthesis of pro-inflammatory cytokines [6]. Active vitamin D is used to increase tight junction proteins, which helps to protect the intestinal mucosal barrier [6,30]. Vitamin D receptor knockout mice have a tendency to cause infection, cancer, and inflammation [31]. Expression and localization of tight junction proteins are inhibited during inflammation, causing intestinal permeability and bacterial translocation [32,33]. Thus, the immature immune system, weak gastrointestinal mucosal barrier, and the abnormal colonization of the intestine predispose it to intestinal necrosis caused by progressive inflammation and bacterial invasion [34,35]. Increasing gut permeability and active immune response promotes transepithelial migration of neutrophils, which induces high fecal calprotectin in intestinal lumen [28]. Vitamin D may play a vital role as an immunomodulator in processing the regulation of migration and accumulation of fecal calprotectin.

The fecal calprotectin concentrations of infants diagnosed as having NEC stage III were reported as 32.3 μg/g, and 86.0 μg/g, respectively. The results were relatively lower than the median value of all infants in the study group, as well as those of infants with intestinal distress. The association between significantly low meconium calprotectin concentrations and developed fulminant NEC in preterm infants was also previously reported [36]. It can therefore be understood that under extremely severe inflammatory conditions, the impaired function of granulocytes in the intestinal lumen causes the decreased migration and release of calprotectin [36]. In the present study, the cut-off value of 359.8 μg/g with a sensitivity of 0.53 and a specificity of 0.82 indicated the development of intestinal distress in the first two weeks of life. This result represents similar fecal calprotectin levels and lower sensitivity than a previous study which had a cut-off value of 363 μg/g with a sensitivity of 0.65 and a specificity of 0.82 set for mild digestive symptoms [37]. Higher gestational age and strict criteria for intestinal distress may lead to the representation of a relatively high proportion of infants with mild distress signs.

To the best of our knowledge, the present study is the first of its kind to present a significant correlation between vitamin D and calprotectin in newborns, which suggests that the role of vitamin D functions as an immune modulator with anti-inflammatory effects. When considered in connection with a previous study found to have low maternal vitamin D levels in NEC infants [11], it is thought that maintaining adequate vitamin D levels during pregnancy may affect intestinal conditions in the early neonatal period. Abnormal intestinal colonization and an undeveloped balance of immune system response may cause feeding intolerance in the early postnatal period [38], which is also a known association with the migration of high fecal calprotectin into the gut lumen. The present study found that fecal calprotectin was significantly higher in infants with intestinal distress signs. Through these results, fecal calprotectin in meconium can be considered to be a predictive factor of feeding intolerance and also of inflammatory changes of the intestine which can cause feeding interruption. In inflammatory bowel disease patients, it remains unclear whether vitamin D deficiency can lead to or result in severe disease activity. Nonetheless, fecal calprotectin in meconium can be used to find accurate correlations between fecal calprotectin and 25-OHD levels, as it is a component that is measured before disease progression.

The present study is observational, and we reviewed all participants belonging to the inclusion criteria, which may affect the disproportion of the study group. We analyzed the distribution of each variable and between groups to minimize statistical flaws. The distribution of fecal calprotectin in meconium was similar to that of a previous study [27]. However, the participants of the present study included more moderate-to-late preterm infants compared with extremely preterm infants, so the incidence of NEC was reported to be low. Therefore, it has a limited ability to evaluate the role of fecal calprotectin as a predictor of NEC. Considering previous reports found that fecal calprotectin tends to vary widely in the first month, the present study only investigated the correlation with intestinal distress in the early neonatal period. The present study suggests that fecal calprotectin in meconium can predict early intestinal distress but requires the further exploration of longitudinal changes according to the time of intestinal signs. The factors affecting fecal calprotectin in infants have not been thoroughly understood and different results have previously been reported on the correlation with gestational age, birth weight, hypoxic condition, and maternal diseases. Further research is necessary to investigate the association between maternal and neonatal demographics, and clinical factors, along with fecal calprotectin levels.

5. Conclusions

Infants with intestinal distress had higher fecal calprotectin levels compared with infants without intestinal distress. Serum 25-OHD levels in cord blood were inversely correlated with fecal calprotectin concentrations in meconium, which suggests maintaining appropriate vitamin D status during the fetal period may prevent intestinal distress after birth.

Author Contributions: Conceptualization, S.H.P.; methodology, S.H.P.; validation, S.H.P.; formal analysis, S.H.P.; investigation, S.H.P.; data curation, S.H.P.; writing—original draft preparation, J.H.J., and S.H.P.; writing—review and editing, J.H.J., and S.H.P.; visualization, S.H.P.; supervision, S.H.P.; project administration, S.H.P.; funding acquisition, S.H.P. All authors have read and agreed to the published version of the manuscript.

References

1. González-Molero, I.; Rojo-Martínez, G.; Morcillo, S.; Gutierrez, C.; Rubio, E.; Pérez-Valero, V.; Esteva, I.; de Adana, M.S.R.; Almaraz, M.C.; Olveira, G.; et al. Hypovitaminosis D and incidence of obesity: A prospective study. *Eur. J. Clin. Nutr.* **2013**, *67*, 680–682. [CrossRef] [PubMed]
2. Sloka, S.; Silva, C.; Wang, J.; Yong, V.W. Predominance of Th2 polarization by vitamin D through a STAT6-dependent mechanism. *J. Neuroinflamm.* **2011**, *8*, 56. [CrossRef] [PubMed]
3. Hossein-Nezhad, A.; Mirzaei, K.; Keshavarz, S.A.; Ansar, H.; Saboori, S.; Tootee, A. Evidences of dual role of vitamin D through cellular energy homeostasis and inflammation pathway in risk of cancer in obese subjects. *Minerva Med.* **2013**, *104*, 295–307. [PubMed]
4. Talsness, C.E.; Penders, J.; Jansen, E.H.J.M.; Damoiseaux, J.; Thijs, C.; Mommers, M. Influence of vitamin D on key bacterial taxa in infant microbiota in the KOALA Birth Cohort Study. *PLoS ONE* **2017**, *12*, e0188011. [CrossRef]
5. Schwalfenberg, G.K. A review of the critical role of vitamin D in the functioning of the immune system and the clinical implications of vitamin D deficiency. *Mol. Nutr. Food Res.* **2011**, *55*, 96–108. [CrossRef]
6. Limketkai, B.N.; Bechtold, M.L.; Nguyen, D.L. Vitamin D and the pathogenesis of inflammatory bowel disease. *Curr. Gastroenterol. Rep.* **2016**, *18*, 52. [CrossRef]
7. Lagishetty, V.; Misharin, A.V.; Liu, N.Q.; Lisse, T.S.; Chun, R.F.; Ouyang, Y.; McLachlan, S.M.; Adams, J.S.; Hewison, M. Vitamin D deficiency in mice impairs colonic antibacterial activity and predisposes to colitis. *Endocrinology* **2010**, *151*, 2423–2432. [CrossRef]
8. Del Pinto, R.; Pietropaoli, D.; Chandar, A.K.; Ferri, C.; Cominelli, F. Association between inflammatory bowel disease and vitamin D deficiency: A systematic review and meta-analysis. *Inflamm. Bowel. Dis.* **2015**, *21*, 2708–2717. [CrossRef]
9. Kong, J.; Zhang, Z.; Musch, M.W.; Ning, G.; Sun, J.; Hart, J.; Bissonnette, M.; Li, Y.C. Novel role of the vitamin D receptor in maintaining the integrity of the intestinal mucosal barrier. *Am. J. Physiol. Gastrointest Liver Physiol.* **2008**, *294*, 208–216. [CrossRef]
10. Garg, M.; Hendy, P.; Ding, J.N.; Shaw, S.; Hold, G.; Hart, A. The effect of vitamin D on intestinal inflammation and faecal microbiota in patients with ulcerative colitis. *J. Crohns Colitis* **2018**, *12*, 963–972. [CrossRef]
11. Cetinkaya, M.; Erener-Ercan, T.; Kalayci-Oral, T.; Babayiğit, A.; Cebeci, B.; Semerci, S.Y.; Buyukkale, G. Maternal/neonatal vitamin D deficiency: A new risk factor for necrotizing enterocolitis in preterm infants? *J. Perinatol.* **2017** *37*, 673–678. [CrossRef] [PubMed]

12. Berstad, A.; Arslan, G.; Folvik, G. Relationship between intestinal permeability and calprotectin concentration in gut lavage fluid. *Scand. J. Gastroenterol.* **2000**, *35*, 64–69. [PubMed]
13. Kristinsson, J.; Røseth, A.; Fagerhol, M.K.; Aadland, E.; Schjønsby, H.; Børmer, O.P.; Raknerud, N.; Nygaard, K. Fecal calprotectin concentration in patients with colorectal carcinoma. *Dis. Colon Rectum* **1998**, *41*, 316–321. [CrossRef]
14. Lee, Y.M.; Min, C.Y.; Choi, Y.J.; Jeong, S.J. Delivery and feeding mode affects fecal calprotectin levels in infants <7 months old. *Early Hum. Dev.* **2017**, *108*, 45–48.
15. Røseth, A.G.; Schmidt, P.N.; Fagerhol, M.K. Correlation between faecal excretion of indium-111-labelled granulocytes and calprotectin, a granulocyte marker protein, in patients with inflammatory bowel disease. *Scand. J. Gastroenterol.* **1999**, *34*, 50–54. [PubMed]
16. van Zoonen, A.G.J.F.; Hulzebos, C.V.; Kobold, A.C.M.; Kooi, E.M.W.; Bos, A.F.; Hulscher, J.B.F. Serial fecal calprotectin in the prediction of necrotizing enterocolitis in preterm neonates. *J. Pediatr. Surg.* **2019**, *54*, 455–459. [CrossRef]
17. D'Incà, R.; Dal Pont, E.; Di Leo, V.; Ferronato, A.; Fries, W.; Vettorato, M.G.; Martinez, D.; Sturniolo, G.C. Calprotectin and lactoferrin in the assessment of intestinal inflammation and organic disease. *Int. J. Colorectal Dis.* **2007**, *22*, 429–437. [CrossRef]
18. Fagerhol, M.K. Calprotectin, a faecal marker of organic gastrointestinal abnormality. *Lancet* **2000**, *356*, 1783–1784. [CrossRef]
19. Aydemir, O.; Aydemir, C.; Sarikabadayi, Y.U.; Canpolat, F.E.; Erdeve, O.; Biyikli, Z.; Dilmen, U. Fecal calprotectin levels are increased in infants with necrotizing enterocolitis. *J. Matern. Fetal Neonatal Med.* **2012**, *25*, 2237–2241. [CrossRef]
20. Yang, Q.; Smith, P.B.; Goldberg, R.N.; Cotton, C.M. Dynamic change of fecal calprotectin in very low birth weight infants during the first month of life. *Neonatology* **2008**, *94*, 267–271. [CrossRef]
21. Nakayuenyongsuk, W.; Christofferson, M.; Stevenson, D.K.; Sylvester, K.; Lee, H.C.; Park, K.T. Point-of-care fecal calprotectin monitoring in preterm infants at risk for necrotizing enterocolitis. *J. Pediatr.* **2018**, *196*, 98–103. [CrossRef] [PubMed]
22. Beşer, O.F.; Sancak, S.; Erkan, T.; Kutlu, T.; Cokuğraş, H.; Cokuğraş, F.Ç. Can fecal calprotectin level be used as a markers of inflammation in the diagnosis and follow-up of cow's milk protein allergy? *Allergy Asthma Immunol. Res.* **2014**, *6*, 33–38. [CrossRef] [PubMed]
23. Orivuori, L.; Mustonen, K.; de Goffau, M.C.; Hakala, S.; Paasela, M.; Roduit, C.; Dalphin, J.C.; Genuneit, J.; Lauener, R.; Riedler, J.; et al. High level of fecal calprotectin at age 2 months as a marker of intestinal inflammation predicts atopic dermatitis and asthma by age 6. *Clin. Exp. Allergy J.* **2015**, *45*, 928–939. [CrossRef] [PubMed]
24. Moussa, R.; Khashana, A.; Kamel, N.; Elsharqawy, S.E. Fecal calprotectin levels in preterm infants with and without feeding intolerance. *J. Pediatr.* **2016**, *92*, 486–492. [CrossRef]
25. Fenton, T.R.; Kim, J.H. A systematic review and meta-analysis to revise the Fenton growth chart for preterm infants. *BMC Pediatr.* **2013**, *13*, 59. [CrossRef]
26. Walsh, M.C.; Kliegman, R.M. Necrotizing enterocolitis: Treatment based on staging criteria. *Pediatr. Clin. N. Am.* **1986**, *33*, 179–201. [CrossRef]
27. Laforgia, N.; Baldassarre, M.E.; Pontrelli, G.; Indrio, F.; Altomare, M.A.; Di Bitonto, G.; Mautone, A. Calprotectin levels in meconium. *Acta Paediatr.* **2003**, *92*, 463–466. [CrossRef]
28. Rougé, C.; Butel, M.J.; Piloquet, H.; Ferraris, L.; Legrand, A.; Vodovar, M.; Voyer, M.; de la Cochetière, M.F.; Darmaun, D.; Rozé, J.C. Fecal calprotectin excretion in preterm infants during the neonatal period. *PLoS ONE* **2010**, *5*, e11083. [CrossRef]
29. de Souza Rugolo, L.M.S.; Bentlin, M.R.; Trindade, C.E.P. Preeclampsia: Effect on the fetus and newborn. *NeoReviews* **2011**, *12*, 198–206. [CrossRef]
30. Gregori, S.; Giarratana, N.; Smiroldo, S.; Uskokovic, M.; Adorini, L. A 1alpha, 25-dihydroxyvitamin D(3) analog enhances regulatory T-cells and arrests autoimmune diabetes in NOD mice. *Diabetes* **2002**, *51*, 1367–1374. [CrossRef]
31. Jin, D.; Wu, S.; Zhang, Y.G.; Lu, R.; Xia, Y.; Dong, H.; Sun, J. Lack of vitamin D receptor causes dysbiosis and changes the functions of the murine intestinal microbiome. *Clin. Ther.* **2015**, *37*, 996–1009. [CrossRef] [PubMed]

32. Anand, R.J.; Leaphart, C.L.; Mollen, K.P.; Hackam, D.J. The role of the intestinal barrier in the pathogenesis of necrotizing enterocolitis. *Shock* **2007**, *27*, 124–133. [CrossRef] [PubMed]
33. Torrazza, R.M.; Neu, J. The altered gut microbiome and necrotizing enterocolitis. *Clin. Perinatol.* **2013**, *40*, 93–108. [CrossRef] [PubMed]
34. Kastenberg, Z.J.; Sylvester, K.G. The surgical management of necrotizing enterocolitis. *Clin. Perinatol.* **2013**, *40*, 135–148. [CrossRef]
35. De Plaen, I.G. Inflammatory signaling in necrotizing enterocolitis. *Clin. Perinatol.* **2013**, *40*, 109–124. [CrossRef]
36. Zoppelli, L.; Güttel, C.; Bittrich, H.J.; Andrée, C.; Wirth, S.; Jenke, A. Fecal calprotectin concentrations in premature infants have a lower limit and show postnatal and gestational age dependence. *Neonatology* **2012**, *102*, 68–74. [CrossRef]
37. Campeotto, F.; Baldassarre, M.; Butel, M.J.; Viallon, V.; Nganzali, F.; Soulaines, P.; Kalach, N.; Lapillonne, A.; Laforgia, N.; Moriette, G.; et al. Fecal calprotectin: Cutoff values for identifying intestinal distress in preterm infants. *J. Pediatr. Gastroenterol. Nutr.* **2009**, *48*, 507–510.
38. Indrio, F.; Riezzo, G.; Cavallo, L.; Di Mauro, A.; Francavilla, R. Physiological basis of food intolerance in VLBW. *J. Matern. Fetal Neonatal Med.* **2011**, *24*, 64–66. [CrossRef]

7

The Impact of Sample Type on Vitamin D Quantification and Clinical Classification during Pregnancy

Soriah M. Harvey [1], Vanessa E. Murphy [1], Peter G. Gibson [2,3], Michael Clarke [4,5] and Megan E. Jensen [1,*]

1 Priority Research Centre Grow Up Well, Hunter Medical Research Institute, School of Medicine and Public Health, University of Newcastle, Callaghan, NSW 2305, Australia; soriah.harvey@uon.edu.au (S.M.H.); vanessa.murphy@newcastle.edu.au (V.E.M.)

2 Priority Research Centre for Healthy Lungs, University of Newcastle and Hunter Medical Research Institute, Callaghan, NSW 2305, Australia; peter.gibson@newcastle.edu.au

3 Department of Respiratory and Sleep Medicine, John Hunter Hospital, New Lambton Heights, NSW 2305, Australia

4 Metabolomics Australia, Centre for Microscopy, Characterisation and Analysis, The University of Western Australia, Perth, WA 6000, Australia; michael.clarke@uwa.edu.au

5 School of Molecular Sciences, The University of Western Australia, Perth, WA 6000, Australia

* Correspondence: megan.jensen@newcastle.edu.au

Abstract: Measurement of vitamin D status has significant use in clinical and research settings, including during pregnancy. We aimed to assess the agreement of total 25-hydroxyvitamin D (25(OH)D) concentration, and its three analytes (25-hydroxyvitamin D_3 (25(OH)D_3), 25-hydroxyvitamin D_2 (25(OH)D_2) and Epi-25-hydroxyvitamin D_3 (Epi-25(OH)D_3)), in plasma and serum samples collected during pregnancy, and to examine the proportion of women who change vitamin D status category based on sample type. Matching samples were collected from n = 114 non-fasting women between 12–25 weeks gestation in a clinical trial in Newcastle, Australia. Samples were analysed by liquid chromatography-tandem mass-spectrometry (LC-MS/MS) to quantify total 25(OH)D and its analytes and examined using Bland-Altman plots, Pearson correlation (r), intraclass correlation coefficient and Cohen's Kappa test. Serum total 25(OH)D ranged from 33.8–169.8 nmol/L and plasma ranged from 28.6–211.2 nmol/L. There was a significant difference for total 25(OH)D based on sample type (measurement bias 7.63 nmol/L for serum vs plasma (95% Confidence Interval (CI) 5.36, 9.90, $p \leq 0.001$). The mean difference between serum and plasma concentrations was statistically significant for 25(OH)D_3 (7.38 nmol/L; 95% CI 5.28, 9.48, $p \leq 0.001$) and Epi-25(OH)D_3 (0.39 nmol/L; 95% CI 0.14, 0.64, $p = 0.014$). Of 114 participants, 28% were classified as vitamin D deficient (<50 nmol/L) or insufficient (<75 nmol/L) based on plasma sample and 36% based on serum sample. Nineteen (16.7%) participants changed vitamin D status category based on sample type. 25-hydroxyvitamin D quantification using LC-MS/MS methodology differed significantly between serum and plasma, yielding a higher value in plasma; this influenced vitamin D status based on accepted cut-points, which may have implications in clinical and research settings.

Keywords: vitamin D; pregnancy; quantification; clinical; 25OHD; asthma; analytes; spectrophotometry; sample; plasma; serum; LC-MS/MS

---

1. Introduction

The circulating concentration of 25-hydroxyvitamin D (25(OH)D) is considered the accepted clinical biomarker of vitamin D status [1]. With increasing awareness of the importance of vitamin D for maintaining optimal health by healthcare professionals, researchers and the public, requests for vitamin D quantification in human samples has increased in recent years [2,3], therefore ensuring the accuracy of analyses is highly relevant and important.

Testing is most commonly conducted through measurement of 25(OH)D via assay and quantification of 25(OH)D is routinely outsourced to be completed in external laboratories for clinical and research requirements. Previous studies have examined vitamin D in serum vs. plasma in small sample sizes, using assay techniques, and found serum and plasma to be mostly agreeable [4–7], but with evidence that 25(OH)D concentration may be higher in heparinised plasma compared to serum or ethylenediamine tetraacetic acid (EDTA) plasma [5]. However, this methodology has significant limitations to the usefulness and interpretation of the results, as assays have high result variability due to issues with standardisation, precision and accuracy [8]. Unlike immunoassays or high-pressure liquid chromatography (HPLC) methods, liquid chromatography tandem mass spectrophotometry (LC-MS/MS) offers higher specificity of detection, lower matrix interferences and high detectability of molecules present in low concentrations. This method is considered the gold standard method for vitamin D analysis, with the capability to measure 25(OH)D_2, 25(OH)D_3, and Epi-25(OH)D_3 separately [9–13].

Four previous studies have compared sample type for 25(OH)D quantification using LC-MS/MS; however, the samples were collected from non-pregnant populations of small sample sizes. Zhang et al. ($n = 25$) and Abu Kassim et al. ($n = 10$) did not find a significant difference between EDTA plasma, heparin plasma and serum for 25(OH)D_2 and 25(OH)D_3 concentrations in healthy adults [14,15]. Differences between sample type for Epi-25(OH)D_3 or total 25(OH)D were not examined. Albarhani et al. examined the usefulness of diluted plasma for quantification of 25(OH)D_3 and Epi-25(OH)D_3 compared to serum in umbilical cord blood samples ($n = 20$), and although their findings demonstrated close agreement for 25(OH)D_3 in serum and plasma across two independent laboratories ($r = 0.983$) issues with analytical sensitivity in regards to limits of detection (LoD) for Epi-25(OH)D_3 quantification highlighted issues with the use of diluted plasma instead of serum in other analytes of vitamin D [16]; 25(OH)D_2 and total vitamin D were not reported. In a study of 13 healthy adults, Mena-Bravo et al. found that plasma and serum provided similar levels for 24,25(OH)D_3, 25(OH)D_3 and cholecalciferol (D_3), while significantly higher concentrations of 1,25(OH)D_3 were detected in plasma versus serum [17]. However, no study has compared quantification of vitamin D analytes in plasma and serum samples collected during pregnancy. Comparing these sample types is of benefit to the Vitamin D Standardisation Program (VDSP) that aims to promote 25(OH)D concentration measurements that are accurate (precise and true) and comparable over time, location and laboratory to improve clinical and public health practice world-wide [18].

It is noted that none of the previous studies examined comparability of total 25(OH)D serum and plasma concentrations, and no study has examined changes in clinical vitamin D status based on sample type during pregnancy. The effect of the sample type on resulting concentrations of 25(OH)D and its analytes during pregnancy needs to be identified clearly to ascertain the suitability of using serum and plasma interchangeably in clinical and research settings. Pregnancy is associated with various hormonal and physiological changes in the body, and with vitamin D also acting as a hormone, adaptive changes of vitamin D homeostasis and metabolite concentrations in pregnancy may have implications for the systemic circulation of total 25(OH)D and its analytes [19]. Vitamin D-Binding Protein levels increase drastically during pregnancy, and this can influence the concentration of free 25(OH)D as well as other analytes [20]. A 2019 study examined serum samples in pregnant ($n = 88$) and non-pregnant women ($n = 20$) and found differences in vitamin D metabolism across a range of analytes in pregnancy, as well as across gestation [21]. Whether there are important differences in vitamin D analyte concentrations, as well as clinical vitamin D status, based on sample type, is unknown.

The primary aim of this study was to investigate the comparability of vitamin D quantification using LC-MS/MS between serum and plasma samples collected during pregnancy in a large well-defined cohort of women enrolled in a clinical asthma trial. The secondary aim was to examine the proportion of women who change vitamin D category based on sample type.

2. Materials and Methods

Serum and plasma samples were collected from pregnant women who were enrolled in a clinical trial of asthma management during pregnancy, conducted in Newcastle, Australia. Details of the trial are previously described [22]. Briefly, women with current asthma, aged 18 years and older, were enrolled via antenatal clinics at the John Hunter Hospital in Newcastle, Australia. Written consent was obtained from participants before trial participation and ethics approval was granted by Hunter New England Health Human Research Ethics Committee (12/10/17/3.04, NSW HREC Reference No: HREC/12/HNE/357).

A non-fasting peripheral blood sample was collected by venepuncture (by a research nurse trained in phlebotomy) into a 6ml EDTA (1.8 mg/mL) plasma tube and 6mL plain serum tube at enrolment (between 12–25 weeks gestation), and processed within 60 min. All samples were centrifuged (3000 rpm) at 4 °C for ten minutes, aliquoted into Eppendorf tubes, and stored at −80 °C. All samples were collected between 2017–2019 and analysed in 2019. Samples were transported by courier on dry ice to the Centre for Microscopy, Characterisation & Analysis in Western Australia, for quantification of vitamin D via LC-MS/MS; this laboratory is certified by the Vitamin D Standardisation Program (VDSP) [18]. LC-MS/MS has been previously described [12]; briefly, samples were extracted using liquid-liquid extraction then separated using a 2D liquid chromatography UPLC system, followed by detection using tandem mass spectrometry. Total vitamin D was comprised of 25(OH)D_2, 25(OH)D_3 and Epi-25(OH)D_3. The LoD for both 25(OH)D_3 and Epi-25(OH)D_3 was 2.0 nmol/L, and 3.0 nmol/L for 25(OH)D_2. For blood samples with values below the LoD, a level equal to the detection limit was used, then divided by the square root of 2 (equal to 1.4 nmol/L for Epi-25(OH)D_3 and 2.12 nmol/L for 25(OH)D_2) [23]. Vitamin D sufficiency was defined as total 25OHD ≥75 nmol/L. Cut points for vitamin D insufficiency and deficiency were 50- <75 nmol/L and <50 nmol/L of total 25(OH)D, respectively [24].

Statistical Analysis

The Shapiro Wilks test was used to determine normality of the data. Bland-Altman plots were used to compare the difference between plasma and serum concentrations of total 25(OH)D, 25(OH)D_2, 25(OH)D_3, epi-25(OH)D_3 and detect proportional bias [25]. Pearson correlation (r) and intraclass correlation coefficient (ICC) was used to examine the agreement between the concentrations. The difference in mean values for total 25(OH)D, 25(OH)D_2, 25(OH)D_3 and Epi-25(OH)D_3 were examined using the paired t-test with 95% confidence intervals (CI). A p-value < 0.05 was considered statistically significant. The mean, range, standard deviation (SD) and coefficient of variation (CV) were reported for each analyte by sample type. The proportion of participants that were vitamin D sufficient, insufficient and deficient were determined based on sample type, as well as any participants that changed category based on the use of plasma compared to serum for total 25(OH)D quantification. Cohen's Kappa test was used to explore interrater reliability between participants vitamin D status and sample type. Statistics were computed with STATA IC v15.1 (StataCorp, College Station, TX, USA), and Microsoft Excel (v16.0.5083.1000, Microsoft Corporation, Santa Rosa, CA, USA).

3. Results

There were 114 matching serum and plasma samples. In total, 96.9% (221/228) samples were below the LoD for 25(OH)D_2 and 11.8% (27/228) samples were below the LoD for Epi-25(OH)D_3 (Table 1). The mean (±SD) for total 25(OH)D in serum was 86.77 ± 24.91 nmol/L (range 33.8–169.8 nmol/L). The mean for total 25(OH)D in plasma was 94.4 ± 28.8 nmol/L (range 28.6–211.2 nmol/L) (Table 1).

Table 1. Mean, range, standard deviation and coefficient of variation for $n = 114$ matched serum and plasma samples collected from pregnant women.

Total 25(OH)D	Minimum (nmol/L)	Maximum (nmol/L)	Mean (nmol/L)	SD (nmol/L)	CV%	*p*-Value *
PLASMA	28.60	211.2	94.40	28.80	30.51	
SERUM	33.80	169.8	86.77	24.91	28.71	<0.001
25(OH)D_3						
PLASMA	24.50	200.80	87.83	27.10	30.9	
SERUM	30.3	161.7	80.45	23.65	29.4	<0.001
25(OH)D_2 ‡						
PLASMA	<3.0	6.3	2.23	0.54	24.22	
SERUM	<3.0	4.5	2.15	0.24	11.16	0.112
Epi-25(OH)D_3 ‡						
PLASMA	<2.0	20.2	4.44	2.81	63.29	
SERUM	<2.0	16.8	4.05	2.28	56.30	0.003

* Paired *t*-test *p*-value comparing mean difference between serum and plasma for each analyte and total 25-hydroxyvitamin D (25(OH). Dusing liquid chromatography-tandem mass-spectrometry. Minimum, maximum, mean and SD are expressed in nmol/L. CV, coefficient of variation, expressed as percentage. SD, standard deviation. ‡: 96.9% of 25-hydroxyvitamin D_2 (25(OH)D_2) and 11.8% of Epi-25-hydroxyvitamin D_3 (25(OH)D_3) results were below the LoD's and therefore imputed values were used.

Figure 1 illustrates the agreement between plasma and serum concentrations of total 25(OH)D ($r^2 = 0.903$), 25(OH)D_3 ($r^2 = 0.910$) and Epi-25(OH)D_3 ($r^2 = 0.862$); correlation analyses were not conducted for 25OHD_2 given the high percentage of samples below the LoD.

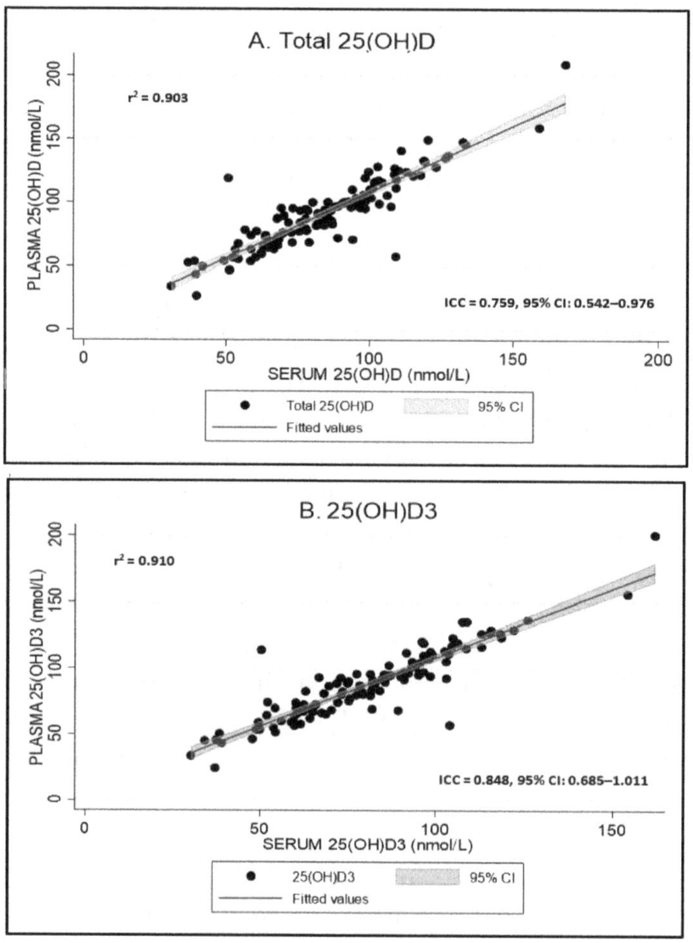

Figure 1. *Cont.*

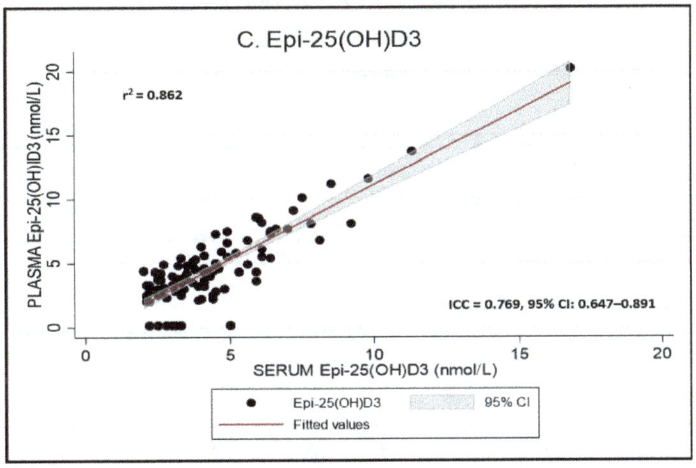

Figure 1. 25(OH)D: 25-hydroxyvitamin D. (**A–C**) Scatter plot with Pearson (r^2) and intraclass correlation coefficients (ICC) between serum and plasma concentrations of vitamin D analogues, quantified using LC-MS/MS. (**A**) Total 25(OH)D, (**B**) 25(OH)D_3 and (**C**): Epi-25(OH)D_3. 95% CI, 95% confidence interval. All results expressed as nmol/L.

The Bland-Altman plot shows a mean total concentration bias for serum vs. plasma of 7.63 mol/L (95% CI 5.36, 9.90, $p = < 0.001$) for total 25(OH)D, 7.38 nmol/L (95% CI 5.28, 9.48 $p = < 0.001$) for 25(OH)D_3, and 0.39 nmol/L (95% CI 0.14, 0.64, $p = 0.003$) for Epi-25(OH)D_3 (Figure 2).

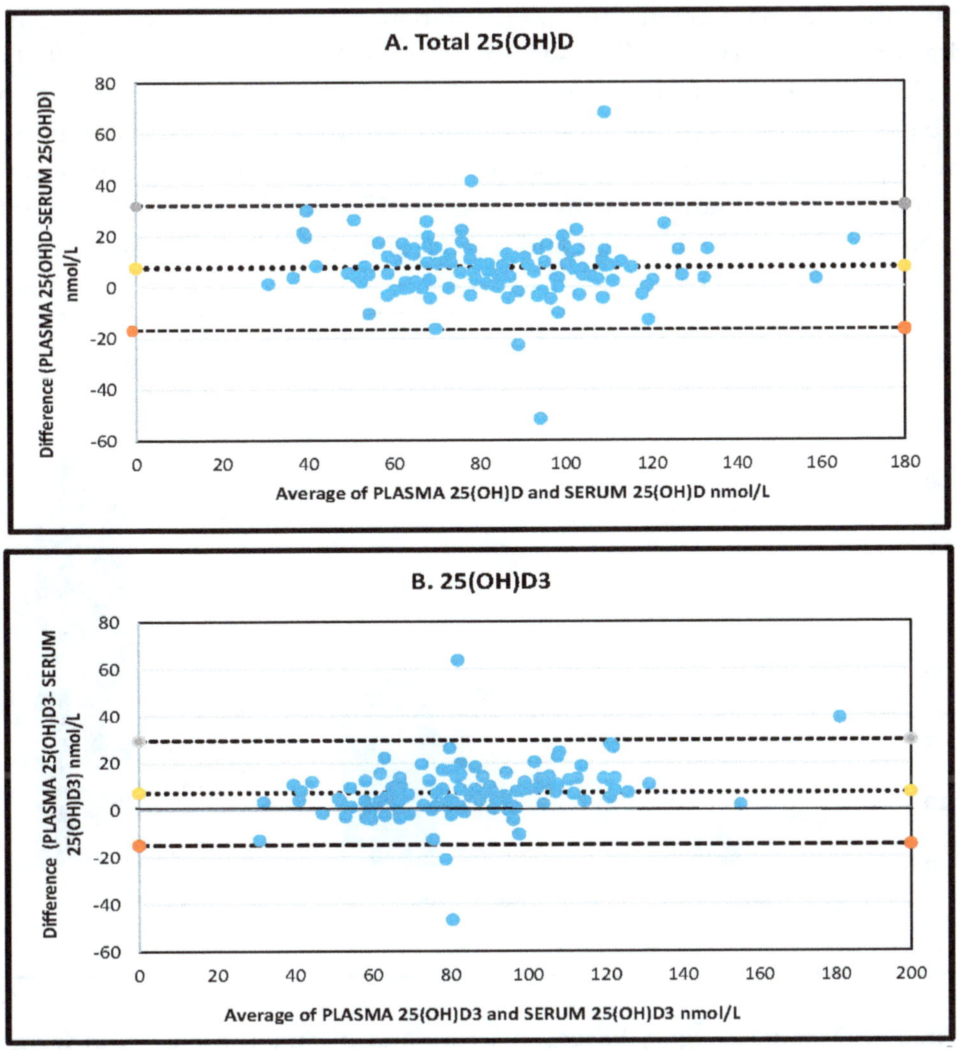

Figure 2. *Cont.*

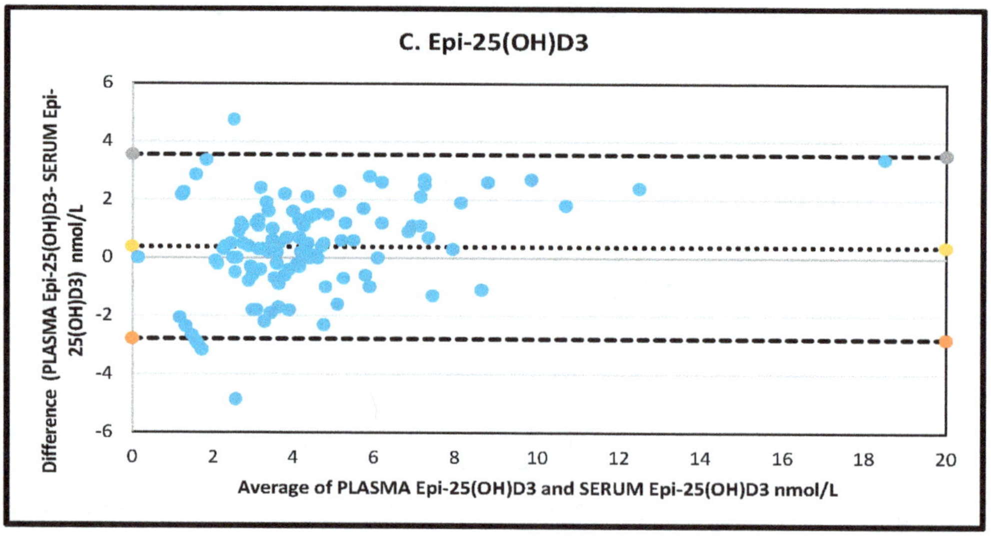

Figure 2. 25(OH)D: 25-hydroxyvitamin D. (**A–C**) Bland-Altman Plot comparison between plasma and serum concentrations of vitamin D analytes quantified using liquid chromatography-tandem mass-spectrometry. (**A**) Total 25-hydroxyvitamin D (25(OH)D), (**B**) 25-hydroxyvitamin D_3 (25(OH)D_3) and (**C**) Epi-25-hydroxyvitamin D_3 (25(OH)D_3). Dotted line: mean difference (bias); dashed line: upper and lower 95% confidence intervals. All results expressed as nmol/L.

In regards to vitamin D status based on sample type, for total 25(OH)D; results are shown in Figure 3 for serum and plasma. Cohen's Kappa (κ) statistic showed moderate agreement between the participants' vitamin D category based on serum compared to plasma ($\kappa = 0.639$, 95% CI 0.48, 0.80, $p \leq 0.001$) with 83.3% agreement found. In total, 16.7% ($n = 19$) of participants changed vitamin D status category based on which sample type was used. Of the $n = 19$ that changed vitamin D status based on serum vs plasma samples; $n = 12$ participants changed from insufficient (<75 nmol/L) to sufficient (≥75 nmol/L), $n = 3$ changed from deficient (<50 nmol/L) to insufficient (50- <75 nmol/L), $n = 1$ changed from insufficient to deficient and $n = 3$ changed from sufficient to insufficient.

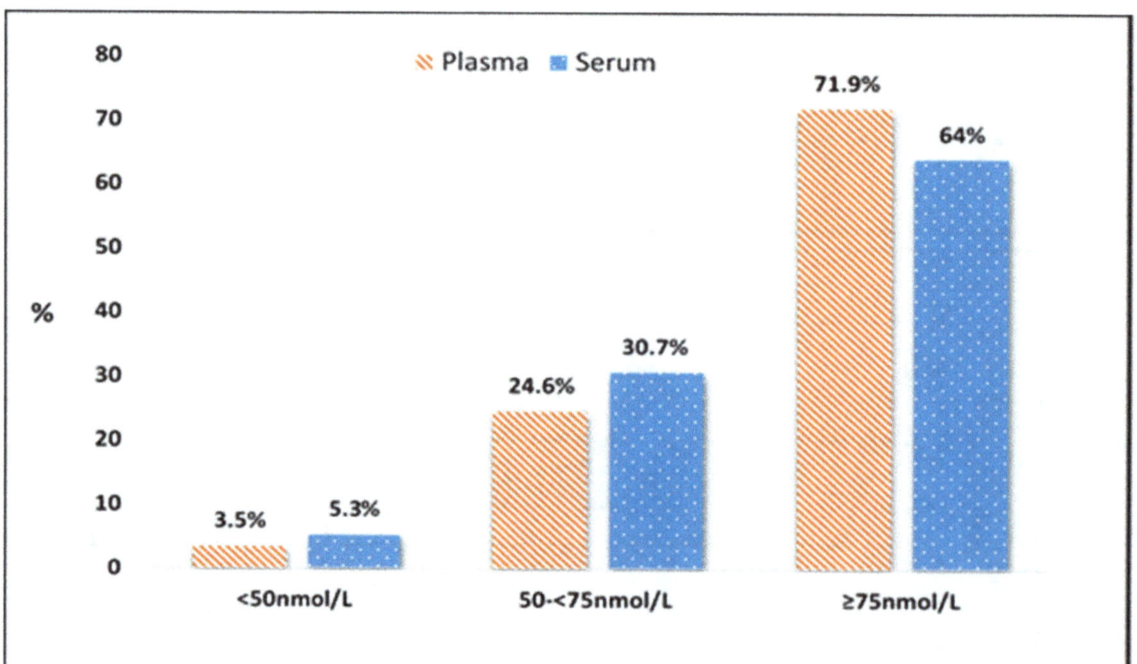

Figure 3. Vitamin D status category based on serum and plasma samples from women between 12–25 weeks gestation using LC-MS/MS.

4. Discussion

This study is the first to examine the comparability of vitamin D quantification by LC-MS/MS in serum and plasma samples collected during pregnancy, and the first to examine the impact of sample type on vitamin D adequacy. Despite a relatively high Pearson and intraclass correlation between serum and plasma concentrations, examination of the concentration bias revealed a significant difference in the mean concentrations of total 25(OH)D in serum vs. plasma. Furthermore, we found 16.7% of participants changed category based on sample type, with 13% changing from deficient to insufficient or insufficient to sufficient with the use of plasma instead of serum.

These results are of concern in a clinical context, especially for pregnant women, as even small differences for patients close to cut-off points for vitamin D deficiency or insufficiency may result in misclassification of their vitamin D status, and may influence subsequent treatment decisions. The current national Australian pregnancy guidelines state that vitamin D supplementation may be considered for women with vitamin D levels <50 nmol/L, highlighting the impact this may have on recommended maternal supplementation, based on the vitamin D test result obtained [26]. Cut-points for vitamin D status and appropriate levels for optimal health have been highly controversial in recent years [27,28]. The Institute of Medicine recommends optimal levels of serum 25(OH)D to be >50 nmol/L based on requirements for bone health [29]. The Endocrine Society has opposed this as an adequate target level, and has identified a target 25(OH)D concentration for optimal health to be >75 nmol/L, based on a large body of evidence highlighting associated outcomes [27], with clinical guidelines recommending supplementation in children and adults to obtain this level [24].

Due to our large sample size, we were able to use Kappa statistic to explore participant's vitamin D status category based on sample type [30,31]. Our resulting Kappa can be interpreted as moderate agreement between the participants resulting vitamin D status (deficient, insufficient or sufficient) based on serum or plasma sample type [31]. Whether a moderate level of agreement is adequate for the use of plasma and serum interchangeably has not been established, but our result does elucidate possible issues, as 13% of participants results could be categorised as false negatives for vitamin D insufficiency or deficiency when plasma was used instead of serum. A 2009 paper examined numerical specifications for trueness and analytical precision for routine analysis of serum/plasma 25(OH)D via immunoassay and LC-MS/MS for establishment of a reference measurement system [32]. Running several models for stringency and practical achievability; they found that, assuming a maximum tolerable limit of 20% clinical misclassifications, the quality goal for bias must be significantly less than 10% [32]. It is noted that the rate of 20% was chosen on an arbitrary basis and data are currently inadequate to ascertain a rate that could be considered acceptable to limit misclassification risk to the population [32]. Further research into acceptable agreement rates of vitamin D category based on sample type is warranted.

Assessing the comparability of sample types for results is important for future research and to assist in the VDSP's goal of standardising vitamin D analysis. These results provide evidence of an important difference in vitamin D quantification, and assessment of vitamin D status, during pregnancy, based on sample type. These results are applicable to LC-MS/MS methods; whether there are differences with nonchromatographic methods based on radioimmunoassay's, such as antibody assays, is unknown. Whether the results would be altered with different anticoagulants used is unknown and requires further investigation. Although serum and plasma are commonly used blood specimen types; they are not equivalent biological matrices [33]. Serum and plasma are used interchangeably for the quantification of vitamin D in some clinical and research settings, and this is the first study to supply evidence that there may be a significant difference in resulting vitamin D concentration using LC-MS/MS and status during pregnancy based on sample type. These results are applicable to pregnant populations; whether these differences in total 25(OH)D quantification by sample type, and subsequent categorisation of vitamin D status, are also seen in non-pregnant populations would require further research. Whilst evidence based recommendations are in place supporting the use of serum and plasma for other nutrients, such as vitamin A and E [16,34,35], similar recommendations are not in place for vitamin D. Serum is considered the appropriate sample type to use for vitamin D analysis and vitamin D reference ranges are based on serum levels, not plasma levels [24]. Our data further support this recommendation; however, where the use of plasma is unavoidable, development of a conversion factor would allow serum and plasma to be used interchangeably with more confidence in regards to the accuracy and precision of the results.

Author Contributions: Conceptualization, S.M.H., V.E.M. and M.E.J.; methodology, S.M.H., V.E.M. and M.E.J.; software, S.M.H.; validation, M.C.; formal analysis, S.M.H.; resources, M.E.J.; data curation, M.E.J., V.E.M.; writing—original draft preparation, S.M.H.; writing—review and editing, V.E.M., P.G.G., M.C. and P.G.G.; visualization, S.M.H., M.E.J. and V.E.M.; supervision, V.E.M., M.E.J. and P.G.G.; funding acquisition, M.E.J. All authors have read and agreed to the published version of the manuscript.

Acknowledgments: The authors would like to thank Kelly Steel for clinical support and Lakshitha Gunawardhana for laboratory assistance for this study.

References

1. National Institutes of Health. Vitamin D: Fact Sheet for Health Professionals. 2014. Available online: https://ods.od.nih.gov/factsheets/VitaminD-HealthProfessional (accessed on 1 October 2020).
2. Zhao, S.; Gardner, K.; Taylor, W.; Marks, E.; Goodson, N. Vitamin D assessment in primary care: Changing patterns of testing. *Lond. J. Prim. Care (Abingdon)* **2015**, *7*, 15–22. [CrossRef]
3. Gordon, L.; Waterhouse, M.; Reid, I.R.; Neale, R.E. The vitamin D testing rate is again rising, despite new MBS testing criteria. *Med. J. Aust.* **2020**, 213. [CrossRef]
4. Colak, A.; Toprak, B.; Dogan, N.; Ustuner, F. Effect of sample type, centrifugation and storage conditions on vitamin D concentration. *Biochem. Med.* **2013**, *23*, 321–325. [CrossRef] [PubMed]
5. Yu, C.-L.; Falk, R.T.; Kimlin, M.G.; Rajaraman, P.; Sigurdson, A.J.; Horst, R.L.; Cosentino, L.M.; Linet, M.S.; Freedman, D.M. The impact of delayed blood centrifuging, choice of collection tube, and type of assay on 25-hydroxyvitamin D concentrations. *Cancer Causes Control CCC* **2010**, *21*, 643–648. [CrossRef] [PubMed]
6. Lissner, D.; Mason, R.S.; Posen, S. Stability of vitamin D metabolites in human blood serum and plasma. *Clin. Chem.* **1981**, *27*, 773–774. [CrossRef]
7. Norris, R.L.; Thomas, M.J.; Craswell, P.W. Assessment of a two-step high-performance liquid chromatographic assay using dual-wavelength ultraviolet monitoring for 25-hydroxyergocalciferol and 25-hydroxycholecalciferol in human serum or plasma. *J. Chromatogr.* **1986**, *381*, 53–61. [CrossRef]
8. Farrell, C.-J.L.; Martin, S.; McWhinney, B.; Straub, I.; Williams, P.; Herrmann, M. State-of-the-Art Vitamin D Assays: A Comparison of Automated Immunoassays with Liquid Chromatography-Tandem Mass Spectrometry Methods. *Clin. Chem.* **2012**, *58*, 531–542. [CrossRef]
9. Yetley, E.A.; Pfeiffer, C.M.; Schleicher, R.L.; Phinney, K.W.; Lacher, D.A.; Christakos, S.; Eckfeldt, J.H.; Fleet, J.C.; Howard, G.; Hoofnagle, A.N.; et al. NHANES monitoring of serum 25-hydroxyvitamin D: A roundtable summary. *J. Nutr.* **2010**, *140*, 2030s–2045s.
10. de la Hunty, A.; Wallace, A.M.; Gibson, S.; Viljakainen, H.; Lamberg-Allardt, C.; Ashwell, M. UK Food Standards Agency Workshop Consensus Report: The choice of method for measuring 25-hydroxyvitamin D to estimate vitamin D status for the UK National Diet and Nutrition Survey. *Br. J. Nutr.* **2010**, *104*, 612–619. [CrossRef]
11. Chen, H.; McCoy, L.; Schleicher, R.; Pfeiffer, C. Measurement of 25-hydroxyvitamin D-3 (25OHD(3)) and 25-hydroxyvitamin D-2 (25OHD(2)) in human serum using liquid chromatography-tandem mass spectrometry and its comparison to a radioimmunoassay method. *Clin. Chim. Acta Int. J. Clin. Chem.* **2008**, *391*, 6–12. [CrossRef]

12. Clarke, M.W.; Tuckey, R.C.; Gorman, S.; Holt, B.; Hart, P.H. Optimized 25-hydroxyvitamin D analysis using liquid-liquid extraction with 2D separation with LC/MS/MS detection, provides superior precision compared to conventional assays. *Metabolomics* **2013**, *9*, 1031–1040. [CrossRef]
13. Wise, S.A.; Phinney, K.W.; Tai, S.S.; Camara, J.E.; Myers, G.L.; Durazo-Arvizu, R.; Tian, L.; Hoofnagle, A.N.; Bachmann, L.M.; Young, I.S.; et al. Baseline Assessment of 25-Hydroxyvitamin D Assay Performance: A Vitamin D Standardization Program (VDSP) Interlaboratory Comparison Study. *J. AOAC Int.* **2017**, *100*, 1244–1252. [CrossRef]
14. Zhang, S.W.; Jian, W.; Sullivan, S.; Sankaran, B.; Edom, R.W.; Weng, N.; Sharkey, D. Development and validation of an LC-MS/MS based method for quantification of 25 hydroxyvitamin D2 and 25 hydroxyvitamin D3 in human serum and plasma. *J. Chromatogr. B Anal. Technol. Biomed. Life Sci.* **2014**, *961*, 62–70. [CrossRef] [PubMed]
15. Abu Kassim, N.S.; Gomes, F.P.; Shaw, P.N.; Hewavitharana, A.K. Simultaneous quantitative analysis of nine vitamin D compounds in human blood using LC-MS/MS. *Bioanalysis* **2016**, *8*, 397–411. [CrossRef] [PubMed]
16. Albarhani, A.A.; Collier, F.; Greaves, R.F.; Ponsonby, A.L.; Allen, K.J.; Vuillermin, P.J.; Roche, P.; Clarke, M.W.; BIS Steering Committee. Vitamins D and A can be successfully measured by LC-MS/MS in cord blood diluted plasma. *Clin. Biochem.* **2015**, *48*, 1105–1112. [CrossRef] [PubMed]
17. Mena-Bravo, A.; Priego-Capote, F.; Luque de Castro, M.D. Study of blood collection and sample preparation for analysis of vitamin D and its metabolites by liquid chromatography-tandem mass spectrometry. *Anal. Chim. Acta* **2015**, *879*, 69–76. [CrossRef]
18. Sempos, C.T.; Vesper, H.W.; Phinney, K.W.; Thienpont, L.M.; Coates, P.M. Vitamin D status as an international issue: National surveys and the problem of standardization. *Scand. J. Clin. Lab. Investig. Suppl.* **2012**, *243*, 32–40.
19. Karras, S.N.; Wagner, C.L.; Castracane, V.D. Understanding vitamin D metabolism in pregnancy: From physiology to pathophysiology and clinical outcomes. *Metabolism* **2018**, *86*, 112–123. [CrossRef]
20. Fernando, M.; Ellery, S.J.; Marquina, C.; Lim, S.; Naderpoor, N.; Mousa, A. Vitamin D-Binding Protein in Pregnancy and Reproductive Health. *Nutrients* **2020**, *12*, 1489. [CrossRef]
21. Beentjes, C.H.L.; Taylor-King, J.P.; Bayani, A.; Davis, C.N.; Dunster, J.L.; Jabbari, S.; Mirams, G.; Jenkinson, C.; Kilby, M.; Hewison, M.; et al. Defining vitamin D status using multi-metabolite mathematical modelling: A pregnancy perspective. *J. Steroid Biochem. Mol. Biol.* **2019**, *190*, 152–160. [CrossRef]
22. Murphy, V.E.; Jensen, M.E.; Mattes, J.; Hensley, M.J.; Giles, W.B.; Peek, M.J.; Bisits, A.; Callaway, L.K.; McCaffery, K.; Barrett, H.L.; et al. The Breathing for Life Trial: A randomised controlled trial of fractional exhaled nitric oxide (FENO)-based management of asthma during pregnancy and its impact on perinatal outcomes and infant and childhood respiratory health. *BMC Pregnancy Childbirth* **2016**, *16*. [CrossRef] [PubMed]
23. Bartolucci, A.A. *Limits of Calibration. Introduction to Statistical Analysis of Laboratory Data*; John Wiley & Sons: New Jersey, NJ, USA, 2016; Chapter 6.
24. Holick, M.F.; Binkley, N.C.; Bischoff-Ferrari, H.A.; Gordon, C.M.; Hanley, D.A.; Heaney, R.P.; Hassan Murad, M.; Weaver, C.M. Evaluation, Treatment, and Prevention of Vitamin D Deficiency: An Endocrine Society Clinical Practice Guideline. *J. Clin. Endocrinol. Metab.* **2011**, *96*, 1911–1930. [CrossRef] [PubMed]
25. Bland, J.M.; Altman, D.G. Statistical methods for assessing agreement between two methods of clinical measurement. *Lancet* **1986**, *1*, 307–310. [CrossRef]
26. Department of Health. *Clinical Practice Guidelines: Pregnancy Care*; Australian Government, Department of Health: Canberra, Australia, 2018.
27. Vieth, R.; Holick, M.F. The IOM—Endocrine Society Controversy on Recommended Vitamin D Targets. In *Support of the Endocrine Society Position*, 4th ed.; Feldman, D., Ed.; Academic Press: Cambridge, MA, USA, 2018; Chapter 57B; pp. 1091–1107.
28. Bouillon, R.; Rosen, C. The IOM—Endocrine Society Controversy on Recommended Vitamin D Targets. In *Support of the IOM Position*, 4th ed.; Feldman, D., Ed.; Academic Press: Cambridge, MA, USA, 2018; Chapter 57A; pp. 1065–1089.
29. Del Valle, H.B.; Yaktine, A.L.; Taylor, C.L.; Ross, A.C. *Dietary Reference Intakes for Calcium and Vitamin D*; National Academies Press: Washington, DC, USA, 2011.

30. Sim, J.; Wright, C.C. The Kappa Statistic in Reliability Studies: Use, Interpretation, and Sample Size Requirements. *Phys. Ther.* **2005**, *85*, 257–268. [CrossRef]
31. McHugh, M.L. Interrater reliability: The kappa statistic. *Biochem. Med.* **2012**, *22*, 276–282. [CrossRef]
32. Stöckl, D.; Sluss, P.M.; Thienpont, L.M. Specifications for trueness and precision of a reference measurement system for serum/plasma 25-hydroxyvitamin D analysis. *Clin. Chim. Acta* **2009**, *408*, 8–13. [CrossRef]
33. Sapan, C.V.; Lundblad, R.L. Considerations regarding the use of blood samples in the proteomic identification of biomarkers for cancer diagnosis. *Cancer Genom. Proteom.* **2006**, *3*, 227–230.
34. Castle, M.C.; Cooke, W.J. Measurement of vitamin E in serum and plasma by high performance liquid chromatography with electrochemical detection. *Ther. Drug Monit.* **1985**, *7*, 364–368. [CrossRef]
35. Greaves, R.F.; Woollard, G.A.; Hoad, K.E.; Walmsley, T.A.; Johnson, L.A.; Briscoe, S.; Koetsier, S.; Harrower, T.; Gill, J.P. Laboratory medicine best practice guideline: Vitamins a, e and the carotenoids in blood. *Clin. Biochem. Rev.* **2014**, *35*, 81–113.

8

Vitamin D in Neurological Diseases: A Rationale for a Pathogenic Impact

Rita Moretti *, Maria Elisa Morelli and Paola Caruso

Neurology Clinic, Department of Medical, Surgical and Health Sciences, University of Trieste, Strada di Fiume, 447, 34149 Trieste, Italy; mariaelisa.morelli@gmail.com (M.E.M.); caruso.paola1983@libero.it (P.C.)

* Correspondence: moretti@units.it

Abstract: It is widely known that vitamin D receptors have been found in neurons and glial cells, and their highest expression is in the hippocampus, hypothalamus, thalamus and subcortical grey nuclei, and substantia nigra. Vitamin D helps the regulation of neurotrophin, neural differentiation, and maturation, through the control operation of growing factors synthesis (i.e., neural growth factor [NGF] and glial cell line-derived growth factor (GDNF), the trafficking of the septohippocampal pathway, and the control of the synthesis process of different neuromodulators (such as acetylcholine [Ach], dopamine [DA], and gamma-aminobutyric [GABA]). Based on these assumptions, we have written this review to summarize the potential role of vitamin D in neurological pathologies. This work could be titanic and the results might have been very fuzzy and even incoherent had we not conjectured to taper our first intentions and devoted our interests towards three mainstreams, demyelinating pathologies, vascular syndromes, and neurodegeneration. As a result of the lack of useful therapeutic options, apart from the disease-modifying strategies, the role of different risk factors should be investigated in neurology, as their correction may lead to the improvement of the cerebral conditions. We have explored the relationships between the gene-environmental influence and long-term vitamin D deficiency, as a risk factor for the development of different types of neurological disorders, along with the role and the rationale of therapeutic trials with vitamin D implementation.

Keywords: neuro-degeneration; MS; demyelination; vascular disease; stroke; AD; vitamin D-OH 25; VDR; VDH; calcium

---

1. Introduction

Low levels of vitamin D, considering serum 25-hydroxyvitamin D (25(OH)D), have been recognized as a widespread health problem, affecting approximately one billion people worldwide [1]. Latitude, season, cultural norms, religious practices, limited awareness, lack of knowledge, indoor lifestyles, urban living, skin pigmentation, malnutrition, diet, co-morbidities (like tuberculosis, malnutrition, chronic inflammatory conditions, etc.), and drugs, may contribute to vitamin D deficiency, especially in the developing world, even if some genetic predispositions can interfere with it (i.e., blacks tend to have lower levels of 25(OH)D compared to whites) [2,3].

Vitamin D is a lipid-soluble vitamin, which can be synthesized and act as a hormone [4]. The active form of vitamin D, 1,25(OH)$_2$D, known as calcitriol, has chemical similarities to typical hormones, such as testosterone, estrogen, and cortisol.

Vitamin D yields both genomic and non-genomic actions; the Vitamin D Receptors (VDR) mediates the former, one of the representative of the steroid hormone superfamily, which are evident in more than 30 human tissues, therefore regulating 3% of the human genome (approximately 700 genes) [5]. Nuclear VDRs are found in most cells, and support the role for the extra-skeletal benefits of vitamin D. The VDR are found in almost all human tissues, participating in the classic actions of vitamin D in the bone, gut, and kidney, but are also involved in immune functions, hormone secretion, and cellular proliferation and differentiation [6]. To be biologically active, vitamin D undergoes hydroxylations in the liver, mediated by the 25-hydroxylase, and in the kidney, mediated by 1α-hydroxylase. The 1,25$(OH)_2$D is recognized by VDR, in various cells, mainly in the intestine. As vitamin D plays a significant role in modulating the immune system in the intestine, it is possible that its deficiency could deteriorate the gut barrier function, favoring the translocation of endotoxins. Vitamin D deficiency has been associated with intestinal dysbiosis and increased susceptibility to intestinal diseases; moreover, vitamin D could be contributing to disturbances of the glucose metabolism by modulating the composition of the gut microbiota. The changed intestinal microbiome has become epidemic, in parallel with the epidemic of vitamin D deficiency, suggesting that they might be linked. Proper supplemental doses of vitamin D plus all of the B vitamins appears to return the intestinal microbiome back to normal after few months [7,8]. Moreover, there are more and more evidence that links the microbiome to neurologic disorders [9], which can share a common auto-immune involvement; the potential link between the three actors (VDR, neurological disorders, and vitamin D) is quite fascinating and many studies should be done to gain knowledge on them.

The non-genomic actions of vitamin D help to cooperate with the classical genomic pathway, to transactivate VDR, and exert the effects of calcitriol; the signal does not depend on the transcription phases, but it can operate via cross-talk with different signaling pathways, such as rapid membrane response binding proteins (see later). The genomic and the non-genomic pathways support the emerging not calcemic effects of the vitamin D metabolites, trying to define a role in the autoimmune pathologies, infectious diseases, diabetes mellitus, obesity, and cardio-metabolic disorders [10].

It has also been demonstrated that Vitamin D is involved in different neurological disorders, such as multiple sclerosis, Alzheimer's disease, Parkinson's disease, and stroke [11–14].

The presence of VDR in the hippocampus, hypothalamus, thalamus, cortex, and substantia nigra [15] prompted many studies on the possible determinant role of vitamin D in different neurological conditions [16,17]. It has been evidenced that calcitriol is a fundamental actor in the neuronal differentiation and the neural maturation [18]. Vitamin D normalizes the trafficking of the septo-hippocampal pathways, mainly via the neural growth factor (NGF); moreover, it is an active controller of the genetic regulation of the synthesis of acetylcholine (Ach), dopamine (DA), serotonin (5HT3), and gamma-aminobutyric (GABA) [19–21].

The knock-out model of $VDR^{-/-}$ has an accelerated aging process in all of the organs, as well as in the brain [22,23], with a significant in-brain decrease of NGF [24] and other neurotransmitters, such as Ach [25,26]. The congenital deficiency of vitamin D significantly reduces the activity of glutamic acid decarboxylase (GAD) 65/67 (critical enzymes in GABAergic inter-neurons) and the levels of glutamate and glutamine in the brain tissue [27].

For these reasons, we reckon that a vitamin D deficiency could contribute to the complex relationship between genetics and the environment, the two common poles that many neurological pathologies debate between. It could intervene in the exacerbation of precipitating factors or in demodulating the repair process; therefore, we consider that this topic should be approached from a neurological perspective. Therefore, we have started this review. We searched MEDLINE using the following search terms: "vitamin D central nervous system", both "vitamin D" and "central nervous system"; "vitamin D immune system/response", both "vitamin D" and "immune system" or "immune response"; "vitamin D multiple sclerosis risk", both "vitamin D" and "multiple sclerosis risk"; "vitamin D multiple sclerosis relapse", both "vitamin D" and "multiple sclerosis relapse"; "vitamin D multiple sclerosis magnetic resonance imaging", both "vitamin D" and "multiple sclerosis magnetic resonance imaging"; "vitamin D multiple sclerosis disability", both "vitamin D" and "multiple sclerosis disability"; "vitamin D supplementation/therapy/treatment multiple sclerosis", both "vitamin D supplementation" or "vitamin D therapy" or "vitamin D treatment" and "multiple sclerosis"; "vascular dementia", both "vascular" and "dementia"; "subcortical vascular dementia", both "subcortical" and "dementia"; "Alzheimer's disease"; "pathogenesis neural-degeneration"; "amyloid"; "cholinergic afferents"; "arteriolosclerosis"; "cerebral flow regulation"; and "stroke". The publications that were selected were mostly from the past 20 years, but they did not exclude the frequently referenced and highly regarded older publications. The research has been extended, with the same strings, EMBASE, COCHRANE LIBRARY, and LILACS. All of the searches were done from 1 January 1993 up to 31 May 2018. We considered papers published in English, French, German, and Italian. Congress abstracts and isolated case reports (even if the total cases were under 10) were not considered. Review articles and book chapters are cited to provide additional details. The authors carefully read all of the selected articles.

2. Vitamin D Deficiency and Multiple Sclerosis: Role in the Susceptibility, Activity, and Treatment of the Disease

Multiple Sclerosis (MS) is a multifactorial demyelinating pathology affecting the brain and the spinal cord, firmly relying on an altered immune response. Activated autoreactive T cells invade the blood–brain barrier and initiate an inflammatory response that leads to myelin destruction and axonal loss. The etiology of MS, the mechanisms associated with its onset, the unpredictable clinical course, and the different rates of progression leading to disability over time, remain unresolved questions [28].

Immunological research makes two significant observations to explain the link between vitamin D and the immune system.

Firstly, most immune cells, of both the innate and the adaptive immune system, express the VDR [29,30]. Secondly, the immune cells exhibit an active vitamin D metabolism, with the expression of the rate-limiting enzyme for vitamin D synthesis, 1α-hydroxylase (CYP27B1) [31]. Immune cells are, therefore, able to synthesize and secrete vitamin D in an autocrine and paracrine condition [32]. The immune cell types, targeted by vitamin D, include monocytes and macrophages, dendritic cells (DCs), and T and B cells [33]. 1,25(OH)$_2$ vitamin D induces monocytes proliferation and differentiation into macrophages [34], the potentiate the expression of interleukin-1 (IL-1), and the antimicrobial peptides (cathelicidin, β-defensin-2, and hepcidin) [35]. Vitamin D inhibits DC differentiation and maturation, their major histocompatibility complex (class II) expression (MHC), CD40, CD80, CD86, and IL-12 (while inducing the production of IL-10), leading to reduced T cell stimulatory capacity [36,37]. Vitamin D decreases the production of nitric oxide (NO), mediating the downregulation of the inducible nitric oxide synthase (iNOS) expression [38]. Moreover, it stimulates the development of natural killer T (NKT) cells, and it increases IL-4 and interferon (IFN)-γ production [39]; vitamin D attenuates the proliferation of CD8+ T cells and reduces their cytotoxic activity by decreasing the production of IL-2, IL-17, and IFN-γ.

Vitamin D exerts its immunomodulatory effects on T lymphocytes, by inhibiting the production of pro-inflammatory Th1 cytokines (IL-1, IL-2, IL-6, IL-12, IFN-γ, TNF-α, and TNF-β), and stimulating the production of anti-inflammatory regulatory Th2 cytokines (IL-4, IL-5, and IL-10) [40,41].

Thus, vitamin D potentiates the innate immune system and regulates the adaptive immune system, mainly by inducing the split to Th2 and regulatory T cells (Tregs), over the Th1 and Th17 lymphocytes differentiation [42], via direct and indirect actions on naive CD4+ cells. The general result is an evident effect of switching capacity, from a pro-inflammatory autoimmune to an anti-inflammatory tolerogenic immunological response.

In multiple sclerosis (MS) patients, the blood level of 25(OH)D or 1,25(OH)$_2$D has been linked with the suppressive activity of Tregs [43], and the number of Tregs has been correlated with the serum levels of 25(OH)D or 1,25(OH)$_2$D. The Tregs are increased in the MS patients that have supplemented with vitamin D [44,45].

According to many studies, vitamin D may have an impact on the balance between the inflammatory and anti-inflammatory mechanisms, which might help/regulate the remyelination process. Vitamin D increases the microglial activation, promoting the clearance of myelin debris, and consequently activating the remyelination process [46]. In the oligodendrocyte precursor cells (OPC) cultures, vitamin D up-regulates the transcription of VDR and NGF mRNA, but not of myelin basic protein (MBP) [47–49]. The remyelination of demyelinated lesions has been observed in the early stages of MS [50,51], and it has been supported by neuroimaging findings [52,53]. However, remyelination might be incomplete [54], and eventually, it might cease [55], because of the OPC inability to migrate and reach the site of demyelination [56], or for the OPC differentiation inability [57]. In fact, an inflammatory microenvironment prevents OPC maturation and the differentiation into oligodendrocytes, and subsequently prevents axon remyelination. This is relevant for MS treatment, as current treatments are only useful for controlling immune mechanisms (i.e., in the early stages of the disease), but do not affect remyelination. In vitro studies show that when blocking VDR, there is a reduction of OPC differentiation, with a consequent blockage of myelination and remyelination; on the other hand, by activating VDR, via vitamin D, there is an increase in the differentiation of OPC and the consequent remyelination [58]. Likewise, neural stem cells (NSC) express VDR and 1,25$(OH)_2$D, which seems to promote the NCS proliferation and differentiation into neurons and oligodendrocytes, and to reduce astrogliosis [59,60].

As vitamin D deficiency has been proposed as a significant risk factor in MS development, most epidemiologic observational studies have suggested that adequate vitamin D levels may reduce the risk of MS onset and modify the course of the disease. MS is a disease that is virtually unknown at the equator, and the prevalence of the disease increases in populations that live farther away from the equator [61]. The prevalence of MS is higher at higher latitudes, and tends to peak in the areas with the lowest exposure to ultraviolet (UV) light [62,63]; however, in these areas, diets rich in vitamin D-containing oily fish may offset this risk to some degree [62–65]. Moreover, the risk of MS has been found to decrease among people who migrate from higher to lower latitudes [66]. This latitudinal finding has been declining in recent decades, instead of an associated increasing trend towards avoiding sun exposure by staying indoors for more extended periods of the day, even in warmer climates [67,68]. In fact, higher levels of sun exposure (past, recent, and cumulative) were independently associated with higher levels of vitamin D and with a significantly reduced risk of developing demyelinating events [69]. Sunlight seems to have an immunosuppressive effect and, therefore, the effects of sunlight on MS risk could be related to the sunlight itself, or to an increase of vitamin D [70]. The association between the calculated vitamin D intake from diet or supplements, and the risk of developing MS has been prospectively evaluated in two large cohorts involving more than 187,000 women [71]. Women who had a higher intake of dietary vitamin D (approximately 700 IU/day) had a 33% lower incidence of MS compared with those with a lower intake. Moreover, the women who used vitamin D supplements (more than 400 UI/day) had a 41% reduced risk of developing MS compared with non-users. Higher levels of 25(OH)D (independently, from dietary vitamin D intake) also seem to predict a lower risk of MS onset. A more recent prospective study confirmed these findings and reported that the levels of vitamin D over 30 ng/mL were associated with a decreased MS risk [72]. Adiposity has been associated with lower vitamin D levels [73,74], and a higher body mass index (BMI) has been associated with higher incidence of MS in adolescent women, but not in adult women [75].

A crucial question related to a primary prevention trial or from vitamin D supplementation in MS is the relevant age of exposure, which can range from in utero to adolescence and adulthood [76]. Mirzaei et al. studied a large cohort and analyzed the association between maternal dietary vitamin D intake and the predicted maternal serum 25(OH)D during pregnancy, and their daughters' risk of developing MS [77]. The study showed that the relative risk of MS was significantly lower in the women whose mothers had high vitamin D intake during pregnancy compared with the women born to low-intake mothers. A diminished in utero exposure to vitamin D, coupled with the solar cycle and latitudinal differences, may be an environmental risk factor for the development of MS. Similarly, albeit not statistically significant, a reduced MS risk was reported among the women reporting an increased vitamin D intake from supplements in adolescence [78]. These results suggest that MS risk is related not only to new vitamin D levels, but it might also be related to its levels during childhood or even in utero. Several studies, including a meta-analysis, demonstrated that spring-born have a significantly higher lifetime MS risk than autumn-born, which has been attributed, at least in part, to insufficient in utero vitamin D levels, because of low maternal serum vitamin D levels during winter [79,80].

In a large population-based case-control study [81], children born with 25(OH)D levels <10 ng/mL seemed to be at a high risk of developing MS. Likewise, the level of sun exposure in childhood and adolescence (e.g., by outdoor leisure activities), which may serve as a proxy for vitamin D supply in early life, has been inversely linked to the risk of MS in adulthood [82,83]. In a recent longitudinal Canadian study of 302 children with the acute demyelinating syndrome, low vitamin D levels were significantly associated with MS risk in the subsequent three years [84]. One report showed that children with higher serum 25(OH)D concentrations at presentation, with an acquired demyelinating syndrome, had a lower risk of early MS diagnosis [85]. Gender- and sex-related immunological differences may influence the association between vitamin D and MS. The disproportional increase in the incidence of MS in women is likely to be caused by sex-specific exposure or susceptibility to environmental factors [86]. The data supporting an interaction between female sex, possibly mediated by estrogen, and vitamin D for MS risk is accumulating. A protective effect of sun exposure was only observed in female monozygotic twins [87], and the association of sun-sensitive skin types with a disability was only found in untreated female MS patients [88]. In vitro studies of MBP-specific T cell proliferation have shown sex differences in the metabolism of vitamin D, which were confirmed by treating male MBP-specific T cells with 17β-estradiol in the assay [89]. In one animal study, vitamin D resulted in fewer clinical, histopathologic, and immunologic signs of Experimental Autoimmune Encephalomyelitis (EAE) in female mice compared with ovariectomized females and intact or castrated males [90]. A synergy between E_2 and vitamin D occurred through the VDR-mediated enhancement of E_2 synthesis, as well as through the E_2-mediated enhancement of VDR expression due to the inflammation of central nervous system (CNS). In males, E_2 did not enable vitamin D to inhibit EAE [91], possibly suggesting that vitamin D-mediated protection in EAE is female-specific, and that MS tends to have a more aggressive course in men than in women.

Several genome-wide association studies (GWAS) and gene-candidate studies have investigated the influence of the specific genetic polymorphisms of vitamin D metabolites on the 25(OH)D levels, and their susceptibility to MS; one study found [92] an association between the short variant of the VDR protein (F allele) and a genetic predisposition to lower 25(OH)D levels, but not to a higher risk of MS; in a GWAS of 4501 European patients [93], single-nucleotide polymorphisms (SNPs) of the gene encoding components of the vitamin D binding protein were associated with 25(OH)D concentrations, or with the genes involved in vitamin D synthesis or activation; moreover, a genetically lowered 25(OH)D level was strongly associated with increased MS risk and progression in two studies [94,95].

The role of vitamin D in MS disease progression has also been assessed: it has been hypothesized that 25(OH)D levels can predict a later development of MS in acute optic neuritis (ON) [96], but the result is inconclusive. A discrete quantity of studies demonstrated that vitamin D levels affect clinical relapses and MS disease activity. In a retrospective study of 110 patients with pediatric-onset MS, the authors found that each increase of 10 ng/mL in the 25(OH)D level was associated with a 34% decrease in the relapse risk [97]. Similar findings were seen in a prospective cohort study, whose authors concluded that raising 25(OH)D by 20 ng/mL could decrease the hazard of relapse by up to 50% [98]. In a prospective longitudinal study, the relapse risk was significantly reduced in those patients with medium (20–40 ng/mL) and high (>40 ng/mL) serum vitamin D levels, compared with those with low levels (<20 ng/mL) [99]. Moreover, the same authors found that for each doubling of the serum vitamin D concentration from a baseline of 10, 20, and 30 ng/mL, MS relapse risk decreased by 27%. In another study, lower vitamin D levels predicted a conversion from Clinically Isolated Syndrome (CIS) to clinically definite MS [100,101]. In the study by Embry et al., low serum 25(OH)D levels predicted an increased likelihood of gadolinium-enhancing lesions (Gd+) in the Magnetic Resonance Imaging (MRI) scans performed in the subsequent two months period [102]. In the EPIC study [103], a five-year MS cohort study in which subjects had clinical and MRI evaluations and gave a blood sample annually. The authors concluded that individuals with CIS/relapsing-remitting multiple sclerosis (RRMS) with higher vitamin D levels have a lower risk of the subsequent development of new T2 lesions and Gd+ lesions on a brain MRI, even after accounting for potential confounding factors. Moreover, an increment of 10 ng/mL of 25(OH)D was associated with a 15% lower risk of new T2 lesions and a 32% lower risk of Gd+ lesions [103]. In a post hoc analysis, including up to two years of follow-up of participants treated with interferon beta (IFNB)-1b in the BENEFIT trial [104], Gd+ lesions development was inversely associated with 25(OH)D levels, those patients whose 25(OH)D levels were >20 ng/mL had a 39% lower risk of new Gd+ lesions. Unfortunately, across all of the analyses, associations with lower vitamin D were generally stronger for MRI than for the clinical outcomes. Moreover, the participants of the Betaferon Efficacy Yielding Outcomes of a New Dose (BEYOND) study (BEYOND study) [105], treated with IFNB-1b, with higher serum 25(OH)D levels, had lower numbers of new T2 and Gd+ lesions during the first 12 months of follow-up. Moreover, a 20 ng/mL higher serum 25(OH)D level was associated with a 31% lower rate of new lesions, and the patients with 25(OH)D $\geq$ 40 ng/mL showed 47% lower rate of new T2 lesions and new Gd+ lesions, when compared with the patients who had serum levels of 20–32 ng/mL. Vitamin D and disease-modifying therapies (DMTs) may positively influence each other and produce an additive, or even synergistic, effect on MS disease activity. In an observational cohort study, which included 178 patients with MS [106], the patients who were treated by IFN had significantly higher 25(OH)D levels than those who were not. Interestingly, the IFN treatment was protective only against relapses among the patients with higher vitamin D levels. The authors hypothesized that treatment with IFNB might increase the serum vitamin D levels through an enhanced responsiveness to sun exposure [106]. The same authors did not find similar associations for glatiramer acetate (GA) therapy and vitamin D. More recently, Laursen et al. [107] found that higher vitamin D levels in CIS may slow neurodegeneration evaluated by brain volume measures. In fact, they found that each 10 ng/mL increase in 25(OH)D was significantly associated with a 7.8 mL higher gray matter volume [108]. Variations in the relapse rate and the number of MRI brain lesions have shown a seasonal pattern that can be related to a variation in Ultra Violet Radiation (UVR) exposure and vitamin D status [109,110], with some exceptions [111,112]. Most cross-sectional studies have concluded a negative correlation between the 25(OH) D level and disability [103,113,114], and, interestingly, even a direct correlation between the 25(OH) D level and poorer memory performance [115]. However, the causality is considered uncertain, at the moment.

Given the previous reviewed findings, the assessment of vitamin D supplementation for a possible disease-modifying course of MS is obviously of crucial interest. Unfortunately, the current evidence does not offer a definite consensus for supplementation. Kimball et al. [115] performed a six-month safety study with escalating doses of vitamin D, and they found a significant reduction in the mean number of Gd+ lesions at the end of the study. In an open-label randomized trial, patients randomized to a vitamin D supplementation had an annualized relapse rate (ARR) significantly lower in the treatment, with a prolonged relapse-free time and with a persistent reduction in the T cell proliferation [44]. In a one year double-blind, randomized placebo-controlled trial with vitamin D3 as an add-on treatment to IFNB-1b, the MRI T2 lesion burden and the new/enlarging T2 lesions, tended to increase more in the placebo group than in the vitamin D group, however, without statistical significance [116]. A preliminary Iranian study assessed the safety and efficacy of high-dose vitamin D supplementation during pregnancy in women with MS [117]. The women in the vitamin D group had significantly fewer relapses during pregnancy, a tendency for fewer relapses up six months after delivery, and a more stable Expanded Disability Status Scale (EDSS) than those without supplementation [107]. In a longitudinal study [118], in which 170 natalizumab-treated patients were followed for one year between two winter seasons, patients with insufficient serum 25(OH)D levels at baseline (<20 ng/mL) were advised to take vitamin D supplements, and a significant inverse relationship with the ARR was found, as, for each nmol/L increase in 25(OH)D, a 0.014 decrease in ARR was observed. The double-blind, multicentre, 48-week study, named SOLAR, of supplementation of high-dose oral vitamin D has been the most extensive study to date [119]. An insignificant trend toward lower ARR in the treatment group was found in vitamin D groupersus placebo, and no statistically significant differences in the disease activity were found between the two groups. Vitamin D3 was associated with a statistically significant reduction in the combined unique lesions (secondary endpoint). The effect of the addition of vitamin D3 to IFNB-1a over 96 weeks was investigated with appropriate cognitive tests [120]. It did not show a significant trend toward a lower ARR (primary endpoint) among those patients receiving vitamin D treatment, which became statistically significant when the analysis was restricted to those who completed the study. Among the completers, there were also significantly fewer new T2 lesions in the vitamin D group. It is unclear whether the findings of these trials are related to insufficient power or other issues leading to an inability to detect a treatment effect for all outcomes [120].

Larger randomized controlled trails (RCTs) are currently underway to reveal the role of vitamin D supplementation as an add-on to IFNB therapy in the treatment of RRMS, and even CIS, patients, namely, the VITADEM study in Spain, EVIDIMS study in Germany, PrevANZ study in Australia, D-Lay-MS study in France, and the VIDAMS trial in the United States. One study investigated the cognitive effects of vitamin D supplementation on patients with MS who were treated with IFNB [121], and after the follow-up period they scored better on the Brief Visuospatial Memory test (BVMT) for delayed recall.

In conclusion, numerous studies suggest that vitamin D supplementation may benefit MS patients, although larger RCTs are needed to establish this supplementation as a standard of care for MS. Moreover, there is no consensus on the definition of 'sufficient' vitamin D levels in MS, and many physicians question whether people with MS should empirically be supplemented while waiting for more conclusive results of vitamin D clinical trials. In the view of the Institute of Medicine (IOM), 25(OH) D levels greater than 20 ng/mL (50 nmol/L) are sufficient. The Endocrine Society, considering skeletal and non-skeletal health, argues for levels of almost 30 ng/mL (75 nmol/L). In the MS field, numerous studies suggest that serum 25(OH)D levels of approximately 40 ng/mL (100 nmol/L) are the lower limit for controlling MRI and clinical activity. Some experts favor maintaining 25(OH)D levels between 30 and 50 ng/mL in MS patients, as immune-modulatory effects have been observed in these ranges in experimental studies. Longitudinal RCTs are needed to establish the recommended levels of vitamin D supplementation necessary to reduce the risk of MS onset and MS pathological activity. According to other authors [122], for individuals with CIS or MS and vitamin D deficiency (<20 ng/mL), an 'attack' supplementation with 50,000 IU/week of vitamin D2 (ergocalciferol) for eight weeks, and a subsequent evaluation of the serum level, is recommended. The continuation of this therapy until the serum 25(OH)D is higher than 30 ng/dL may be necessary. A maintenance supplementation with vitamin D3 (cholecalciferol) at 1000 to 2000 IU/day may be started when the deficiency has been corrected, and at once in case of vitamin D insufficiency (20–29 ng/mL). As current evidence also suggests both an obstetric and pediatric benefit from vitamin D against the risk of developing MS, vitamin D supplementation in children and pregnant women at risk of developing or being affected by MS should be considered [123]. According to other authors, as a goal, the general aim is 25(OH)D levels between 40 and 60 ng/mL, and most patients should take a dose that arises from 2000 to 5000 IU/day vitamin D3 [123]. Many studies have been conducted to show the potential relationships between genome-wide association studies (GWAS) and gene-candidate studies, in order to find out the specific genetic polymorphisms of the vitamin D metabolites on the 25(OH)D levels, and their susceptibility to MS and to vitamin D supplementation efficacy in MS [92–95]. Moreover, the Human Leukocyte Antigen (HLA) haplotype might influence epistasis, trans and cis effects, and parent-of-origin effects, as well as the Epstein Barr Virus (EBV) and vitamin D effects on the course of MS [124]. Le Mokry et al. (2015) identified SNPs associated with 25(OH)D level from SUNLIGHT, the largest (n = 33,996) genome-wide association study to date for vitamin D. Four SNPs were genome-wide significant for 25(OH)D levels, and all four SNPs lay in, or near, genes strongly implicated in separate mechanisms influencing 25(OH)D. The authors found out that the count of the 25(OH)D-decreasing alleles across these four SNPs was strongly associated with a lower 25(OH)D level. Other recent perspectives [95] confirmed the research by Ahn et al. [93]; it seems that there are strong links between the 25(OH)D levels and the genotyping of CYP2R1- and NAD-synthetase (NADSYN1-SNPs) in MS patients. The analysis revealed lower 25(OH)D concentrations in MS patients and an association of rs10766197 CYP2R1 SNP with MS risk. After stratifying the MS patients according to gender, the authors [95] found that the minor allele A of rs10766197 had a higher frequency in men in comparison with the women affected by MS. Additionally, the presence of allele A in men was associated with disease progression, assessed by EDSS and Multiple Sclerosis Severity Score (MSSS) scores [96]. The results are not univocal at all; a recent study focussed on VDR polymorphisms (Fok-I, Bsm-I, Taq-I, and Apa-I) that were genotyped by a polymerase chain reaction (PCR), followed by the restriction fragment length polymorphism (RFLP) analyses in both groups, and the serum 25(OH) D levels were determined in the MS patients by high-performance liquid chromatography (HPLC). The distribution of genotype and allele frequencies of the four VDR polymorphisms did not differ significantly between the MS patients and healthy controls, and were unrelated to the forms and the course of MS. Low serum levels of 25(OH) D were observed in MS patients, but no association was observed between the VDR and 25(OH) D levels, except for Fok-I. Moreover, the MS patients with the *FF* and *Ff* genotype had a significantly lower serum level of 25(OH) D [92]. Moreover, further studies are necessary to develop potential relationships between the genome-wide association studies (GWAS) and gene-candidate studies for determining the influence of specific genetic polymorphisms of the vitamin D metabolites on the 25(OH) D levels, and the susceptibility to MS and to vitamin D supplementation efficacy in MS.

3. Vitamin D Deficiencies and Ischemic Stroke

Stroke is the leading cause of significant long-term disability all over the world, and is an enormous source of global disease burden. Ischemic stroke recognizes a heterogeneous etiology, caused by not modifiable risk factors (genetic, age, and sex), and modifiable risk factors, like hypertension, diabetes mellitus (DM), dyslipidemia, sedentary lifestyle, and smoking [125].

Vitamin D deficiency is found to increase the risk of vascular disease and ischemic stroke in healthy subjects; the risk is higher for ischemic stroke than for hemorrhagic ones. Moreover, vitamin D deficiency is associated with other contributing factors for ischemic stroke (i.e., hypertension, hyperlipidemia, diabetes mellitus, and ischemic heart disease). In a stroke, vitamin D deficiency might relate with higher disease severity and adverse outcomes, including death; moreover, hypovitaminosis D is independently associated with larger ischemic infarct volume [126]; finally, vitamin D deficiency is related to slower recovery after stroke. Moreover, recently, it has been found [125,126] that lower concentrations of 25(OH) D were associated with a higher risk of incident stroke in models adjusted for age, race, age and race interaction, and sex. The magnitude and strength of the associations were unchanged after the adjustment for the season of blood draw; systolic blood pressure; BMI; diabetes; current cigarette smoking; atrial fibrillation; and use of anti-hypertensive medications, aspirin, and statins. In their work, no statistically significant differences in the association of lower 25(OH) D with a higher risk of incident stroke were observed in black subjects when compared with white subjects. Vitamin D can inhibit the development of thrombosis, which may provide a rational explanation for the relationship between vitamin D and ischemic stroke. Nevertheless, vitamin D might induce hemorrhagic stroke through other mechanisms, such as inflammation and endothelium shear stress. Even less is known regarding the relationship between vitamin D deficiency and other cerebrovascular diseases, like vessel dissection. Vianello et al. [127] reported that in acute aortic dissection (AAD), hypovitaminosis D is not associated with changes in bone-related metabolic pathways, but is inversely related to osteocalcin, which could be an exciting molecule that is able to mediate the effect of an inadequate 25(OH) D level at vascular level.

Moderate to strong associations between lower serum 25(OH)D concentrations and stroke were identified in different analytic approaches, even after controlling for traditional demographic and lifestyle covariates. Such associations were most evident among young females, younger than 50 years. The mechanisms behind the associations between vitamin D and cerebrovascular and cardiologic profiles have been widely examined in both animal and human studies. Accumulating evidence has shown adverse regulatory effects of vitamin D on the renin-angiotensin system. Renin expression was significantly increased among the vitamin D receptor knockout mice and suppressed among the wild-type mice after being injected with 1,25$(OH)_2$D. The treatment of vitamin D in rats may lead to increased endothelium-dependent vascular relaxation and the inhibition of vascular smooth muscle cell growth and proliferation. Vitamin D supplementation in human subjects may contribute to improved insulin sensitivity and beta-cell function, as well as lower levels of inflammatory markers [128–130].

Moreover, vitamin D deficiency has been shown in several pathologies related to higher incidence of stroke. Shah Sanket et al. reported that a vitamin D deficiency was observed in a significant number of patients with chronic obstructive pulmonary disease (COPD), and in more than half of the study subjects there is an increasing frequency across the combined COPD class of cardiovascular and cerebrovascular disease [130]. Moreover, the stroke patients with enough vitamin D had more favorable outcomes, including improved muscle strength and bone density. Manouchehri et al. [131] showed that a vitamin D deficiency had an increased risk of ischemic stroke by nearly seven-fold compared to the controls. They reported a 13-fold increase in the risk of large vessel stroke, and a 4.37-folded increase for the small vessel stroke was observed. The risk of stroke increases with a concomitant deficit of vitamin D, vitamin B12, and homocysteine. Serum homocysteine, vitamin B12, and vitamin D levels are associated with baseline first-ever stroke severity, but also contribute, to some extent, to its prognosis in the early period after stroke. The early detection and management of these laboratory parameters may contribute both to primary and to secondary stroke prevention. Hyperhomocysteinemia increases the likelihood of stroke and is mostly dependent on folic acid (vitamin B9), vitamin B12, and vitamin B6 serum levels. Vitamin B12 deficiency can be detected in 10–40% of the general population and may contribute to stroke and cognitive decline. The status of homocysteine, vitamin B12, and vitamin D can go further to assess the importance of these correctable factors during the functional recovery after stroke.

The patients with a low level of serum vitamin D at the onset of the stroke showed more severe disability [126]. Qiu et al. [132] also reported a strict association between lower serum levels of 25(OH) D, and the stroke recurrence and stroke mortality at 24 months. Also, the inverse association between serum 25(OH) D levels and functional outcome in patients with acute ischemic stroke had been reported. Mortality in stroke patients is higher for those subjects <75 years old with a low serum 25(OH) D level at stroke onset [133–135]. Few studies have also reported vitamin D deficiency after a stroke. The mean level of 25(OH) D was lower in the subacute and chronic patients than in the healthy controls; furthermore, the level of 25(OH)D was lower in the patients with a longer duration of illness after stroke, for one month. These data suggest that it might be explained by an exhaustion of vitamin D, stored before stroke onset, and insufficient synthesis after stroke. Finally, the patients with an independent gait have higher levels of vitamin D than the immobilized patients. Restricted outdoor activity may have affected the synthesis of vitamin D after the stroke and resulted in a vitamin D deficiency.

The pathophysiology of stroke is quite complex and still not completely understood. Cerebral ischemic damage is due to the activation of several inflammatory events, including the infiltration of circulating immune cells and the activation of microglia, astrocytes, and endothelial cells [136]. In stroke individuals, the mechanism involved in vessel disease, mediated by a vitamin D deficit, might consist of a release of atherogenic pro-inflammatory cytokines, which foster atherosclerotic vascular changes and might induce plaque instability [137,138]. Vitamin D plays an additional role for the regulation of the inflammation process, through prostaglandin inhibition, reduction of mitogen-activated protein kinase (MAPK), and by reducing the expression of the nuclear factor kappa B (NF-κB) pathways [41,139]. Moreover, the down-regulation of pro-inflammatory cytokines, such as tumor necrosis factor (TNF)-α, interleukin (IL)-6, IL-12, and interferon (IFN)-γ, and the up-regulation of anti-inflammatory T regulatory (Treg) and Th2 cells and their cytokines have been reported [140,141]. Thus, the deficit of vitamin D is responsible for endothelial dysfunction [142] and is considered an independent risk factor for the occurrence of acute ischemic stroke [143,144]. As previously reported, VDD is strictly associated with higher levels of high sensitivity C-reactive protein (hsCRP), remarking the anti-inflammatory activities of vitamin D, including the inhibition of IL-6 synthesis by monocytes. CRP acts on endothelial cells inducing tissue factor expression, and promotes smooth muscle and endothelial cell proliferation [145]. Moreover, CRP increases the plasminogen activator inhibitor–1 expression [146] and induces several inflammatory genes via NF-κB activation in human endothelial cells [147]. Usually, vitamin D deficiency in stroke patients preceded stroke, and the prevalence of vitamin D deficiency is more evident in stroke patients than general medical patients. On the other hand, vitamin D supplementation in post-stroke patients may play a role in the prevention of recurrent stroke and improves the functional outcome after stroke [147–150].

Zhao-Nan Wei reported that a vitamin D deficiency is associated with a 3.2-fold increased risk of poor functional outcome events. The adjustment for established cardiovascular risk factors, including glucose level, age, and National Institute of Health Stroke Scale (NIHSS) score, did not attenuate this association. For the vitamin D deficiency, the adjusted risk of mortality increased by 290% [151]. A high dose oral vitamin D supplementation produced a short-term improvement in the endothelial function in stroke patients, with a better management of blood hypertension. Moreover, a possible cardiovascular protective role of vitamin D has been proposed, in reducing the mortality risk in patients with renal failure.

A meta-analysis of 50 RCTs of supplemental vitamin D, administered for a median of two years, involving predominantly senior women who were mainly in institutions and dependent care, showed that vitamin D decreased mortality [152]. Moreover, vitamin D3 (cholecalciferol) has been shown to decrease mortality significantly. Gupta et al. [152], in a randomized controlled open-label trial, found that patients with acute ischaemic stroke that received vitamin D and calcium supplementation, along with the usual care, compared with those receiving usual care alone, presented a higher probability of survival, achieving a better outcome at six months compared to the controls [153]. Concerning stroke, the VITamin D and Omega-3 triaL (VITAL) studied the effect of supplementation on the total cancer and major cardiovascular events (a composite of myocardial stroke, and death due to cardiovascular events), thus reporting significant effects only on a reduction of bone fractures [154,155]. Similarly, the benefit of vitamin D supplementation for stroke-related depressive symptoms is still being debated [156]. If vitamin D contributes to post-stroke recovery by pathophysiological mechanisms that should still be elucidated (some could be related to a reduction in the volume of the cerebral infarct and to neuroprotective properties), vitamin D supplementation could bring the hope of a benefit that is not known yet.

In summary, the precise relationship between vitamin D and stroke is still unclear, a revision of the data suggests that vitamin D status is associated with ischemic stroke and with the injury volume. The vitamin D levels should be measured in all stroke patients and should be considered as an independent stroke risk factor. The supplementation of vitamin D could be considered as a fundamental part of stroke therapy, but new studies should be done.

4. Vitamin D Deficiency and Neurodegenerative Diseases

Different important studies have implicated amyloid beta accumulation, hyperphosphorylation of tau, oxidative stress, mitochondrial dysfunction, and inflammation as the major responsible factors for a neurodegenerative process, which underlies Alzheimer's disease (AD) [157,158]. Nevertheless, the calcium excitotoxic hypothesis and glutamate currents theories can support and amplify the Alzheimer's cascade of events [159]. Moreover, many doubts still merge, especially for sporadic AD cases pathogenesis. It has been established that the etiology of the sporadic AD might involve multiple gene-environment relationships, and probably many epigenetic mechanisms [158,160]. The most debated aspects are those concerning the reasons for Abeta accumulation and the tauopathy consequences in the aging brain being seriously possible, and the relationship between their accumulation and various environmental risk factors, which the brain gathers throughout its life. Epigenetic modifications can act as first hits, with a consequence that remains latent for many years, until a second hit (probably determined by metabolic factors, i.e., altered nutrition, pro-inflammatory cytokines, and aging by itself) can promote the degenerative progression [161]. As a result of these premises, VDR, the major effector of vitamin D, polymorphisms have been studied in AD [162]. It has been demonstrated that there is a link between the altered gene expression of VDR and 1,25MARRS (membrane-associated rapid response steroid-binding); this association endorses the less active employment of vitamin D inside neurons, and lets them be more prone to degeneration [163]. Brewer et al. [163] and confirmed by Thibault et al. [164] recognized that cultured hippocampal cells treated with adequate concentrations of VDH (1–100 nM) were protected against excitotoxic insults, probably because of a modulation of L-type voltage-sensitive calcium channels, whose increase has been documented in hippocampus aged cells [165], and the aged long-term cultured hippocampus cells [166]. VDH down-regulates mRNA expression for different subunits of L-type voltage-sensitive calcium channels. Consequently, VDH has a fundamental role in the homeostasis of calcium-mediated activities [164], such as neuronal death and apoptosis. The $VDR^{-/-}$ knock-out model shows a higher sensitivity to neuro-degeneration, with a rapid increase of calcium currents and neural death [166,167]. Many different VDR polymorphisms have been described as increasing the susceptibility to AD [168], mainly due to the altered expression of neurotrophins. Genome analyses, transcriptomics, and proteomics have pointed out the role of VDR polymorphism in late-onset AD susceptibility [162]. In fact, even in animal models, vitamin D seems to interfere with cognitive functions, even in other ways, probably through its different polymorphic gene expression of VDR [26]. It seems, for instance, that Bsm I and Taq I altered carriers are more prone to manifest memory and cognitive dysfunctions, as well as a vitamin D defect; on the contrary, the APA-I haplotype is associated with an increased risk of fractures, but not memory alterations [169]. Therefore, in line with Buell and Dawson-Hughes [169], calcium concentrations are not likely to vary in the different haplotypes, indicating a protective effect on the brain, beyond the calcium homeostasis. Thus, in the Alzheimer disease culture models, VDH stimulates the amyloid plaques [170,171], supporting the phagocytosis induced by macrophages of a soluble amyloid beta protein [171,172], and reduces the inflammation response induced by amyloid deposition [21]. Lipopolysaccharide-induced levels of mRNA encoding for macrophage colony stimulating factors and tumor necrosis factors in cultured astrocytes are partially reduced after vitamin D treatment [21]. Additionally, vitamin D has neuroprotective properties against glutamate toxicity [173]. It inhibits the synthesis of inducible nitric oxide synthase and regulates the gamma-glutamyl transpeptidase, fundamental in the metabolism of glutathione [174]. Furthermore, vitamin D enhances the protein phosphatase 2A activity, modulating the redox state, and thus reducing the age-related tau hyperphosphorylation, limiting the cascade of neuronal dying back and the promotions of collateral inflammatory potentiation [175]. To summarize, it seems that vitamin D acts in the brain, through the regulation of NGF and neurotransmitters, regulating calcium homeostasis, promoting anti-inflammatory responses, interfering with amyloid beta metabolism, and implementing a brain oxidative response. On the contrary, clinical practice does not give univocal results. A vitamin D deficit has been widely detected in the frail old population [176,177], and calcium homeostasis is heavily lowered in neurodegenerative pathologies, such as Alzheimer disease [177,178]. In a mild cognitive impairment population, not including Alzheimer disease, a low level of vitamin D was reported [179]. Nevertheless, the vitamin D implementation in clinical practice does not give univocal results. A seven-year follow-up study confirmed that a larger intake of vitamin D is associated with a lower risk of developing AD in normal aging women [180,181]. Some recent works have evidenced that the combined effect of vitamin D and docosahexaenoic acid can enhance the neural protection towards the different effects of beta-amyloid deposition [182,183], and a six-month trial determined that the patient obtains better results, with even limited effects, when the memantine was prescribed in association with vitamin D, rather than alone, in the AD patients [182]. On the other hand, two studies showed the opposite results [183,184]. Even though many different studies are needed to demonstrate a definite role in the real clinical practice of the supplementation of vitamin D, many questions remain without a proper answer, such as:

1. When should the implementation begin?
2. Is it a possible preventive therapy for reducing the cascade of events of the AD?
3. Should it be considered as one of the multifactor agents (along with folate, vitamin B12, and antioxidant substances) that can procrastinate the AD second hit process?

4.1. Vascular Dementia

Emergent evidence from experimental and clinical studies suggests that vitamin D may be a causal effect for neurodegeneration, concerning vascular dementia, supporting the underlying/concomitant atherosclerotic pathology [185]. Some studies link the vitamin defect to an increased risk of hypertension, diabetes, congestive heart failure, myocardial infarction, and stroke [186]. Moreover, some very recent studies link it to small vessel disease and vascular dementia as well [187,188]. The vitamin D receptors are hugely expressed by the endothelial cells, and their activation induces the promotion towards the maturation of immature cells, via Vasoactive Endothelium derived Growth Factor (VEGF) [189]. The vitamin D receptor gene is up-regulated during inflammation in endothelial cells [190–192], and the vitamin D analogs protect against advanced glycation products derived insults [193]. Enriched vitamin D diet models promote an anti-lymphoproliferative effect on the endothelium and a diminished response to inflammatory cytokines [194,195]. Moreover, as previously described, vitamin D regulates the expression of 74 genes and 36 proteins, connected with the correct development of the cytoskeleton and exerting a regulation on post-transcriptional controls for L-type voltage-sensitive calcium channels [196,197]. All of the effects of vitamin D on the vascular system link it to vascular dementia in many different ways, such as: epidemiological [198], based on vascular pressure control [191], based on biological properties of vitamin D, above described [199], or simply considering vitamin D deficiency as a risk-modifiable factor [170,200,201]. It seems quite interesting that the three works that link the vitamin D defect to small vessel disease-related dementia [188,189] stand on two axiomatic biological properties, the anti-oxidative capacity of vitamin D (therefore a loss of protection against Reactive Oxygene Species (ROS), whenever it lacks), and the control of the smooth vessel, which is fundamental for auto-regulation in brain circulation. Many studies evidenced an excess of superoxide by Nicotinamide Adenine Dinucleotide Phosphate Hydrogen (NADPH) oxidase in small vessel disease [202]. This causes an increase of ROS, indirectly evidenced by a hyper-expression of the Nitrogen Oxide (NOX) 2 and NOX 4 oxidase isoforms [202,203]; ROS induced damage is one of the triggers for apoptosis. In vitro, vitamin D down-regulates the activity of NF-κB activity [204] and stimulates the anti-inflammatory cytokines [205]. Additionally, vitamin D-binding proteins are more evident in proximity to endothelium injury [206], inhibiting the expression of Matrix Metalloproteinase (MMP-2, MMP-9), and of the endothelium growth factor [207]; they probably diminish the activity of the platelet-derived growth factor, conversely up-regulating thrombomodulin [208,209]. The second study, entirely dedicated to small vessel disease and vitamin D [198], lights some shadows in a fascinating problem; it presents a public association between bone small vessel disease and osteoporosis. Authors hypothesize a common method of alteration, in the peripheral autonomous nervous system, which deteriorates the small-bone vessels as well as brain vessels [210]. The first and the third study on the topic [188,189], starting from two different perspectives have some common points. Chung et al. [188] demonstrated that vitamin D is inversely associated with lacunes, white matter hyperintensities, and deep micro-bleeding in the deep white matter, not elsewhere, suggesting a high impact on small vessel disease. Moretti et al. [198] hypothesized that vitamin D might act on the altered control of cerebral blood flow (CBF) [211,212] and in the distorted neurovascular coupling system [213,214], both heavily impaired in small vessel dementia. Intracerebral calcium, intimately regulated by vitamin D, interferes with the vessel activation. Vessel relaxation is heavily influenced by ATP-sensitive potassium channels (delayed rectifier and inward rectifier potassium channel), but also by calcium-activated potassium channels [215,216]. Mediated by cAMP, calcium-activated-potassium channels seem to be involved in the negative "feedback system to regulate vascular tone" [215]. It seems that in atherosclerosis models, there is a major impairment of calcium-activated potassium channels in mainstream vessels [215]. On the other hand, the neurovascular coupling system (smooth vascular cells, neurons, and astrocytes) seems to be intimately regulated by vitamin D, which is determinant for the glutamate release. Glutamate passes from the synapse, activating Nicotinamide Adenine Dinucleotide Phosphate Hydrogen- Receptors (NMDAR) in the neurons and metabotropic glutamate receptors in the astrocytes [214]. Moreover, by interfering with the calcium influx, vitamin D indirectly mediates the neural nitric oxide synthase. NO activates phospholipase A2 in the astrocytes, enabling the prostaglandin cascade, which widens the arteries. The presence of vitamin D increases, moreover, acetylcholine, and VIP, which potentiates the mechanism. Low levels of vitamin D might, therefore, interfere with smooth cells control, with NO and neuropeptides synthesis, and with defective neurovascular coupling, leading to some aspects of small vessel disease. There are very few the studies concerning vitamin D supplementation in vascular dementia.

4.2. Parkinson Disease (PD)

A significant concentration of vitamin D receptors were found in the hippocampus, in the prefrontal cortex–brain, and the substantia nigra [217]. There is evidence of low levels of vitamin D and increased bone turnover markers, such as bone alkaline phosphatase, compared to the controls [218]. All of the non-genomic roles of vitamin D are evident in the PD models [219,220]; there is an active regulation of calcium inside the neurons and astrocytes; there is a substantial regulation of L-type voltage-sensitive calcium channels; it has been described an induction and promotion of NGF and other growth factors, with a down-regulation of MMP and other inflammatory activity, such as prostaglandins and COX-2 activity; and there is also a reduction of oxidative stress, by interfering with NO production by lipopolysaccharide-stimulated macrophages [221]. There are many data that even relate the vitamin-related genomic factors to PD progression. Increased levels of MHC class II expressions were detected in the monocytes of the cerebrospinal fluid of the PD patients [222], together with Human Leukocyte Antigen Complex- antigen D related (HLA-DR) positive reactive microglia, found in the *substantia nigra* and in nigro-striatal tract of PD patients [223]. Recent evidence demonstrated that vitamin D suppresses the MHC class II antigens [224] and IFN-gamma induced HLA-DR antigen expression in human cells [225]. Additionally, Cytochrome P450 (CYP), and in particular, CYP2D6, which has a polymorphic expression, and which is expressed in neurons and the gut, has a different expression in PD patients; here, it has been found preponderantly as the CYP2D6*4 allele [226]. CYP2D6 acts as a 25-hydroxylase, which can convert vitamin D3 into 25OHD, being the key enzyme to determine a deficiency of vitamin D. In the mouse MPTP treated model (inducing PD phenotype), Singh et al. [225] reported the stable expression of the animal ortholog of CYP2D6, CYP2D22. Very interestingly, the CYP2D loci are located on chromosome 22, where many genes related to PD are segregated [227,228]. It seems surprising that the deletion of chromosome 22q11 was reported to be associated with PD [228], but also with the reduced serum calcium and a reduced level of vitamin D [228].

Moreover, there are three more links between vitamin D and PD. The first one is the so-called Sp1 transcription factor. The protein encoded by this gene is a zinc finger transcription factor that binds to the guanine-cytosine (GC)-rich motifs of many promoters. The encoded protein is involved in many cellular processes, including cell differentiation, cell growth, apoptosis, immune responses, response to DNA damage, and chromatin remodeling. Post-translational modifications, such as phosphorylation, acetylation, glycosylation, and proteolytic processing, significantly affect the activity of this protein, which can be an activator or a repressor. The Sp1 transcriptions factor is a DNA binding protein that mediates the accurate response to oxidative stress in neurons [229,230], controls the expression of the dopamine transporter gene, and of the dopamine receptor gene [231,232]. The link between vitamin D and Sp1 is represented by the fact that many hormones have different binding sites for the transcription factors for Sp1. In fact, two vitamin D-responsive elements (which act by inducing the expression of CYP24 genes, previously described, and 25-OHD-24 hydroxylase) are helped by the synergic activation of Sp1 [229,233]. As Sp1 controls the expression of the dopamine transporter gene within the dopaminergic neurons, VDR conditions and promotes Sp1 trigger gene expression.

The second genomic link factor between vitamin D and PD is represented by Heme oxygenase, a stress protein with anti-oxidant properties. In the healthy brain, its expression is limited to neuroglia [234], whereas it is overexpressed in PD brains, but not in AD patients [235]. In PD brains, Heme oxygenase 1 is overexpressed in astrocytes within the *substantia nigra* and the deteriorated dopaminergic neurons [236]. Entirely unpredicted, calcitriol seems able to delay the effect of Heme oxygenase, reducing the glial fibrillary immunoreactivity [237].

Finally, vitamin D seems to interfere with the activity of Poly (ADP-Ribose) Polymerase-1, also called PARP1. It is a stress protein, which can, however, promote neuronal death. In fact, there is an overexpression of PARP1 in the *substantia nigra* of PD patients [238]; increased levels of vitamin D down regulate the PARP-1 expression, probably mediated by a diminishment of microglial activation [239]. All of these aspects considered in the clinical trials on vitamin D supplementation in Parkinson's disease have been carried out. Although some data demonstrated that low levels of vitamin D might influence the speed of the disease, the supplementation of vitamin D did not modify the disease outcomes. That conclusion probably lies in a clinical time of supplementation, far from the initial ones of labs models.

5. Conclusions

Accumulating evidence shows that vitamin D is important for accurate brain functioning. Moreover, it is important to note that many important neurological diseases are related to low levels of vitamin D. These expressions are supported by in vivo, in vitro, and in human trials. Unfortunately, at the moment, the results for its supplementation in neurological disorders, in particular concerning data on vitamin supplementation and their progression or eventual real clinical benefits are inconclusive. As such, there is a strong need for randomized clinical trials on neurodegenerative patients and vitamin D supplementation, to optimize time, efficacy, and appropriate monitoring [240,241].

It should be said that vitamin D supplementation might be safe and inexpensive. However, physicians may be uncomfortable recommending larger doses of vitamin D, because of its potential toxicity. The rarity of reports of vitamin D toxicity can be explained, in part, by the kidney's ability to limit the production of active calcitriol. Increased calcitriol levels inhibit parathormone (PTH), causing the calcitriol production in the kidney to decrease. The renal 24-hydroxylase activity further limits the availability of calcitriol by creating inert metabolites of both calcitriol (1,24,25-trihydroxyvitamin D) and calcidiol (24,25-dihydroxyvitamin D). The 24-hydroxylase gene is under the transcriptional control of calcitriol, thereby providing a tight negative feedback.

Concerning vitamin D replacement, several studies have shown that both vitamin D2 and vitamin D3 are effective in maintaining the serum 25(OH)D levels. Both D2 (ergocalciferol) and D3 (cholecalciferol) are available as dietary supplements, and both appear to be effective. A single dose of 50,000 IU of D2 or D3 produces a similar increase in the total 25(OH)D concentration, but the apparent longer half-life of D3 suggests that less frequent dosing may be needed. To replenish the serum 25(OH)D levels in persons with a vitamin D deficiency, one cost-effective regimen is oral ergocalciferol at 50,000 IU per week for eight weeks. The optimal time for rechecking the serum levels after being replenished has not been clearly defined, but the goal is to achieve a minimum level of 30 ng per mL.

Special mention is needed for patients who require tube feeding or parenteral nutrition. In those cases, ergocalciferol capsules containing D2 in oil, which can clog the feeding tube, should not be used. Cholecalciferol capsules and tablets contain D3 in powder form and can be used.

New approaches are emerging in vitamin D deficiency. The combined treatment using bisphosphonates and vitamin D has been suspected to be more effective compared with bisphosphonate or vitamin D alone in the prevention of atherosclerosis. In a recent study, the combination of bisphosphonates and vitamin D has been seen to be safe and effective in systemic lupus erythematosus. Bisphosphonates are expected to inhibit the arterial plaque development and calcification through several mechanisms (mostly inducing decreased levels of inflammatory cytokines and matrix metalloproteinases). Bisphosphonates also decrease a variety of mature vascular cells, which migrate into the vessel walls and injure vascular endothelial cells. Moreover, treatment with statins in combination with bisphosphonates has been shown to be more effective in terms of reducing atherosclerotic plaque, compared with either monotherapy in patients with hypercholesterolemia [242,243].

Reading what the literature has reported, it seems that the supplementation of vitamin D might reduce the risks and improve the pathological features in different neurological conditions, but, because of different and unknown reasons, it seems that its supplementation might not be sufficient to change the outcomes and the disease phenotype. All of this considered, there is a strong need for further research in this field, even to account for the best quality of vitamin implementation.

Author Contributions: R.M. designed the study, supervised the entire project and directly studied neurodegeneration and vitamin D; P.C. revised the manuscript and wrote the vascular paragraphs; M.E.M. wrote the multiple sclerosis paragraph.

Acknowledgments: The authors thank Hellen Davies, for her precious help and assistance.

References

1. Holick, M.F. Vitamin D Deficiency. *N. Engl. J. Med.* **2007**, *357*, 266–281. [CrossRef] [PubMed]
2. Arabi, A.; El Rassi, R.; El-Hajj Fuleihan, G. Hypovitaminosis D in developing countries-prevalence, risk factors and outcomes. *Nat. Rev. Endocrinol.* **2010**, *6*, 550–561. [CrossRef] [PubMed]
3. Prentice, A.; Schoenmakers, I.; Jones, K.; Jarjou, L.A.; Goldberg, G. Vitamin D Deficiency and Its Health Consequences in Africa. *Clin. Rev. Bone Miner. Metab.* **2009**, *7*, 94–106. [CrossRef] [PubMed]
4. Ross, A.C.; Manson, J.E.; Abrams, S.A.; Aloia, J.F.; Brannon, P.M.; Clinton, S.K.; Durazo-Arvizu, R.A.; Gallagher, J.C.; Gallo, R.L.; Jones, G.; et al. The 2011 report on dietary reference intakes for calcium and vitamin D from the Institute of Medicine: What clinicians need to know. *J. Clin. Endocrinol. Metab.* **2011**, *96*, 53–58. [CrossRef] [PubMed]
5. Di Somma, C.; Scarano, E.; Barrea, C.; Zhukouskay, V.V.; Savastano, S.; Mele, C.; Scacchi, M.; Aimaretti, G.; Colao, A.; Marzullo, P. Vitamin D and neurological disease: An endocrine view. *Int. J. Mol. Sci.* **2017**, *18*, 2482. [CrossRef] [PubMed]
6. Yang, L.; Ma, J.; Zhang, X.; Fan, Y.; Wang, L. Protective role of the vitamin D receptor. *Cell. Immunol.* **2012**, *279*, 160–166. [CrossRef] [PubMed]
7. Gominak, S.C. Vitamin D deficiency changes the intestinal microbiome reducing B vitamin production in the gut. The resulting lack of pantothenic acid adversely affects the immune system, producing a "pro-inflammatory" state associated with atherosclerosis and autoimmunity. *Med. Hypotheses* **2016**, *94*, 103–107. [PubMed]
8. Luthold, R.V.; Fernandes, G.R.; Franco-de-Moraes, A.C.; Folchetti, L.G.; Ferreira, S.R. Sandra Roberta G Ferreira. Gut microbiota interactions with the immunomodulatory role of vitamin D in normal individuals. *Metabolism* **2017**, *69*, 76–86. [CrossRef] [PubMed]
9. Tremlett, H.; Bauer, K.C.; Appel-Cresswell, S.; Finlay, B.B.; Waubant, E. The gut microbiome in human neurological disease: A review. *Ann. Neurol.* **2017**, *81*, 369–382. [CrossRef] [PubMed]
10. Holick, M.F.; Chen, T.C. Vitamin D deficiency: A worldwide problem, with health consequences. *Am. J. Clin. Nutr.* **2008**, *87*, 1080S–1086S. [CrossRef] [PubMed]
11. DeLuca, G.C.; Kimball, S.M.; Kolasinski, J.; Ramagopalan, S.V.; Ebers, G.C. Review: The role of vitamin D in nervous system health and disease. *Neuropathol. Appl. Neurobiol.* **2013**, *39*, 458–484. [CrossRef] [PubMed]
12. Wang, L.; Song, Y.; Manson, J.E.; Pilz, S.; März, W.; Michaëlsson, K.; Lundqvist, A.; Jassal, S.K.; Barrett-Connor, E.; Zhang, C.; et al. Circulating 25-hydroxy-vitamin D and risk of cardiovascular disease: A meta-analysis of prospective studies. *Circ. Cardiovasc. Qual. Outcomes* **2012**, *5*, 819–829. [CrossRef] [PubMed]
13. Brondum-Jacobsen, P.; Nordestgaard, B.G.; Schnohr, P.; Benn, M. 25-Hydroxyvitamin D and symptomatic ischemic stroke: An original study and meta-analysis. *Ann. Neurol.* **2013**, *73*, 38–47. [CrossRef] [PubMed]

14. Chowdhury, R.; Stevens, S.; Ward, H.; Chowdhury, S.; Sajjad, A.; Franco, O.H. Circulating vitamin D, calcium and risk of cerebrovascular disease: A systematic review and meta-analysis. *Eur. J. Epidemiol.* **2012**, *27*, 581–591. [CrossRef] [PubMed]
15. Fleet, J.C. Rapid, membrane-initiated actions of 1,25 dihydroxyvitamin D: What are they and what do they mean? *J. Nutr.* **2004**, *134*, 3215–3218. [CrossRef] [PubMed]
16. Veenstra, T.D.; Prufer, K.; Koenigsberger, C.; Brimijoin, S.W.; Grande, J.P.; Kumar, R. 1,25-Dihydroxyvitamin D3 receptors in the central nervous system of the rat embryo. *Brain Res.* **2005**, *804*, 193–205. [CrossRef]
17. Annweiler, C.; Montero-Odasso, M.; Hachinski, V.; Seshadri, S.; Bartha, R.; Beauchet, O. Vitamin D concentration and lateral cerebral ventricle volume in older adults. *Mol. Nutr. Food Res.* **2013**, *57*, 267–276. [CrossRef] [PubMed]
18. Brown, J.I.; Bianco, J.; McGrath, J.; Eyles, D.W. 1,25-Dihydroxyvitamin D3 induces nerve growth factor, promotes neurite outgrowth and inhibits mitosis in embryonic rat hippocampal neurons. *Neurosci. Lett.* **2003**, *343*, 139–143. [CrossRef]
19. Baksi, S.N.; Hughes, M.J. Chronic vitamin D deficiency in the weanling rat alters catecholamine metabolism in the cortex. *Brain Res.* **1982**, *242*, 387–390. [CrossRef]
20. Puchacz, E.; Stumpf, W.E.; Stachowiak, E.K.; Stachowiak, M.K. Vitamin D increases expression of the tyrosine hydroxylase gene in adrenal medullary cells. *Mol. Brain Res.* **1996**, *36*, 193–196. [CrossRef]
21. Garcion, E.; Wion-Barbot, N.; Montero-Menei, C.N.; Berger, F.; Wion, D. New clues about vitamin D functions in the nervous system. *Trends Endocrinol. Metab.* **2002**, *13*, 100–105. [CrossRef]
22. Minasyan, A.; Keisala, T.; Lou, Y.R.; Kalueff, A.V.; Tuohimaa, P. Neophobia, sensory and cognitive functions, and hedonic responses in vitamin D receptor mutant mice. *J. Steroid Biochem. Mol. Biol.* **2007**, *104*, 274–280. [CrossRef] [PubMed]
23. Burne, T.H.J.; Johnston, A.N.B.; McGrath, J.J.; MacKay-Sim, A. Swimming behavior and post-swimming activity in Vitamin D receptor knockout mice. *Brain Res. Bull.* **2006**, *69*, 74–78. [CrossRef] [PubMed]
24. Gezen-Ak, D.; Dursun, E.; Yilmazer, S. The effects of vitamin D receptor silencing on the expression of LVSCC-A1C and LVSCC-A1D and the release of NGF in cortical neurons. *PLoS ONE* **2011**, *6*, e17553. [CrossRef] [PubMed]
25. Eyles, D.W.; Liu, P.Y.; Josh, P.; Cui, X. Intracellular distribution of the of the vitamin D receptor in the brain. A comparison with classical target tissues and redistribution with development. *Neuroscience* **2014**, *268*, 1–9. [CrossRef] [PubMed]
26. Becker, A.; Eyles, D.W.; McGarth, J.J.; Grecksc, G. Transient prenatal vitamin D deficiency is associated with subtle alterations in learning and memory functions in adult rats. *Behav. Brain Res.* **2005**, *161*, 306–312. [CrossRef] [PubMed]
27. Byrne, J.H.; Voogt, M.; Turner, K.M.; Eyles, D.W.; McGrath, J.J.; Burne, T.H. The impact of adult vitamin D deficiency on behavior and brain function in male Sprague-Dawley rats. *PLoS ONE* **2013**, *8*, e71593. [CrossRef] [PubMed]
28. Achiron, A.; Gurevich, M.; Magalashvili, D.; Kishner, I.; Dolev, M.; Mandel, M. Understanding autoimmune mechanisms in multiple sclerosis using gene expression microarrays: Treatment effect and cytokine-related pathways. *Clin. Dev. Immunol.* **2004**, *11*, 299–305. [CrossRef] [PubMed]
29. Bhalla, A.K.; Amento, E.P.; Clemens, T.L.; Holick, M.F.; Krane, S.M. Specific high-affinity receptors for 1,25-dihydroxyvitamin D3 in human peripheral blood mononuclear cells: Presence in monocytes and induction in T lymphocytes following activation. *J. Clin. Endocrinol. Metab.* **1983**, *57*, 1308–1310. [CrossRef] [PubMed]
30. Veldman, C.M.; Cantorna, M.T.; DeLuca, H.F. Expression of 1,25-dihydroxyvitamin D3 receptor in the immune system. *Arch. Biochem. Biophys.* **2000**, *374*, 334–338. [CrossRef] [PubMed]
31. Chun, R.F.; Liu, P.T.; Modlin, R.L.; Adams, J.S.; Hewison, M. Impact of vitamin D on immune function: Lessons learned from genome-wide analysis. *Front. Physiol.* **2014**, *5*, 151. [CrossRef] [PubMed]
32. Gottfried, E.; Rehli, M.; Hahn, J.; Holler, E.; Andreesen, R.; Kreutz, M. Monocyte-derived cells express CYP27A1 and convert vitamin D3 into its active metab-olite. *Biochem. Biophys. Res. Commun.* **2006**, *349*, 209–213. [CrossRef] [PubMed]
33. Mora, J.; Iwata, M.; von Andrian, U. Vitamin effects on the immune system: Vitamins A and D take centre stage. *Nat. Rev. Immunol.* **2008**, *8*, 685–698. [CrossRef] [PubMed]
34. Lips, P. Vitamin D physiology. *Prog. Biophys. Mol. Biol.* **2006**, *92*, 4–8. [CrossRef] [PubMed]

35. Martineau, A.R.; Wilkinson, K.A.; Newton, S.M.; Floto, R.A.; Norman, A.W.; Skolimowska, K.; Davidson, R.N.; Sørensen, O.E.; Kampmann, B.; Griffiths, C.J.; et al. IFN-gamma- and TNF-independent vitamin D-inducible human suppression of mycobacteria: The role of cathelicidin LL-37. *J. Immunol.* **2007**, *178*, 7190–7198. [CrossRef] [PubMed]
36. Penna, G.; Adorini, L. 1 Alpha, 25-dihydroxyvitamin D3 inhibits differentiation, maturation, activation, and survival of dendritic cells leading to impaired alloreactive T cell activation. *J. Immunol.* **2000**, *164*, 2405–2411. [CrossRef] [PubMed]
37. Garcion, E.; Nataf, S.; Berod, A.; Darcy, F.; Brachet, P. 1,25-Dihydroxyvitamin D3 inhibits the expression of inducible nitric oxide synthase in rat central nervous system during experimental allergic encephalomyelitis. *Brain Res. Mol. Brain Res.* **1997**, *45*, 255–267. [CrossRef]
38. Yu, S.; Cantorna, M.T. The vitamin D receptor is required for iNKT cell development. *Proc. Natl. Acad. Sci. USA* **2008**, *105*, 5207–5212. [CrossRef] [PubMed]
39. Van Etten, E.; Mathieu, C. Immunoregulation by 1,25-dihydroxyvitamin D3: Basic concepts. *J. Steroid Biochem. Mol. Biol.* **2005**, *97*, 93–101. [CrossRef] [PubMed]
40. Chen, S.; Sims, G.P.; Chen, X.X.; Gu, Y.Y.; Chen, S.; Lipsky, P.E. Modulatory effects of 1,25-dihydroxyvitamin D3 on human B cell differentiation. *J. Immunol.* **2007**, *179*, 1634–1647. [CrossRef] [PubMed]
41. Boonstra, A.; Barrat, F.J.; Crain, C.; Heath, V.L.; Savelkoul, H.F.; O'Garra, A. 1α,25-Dihydroxyvitamin D3 has a direct effect on naive CD4(+) T cells to enhance the development of Th2 cells. *J. Immunol.* **2001**, *167*, 4974–4980. [CrossRef] [PubMed]
42. Smolders, J.; Thewissen, M.; Peelen, E.; Menheere, P.; Cohen Tervaert, T.W.; Hupperts, R.; Hupperts, R. Vitamin D status is positively correlated with regulatory T cell function in patients with multiple sclerosis. *PLoS ONE* **2009**, *4*, e6635. [CrossRef] [PubMed]
43. Smolders, J.; Menheere, P.; Thewissen, M.; Peelen, E.; Cohen Tervaert, J.W.; Hupperts, R.; Damoiseaux, J. Regulatory T cell function correlates with serum 25-hydroxyvitamin D, but not with 1, 25-dihydroxyvita-min D, parathyroid hormone and calcium levels in patients with relapsing remitting multiple sclerosis. *J. Steroid Biochem. Mol. Biol.* **2010**, *121*, 243–246. [CrossRef] [PubMed]
44. Burton, J.M.; Kimball, S.; Vieth, R.; Bar-Or, A.; Dosch, H.M.; Cheung, R.; Gagne, D.; D'Souza, C.; Ursell, M.; O'Connor, P. A phase I/II dose-escalation trial of vitamin D3 and calcium in multiple sclerosis. *Neurology* **2010**, *74*, 1852–1859. [CrossRef] [PubMed]
45. Mahon, B.D.; Gordon, S.A.; Cruz, J.; Cosman, F.; Cantorna, M.T. Cytokine profile in patients with multiple sclerosis following vitamin D supplementation. *J. Neuroimmunol.* **2003**, *134*, 128–132. [CrossRef]
46. Kotter, M.R.; Li, W.W.; Zhao, C.; Franklin, R.J.M. Myelin impairs CNS remyelination by inhibiting oligodendrocyte precursor cell differentiation. *J. Neurosci.* **2006**, *26*, 328–332. [CrossRef] [PubMed]
47. Newmark, H.L.; Newmark, J. Vitamin D and Parkinson's disease—A hypothesis. *Mov. Disord.* **2007**, *22*, 461–468. [CrossRef] [PubMed]
48. Baas, D.; Prüfer, K.; Ittel, M.E.; Kuchler-Bopp, S.; Labourdette, G.; Sarliève, L.L.; Brachet, P. Rat oligodendrocytes express the vitamin D(3) receptor and respond to 1,25-dihydroxyvitamin D(3). *Glia* **2000**, *31*, 59–68. [CrossRef]
49. Eyles, D.W.; Smith, S.; Kinobe, R.; Hewison, M.; McGrath, J.J. Distribution of the vitamin D receptor and 1-hydroxylase in human brain. *J. Chem. Neuroanat.* **2005**, *29*, 21–30. [CrossRef] [PubMed]
50. Lassmann, H.; Bruck, W.; Lucchinetti, C.; Rodriguez, M. Remyelination in multiple sclerosis. *Mult. Scler.* **1997**, *3*, 33–136. [CrossRef] [PubMed]
51. Patrikios, P.; Stadelmann, C.; Kutzelnigg, A.; Rauschka, H.; Schmidbauer, M.; Laursen, H.; Sorensen, P.S.; Brück, W.; Lucchinetti, C.; Lassmann, H. Remyelination is extensive in a subset of multiple sclerosis patients. *Brain* **2006**, *129*, 3165–3172. [CrossRef] [PubMed]
52. Bruck, W.; Bitsch, A.; Kolenda, H.; Bruck, Y.; Stiefel, M.; Lassmann, H. Inflammatory central nervous system demyelination: Correlation of magnetic resonance imaging findings with lesion pathology. *Neurology* **1997**, *42*, 783–793. [CrossRef] [PubMed]
53. Franklin, R.J.; Ffrench-Constant, C.; Edgar, J.M.; Smith, K.J. Neuroprotection and repair in multiple sclerosis. *Nat. Rev. Neurol.* **2012**, *8*, 624–634. [CrossRef] [PubMed]
54. Ludwin, S.K.; Maitland, M. Long-term remyelination fails to reconstitute normal thickness of central myelin sheaths. *J. Neurol. Sci.* **1984**, *64*, 193–198. [CrossRef]
55. Hanafy, K.A.; Sloane, J.A. Regulation of remyelination in multiple sclerosis. *FEBS Lett.* **2011**, *585*, 3821–3828. [CrossRef] [PubMed]

56. Pluchino, S.; Zanotti, L.; Brini, E.; Ferrari, S.; Martino, G. Regeneration and repair in multiple sclerosis: The role of cell transplantation. *Neurosci. Lett.* **2009**, *456*, 101–106. [CrossRef] [PubMed]
57. Fancy, S.P.; Kotter, M.R.; Harrington, E.P.; Huang, J.K.; Zhao, C.; Rowitch, D.H.; Franklin, R.J. Overcoming remyelination failure in multiple sclerosis and other myelin disorders. *Exp. Neurol.* **2010**, *225*, 18–23. [CrossRef] [PubMed]
58. De la Fuente, A.G.; Errea, O.; van Wijngaarden, P.; Gonzalez, G.A.; Kerninon, C.; Jarjour, A.A.; Lewis, H.J.; Jones, C.A.; Nait-Oumesmar, B.; Zhao, C.; et al. Vitamin D receptor-retinoid X receptor heterodimer signaling regulates oligodendrocyte progenitor cell differentiation. *J. Cell Biol.* **2015**, *211*, 975–985. [CrossRef] [PubMed]
59. Shirazi, H.A.; Rasouli, J.; Ciric, B.; Rostami, A.; Zhang, G.X. 1,25-Dihydroxyvitamin D3 enhances neural stem cell proliferation and oligodendrocyte differentiation. *Exp. Mol. Pathol.* **2015**, *98*, 240–245. [CrossRef] [PubMed]
60. Ferguson, B.; Matyszak, M.K.; Esiri, M.M.; Perry, V.H. Axonal damage in acute multiple sclerosis lesions. *Brain* **1997**, *120*, 393–399. [CrossRef] [PubMed]
61. Hayes, C.E. Vitamin D: A natural inhibitor of multiple sclerosis. *Proc. Nutr. Soc.* **2000**, *59*, 531–535. [CrossRef] [PubMed]
62. Swank, R.; Lerstad, O.; Strøm, A.; Backer, J. Multiple Sclerosis in Rural Norway. *N. Eng. J. Med.* **1952**, *246*, 721–728. [CrossRef]
63. Simpson, S.; Blizzard, L.; Otahal, P.; van der Mei, I.; Taylor, B. Latitude is significantly associated with the prevalence of multiple sclerosis: A meta-analysis. *J. Neurol. Neurosurg. Psychiatry* **2011**, *82*, 1132–1141. [CrossRef] [PubMed]
64. Westlund, K. Distribution and mortality time trend of multiple sclerosis and some other diseases in Norway. *Acta Neurol. Scand.* **1970**, *46*, 455–483. [CrossRef] [PubMed]
65. Baarnhielm, M.; Olsson, T.; Alfredsson, L. Fatty fish intake is associated with decreased occurrence of multiple sclerosis. *Mult. Scler.* **2014**, *20*, 726–732. [CrossRef] [PubMed]
66. Kurtzke, J.; Beebe, G.; Norman, J. Epidemiology of multiple sclerosis in US veterans: III. Migration and the risk of MIS. *Neurology* **1985**, *35*, 672. [CrossRef] [PubMed]
67. Ascherio, A.; Munger, K. Environmental risk factors for multiple sclerosis. Part II: Noninfectious factors. *Ann. Neurol.* **2007**, *61*, 504–513. [CrossRef] [PubMed]
68. Ascherio, A.; Munger, K.; Simon, K. Vitamin D and multiple sclerosis. *Lancet Neurol.* **2010**, *9*, 599–612. [CrossRef]
69. Lucas, R.; Ponsonby, A.; Dear, K.; Valery, P.C.; Pender, M.P.; Taylor, B.V.; Kilpatrick, T.J.; Dwyer, T.; Coulthard, A.; Chapman, C.; et al. Sun exposure and vitamin D are independent risk factors for CNS demyelination. *Neurology* **2011**, *76*, 540–548. [CrossRef] [PubMed]
70. Norval, M.; Halliday, G.M. The consequences of UV-induced immunosuppression for human health. *Photochem. Photobiol.* **2011**, *87*, 965–977. [CrossRef] [PubMed]
71. Munger, K.; Zhang, S.; O'Reilly, E.; Hernán, M.A.; Olek, M.J.; Willett, W.C.; Ascherio, A. Vitamin D intake and incidence of multiple sclerosis. *Neurology* **2004**, *62*, 60–65. [CrossRef] [PubMed]
72. Salzer, J.; Hallmans, G.; Nystrom, M.; Stenlund, H.; Wadell, G.; Sundstrom, P. Vitamin D as a protective factor in multiple sclerosis. *Neurology* **2012**, *79*, 2140–2145. [CrossRef] [PubMed]
73. Dong, Y.; Pollock, N.; Stallmann-Jorgensen, I.S.; Gutin, B.; Lan, L.; Chen, T.C.; Keeton, D.; Petty, K.; Holick, M.F.; Zhu, H. Low 25-hydroxyvitamin D levels in adolescents: Race, season, adiposity, physical activity, and fitness. *Pediatrics* **2010**, *125*, 1104–1111. [CrossRef] [PubMed]
74. Bischof, M.G.; Heinze, G.; Vierhapper, H. Vitamin D status and its relation to age and body mass index. *Hormone Res.* **2006**, *66*, 211–215. [CrossRef] [PubMed]
75. Munger, K.L.; Chitnis, T.; Ascherio, A. Body size and risk of MS in two cohorts of US women. *Neurology* **2009**, *73*, 1543–1550. [CrossRef] [PubMed]
76. Handel, A.E.; Giovannoni, G.; Ebers, G.C.; Ramagopalan, S.V. Environmental factors and their timing in adult-onset multiple sclerosis. *Nat. Rev. Neurol.* **2010**, *6*, 156–166. [CrossRef] [PubMed]
77. Mirzaei, F.; Michels, K.B.; Munger, K.; O'Reilly, E.; Chitnis, T.; Forman, M.R.; Giovannucci, E.; Rosner, B.; Ascherio, A. Gestational vitamin D and the risk of multiple sclerosis in offspring. *Ann. Neurol.* **2011**, *70*, 30–40. [CrossRef] [PubMed]

78. Munger, K.L.; Chitnis, T.; Frazier, A.L.; Giovannucci, E.; Spiegelman, D.; Ascherio, A. Dietary intake of vitamin D during adolescence and risk of multiple sclerosis. *J. Neurol.* **2011**, *258*, 479–485. [CrossRef] [PubMed]
79. Dobson, R.; Giovannoni, G.; Ramagopalan, S. The month of birth effect in multiple sclerosis: Systematic review, meta-analysis and effect of latitude. *J. Neurol. Neurosurg. Psychiatry* **2013**, *84*, 427–432. [CrossRef] [PubMed]
80. Munger, K.; Aivo, J.; Hongell, K.; Soilu-Hänninen, M.; Surcel, H.; Ascherio, A. Vitamin D status during pregnancy and risk of multiple sclerosis in offspring of women in the Finnish maternity cohort. *JAMA Neurol.* **2016**, *73*, 515. [CrossRef] [PubMed]
81. Nielsen, N.; Munger, K.; Stenager, E.; Ascherio, A. Author response: Neonatal vitamin D status and risk of multiple sclerosis: A population-based case-control study. *Neurology* **2017**, *89*, 411. [CrossRef] [PubMed]
82. Van der Mei, I.A.F.; Ponsonby, A.-L.; Dwyer, T.; Blizzard, L.; Simmons, R.; Taylor, B.V.; Butzkueven, H.; Kilpatrick, T. Past exposure to sun, skin phenotype, and risk of multiple sclerosis: Case-control study. *BMJ* **2003**, *327*, 316. [CrossRef] [PubMed]
83. Alter, M.; Kahana, E.; Loewenson, R. Migration and risk of multiple sclerosis. *Neurology* **1978**, *28*, 1089–1093. [CrossRef] [PubMed]
84. Banwell, B.; Bar-Or, A.; Arnold, D.L.; Sadovnick, D.; Narayanan, S.; McGowan, M.; O'Mahony, J.; Magalhaes, S.; Hanwell, H.; Vieth, R.; et al. Clinical, environmental, and genetic determinants of multiple sclerosis in children with acute demyelination: A prospective national cohort study. *Lancet Neurol.* **2011**, *10*, 436–445. [CrossRef]
85. Hanwell, H.; Vieth, R.; Magalhaes, S.; McGowan, M.; Marrie, R.A.; Bar-Or, A.; Sadovnick, A.D.; Arnold, D.; Banwell, B. Vitamin D status as a predictor of MS outcome following an initial paediatric demyelinating event. *Mult. Scler.* **2009**, *15*, S40–S41.
86. Orton, S.M.; Herrera, B.M.; Yee, I.M.; Valdar, W.; Ramagopalan, S.V.; Sadovnick, A.D.; Ebers, G.C. Sex ratio of multiple sclerosis in Canada: A longitudinal study. *Lancet Neurol.* **2006**, *5*, 932–936. [CrossRef]
87. Islam, T.; Gauderman, W.J.; Cozen, W.; Hamilton, A.S.; Burnett, M.E.; Mack, T.M. Differential twin concordance for multiple sclerosis by latitude of birthplace. *Ann. Neurol.* **2006**, *60*, 56–64. [CrossRef] [PubMed]
88. Woolmore, J.A.; Stone, M.; Pye, E.M.; Partridge, J.M.; Boggild, M.; Young, C.; Jones, P.W.; Fryer, A.A.; Hawkins, C.P.; Strange, R.C. Studies of associations between disability in multiple sclerosis, skin type, gender and ultraviolet radiation. *Mult. Scler.* **2007**, *13*, 369–375. [CrossRef] [PubMed]
89. Correale, J.; Ysrraelit, M.C.; Gaitan, M.I. Oestrogens and 1,25 dihydroxyvitamin D3 show synergistic effect on multiple sclerosis immunomodulation. *Mult. Scler.* **2009**, *15*, S196.
90. Eikelenboom, M.J.; Killestein, J.; Kragt, J.J.; Uitdehaag, B.M.; Polman, C.H. Gender differences in multiple sclerosis: Cytokines and vitamin D. *J. Neurol. Sci.* **2009**, *286*, 40–42. [CrossRef] [PubMed]
91. Nashold, F.E.; Spach, K.M.; Spanier, J.A.; Hayes, C.E. Estrogen controls vitamin D3-mediated resistance to experimental autoimmune encephalomyelitis by controlling vitamin D3 metabolism and receptor expression. *J. Immunol.* **2009**, *183*, 3672–3681. [CrossRef] [PubMed]
92. Agnello, L.; Scazzone, C.; Ragonese, P.; Salemi, G.; Lo Sasso, B.; Schillaci, R.; Musso, G.; Bellia, C.; Ciaccio, M. Vitamin D receptor polymorphisms and 25-hydroxyvitamin D in a group of Sicilian multiple sclerosis patients. *Neurol. Sci.* **2016**, *37*, 261–267. [CrossRef] [PubMed]
93. Ahn, J.; Yu, K.; Stolzenberg-Solomon, R.; Simon, K.C.; McCullough, M.L.; Gallicchio, L.; Jacobs, E.J.; Ascherio, A.; Helzlsouer, K.; Jacobs, K.B.; et al. Genome-wide association study of circulating vitamin D levels. *Hum. Mol. Genet.* **2010**, *2739–2745*, 2739–2745. [CrossRef] [PubMed]
94. Mokry, L.E.; Ross, S.; Ahmad, O.S.; Forgetta, V.; Smith, G.D.; Goltzman, D.; Leong, A.; Greenwood, C.M.; Thanassoulis, G.; Richards, J.B. Vitamin D and Risk of Multiple Sclerosis: A Mendelian Randomization Study. *PLoS Med.* **2015**, *12*, e1001866. [CrossRef] [PubMed]
95. Scazzone, C.; Agnello, L.; Ragonese, P.; Lo Sasso, B.; Bellia, C.; Bivona, G.; Schillaci, R.; Salemi, G.; Ciaccio, M. Association of CYP2R1 rs10766197 with MS risk and disease progression. *J. Neurosci. Res.* **2018**, *96*, 297–304. [CrossRef] [PubMed]
96. Pihl-Jensen, G.; Frederiksen, J. 25-Hydroxyvitamin D levels in acute monosymptomatic optic neuritis: Relation to clinical severity, paraclinical findings and risk of multiple sclerosis. *J. Neurol.* **2015**, *262*, 1646–1654. [CrossRef] [PubMed]

97. Mowry, E.; Krupp, L.; Milazzo, M.; Chabas, D.; Strober, J.B.; Belman, A.L.; McDonald, J.C.; Oksenberg, J.R.; Bacchetti, P.; Waubant, E. Vitamin D status is associated with relapse rate in pediatric-onset, M.S. *Ann. Neurol.* **2010**, *67*, 618–624. [PubMed]
98. Simpson, S.; Taylor, B.; Blizzard, L.; Ponsonby, A.L.; Pittas, F.; Tremlett, H.; Dwyer, T.; Gies, P.; van der Mei, I. Higher 25-hydroxyvitamin D is associated with lower relapse risk in, M.S. *Ann. Neurol.* **2010**, *68*, 193–203. [PubMed]
99. Runia, T.; Hop, W.; de Rijke, Y.; Buljevac, D.; Hintzen, R. Lower serum vitamin D levels are associated with a higher relapse risk in multiple sclerosis. *Neurology* **2012**, *79*, 261–266. [CrossRef] [PubMed]
100. Martinelli, V.; Dalla Costa, G.; Colombo, B.; Dalla Libera, D.; Rubinacci, A.; Filippi, M.; Furlan, R.; Comi, G. Vitamin D levels and risk of multiple sclerosis in patients with clinically isolated syndromes. *Mult. Scler. J.* **2013**, *20*, 147–155. [CrossRef] [PubMed]
101. Kuhle, J.; Disanto, G.; Dobson, R.; Adiutori, R.; Bianchi, L.; Topping, J.; Bestwick, J.P.; Meier, U.C.; Marta, M.; Dalla Costa, G.; et al. Conversion from clinically isolated syndrome to multiple sclerosis: A large multicentre study. *Mult. Scler.* **2015**, *21*, 1013–1024. [CrossRef] [PubMed]
102. Embry, A.F.; Snowdon, L.R.; Vieth, R. Vitamin D and seasonal fluctuations of gadolinium-enhancing magnetic resonance imaging lesions in multiple sclerosis. *Ann. Neurol.* **2000**, *48*, 271–272. [CrossRef]
103. Mowry, E.; Waubant, E.; McCulloch, C.; Okuda, D.T.; Evangelista, A.A.; Lincoln, R.R.; Gourraud, P.A.; Brenneman, D.; Owen, M.C.; Qualley, P.; et al. Vitamin D status predicts new brain magnetic resonance imaging activity in multiple sclerosis. *Ann Neurol.* **2012**, *72*, 234–240. [CrossRef] [PubMed]
104. Ascherio, A.; Munger, K.; White, R.; Köchert, K.; Simon, K.C.; Polman, C.H.; Freedman, M.S.; Hartung, H.P.; Miller, D.H.; Montalbán, X.; et al. Vitamin D as an early predictor of multiple sclerosis activity and progression. *JAMA Neurol.* **2014**, *71*, 306–314. [CrossRef] [PubMed]
105. Fitzgerald, K.; Munger, K.; Ko¨chert, K.; Arnason, B.G.; Comi, G.; Cook, S.; Goodin, D.S.; Filippi, M.; Hartung, H.P.; Jeffery, D.R.; et al. Association of Vitamin D Levels With multiple sclerosis activity and progression in patients receiving interferon Beta-1b. *JAMA Neurol.* **2015**, *72*, 1458. [CrossRef] [PubMed]
106. Stewart, N.; Simpson, S.; van der Mei, I.; Ponsonby, A.L.; Blizzard, L.; Dwyer, T.; Pittas, F.; Eyles, D.; Ko, P.; Taylor, B.V. Interferon-and serum 25-hydroxyvitamin D interact to modulate relapse risk in, M.S. *Neurology* **2012**, *79*, 254–260. [CrossRef] [PubMed]
107. Laursen, J.; Søndergaard, H.; Sørensen, P.; Sellebjerg, F.; Oturai, A. Vitamin D supplementation reduces relapse rate in relapsing-remitting multiple sclerosis patients treated with natalizumab. *Mult. Scler. Relat. Dis.* **2016**, *10*, 169–173. [CrossRef] [PubMed]
108. Mowry, E.; Pelletier, D.; Gao, Z.; Howell, M.; Zamvil, S.; Waubant, E. Vitamin D in clinically isolated syndrome: Evidence for possible neuroprotection. *Eur. J. Neurol.* **2015**, *23*, 327–332. [CrossRef] [PubMed]
109. Auer, D.P.; Schumann, E.M.; Kumpfel, T.; Gossl, C.; Trenkwalder, C. Seasonal fluctuations of gadolinium-enhancing magnetic resonance resonance imaging lesions in multiple sclerosis. *Ann. Neurol.* **2000**, *47*, 276–277. [CrossRef]
110. Rovaris, M.; Comi, G.; Sormani, M.P.; Wolinsky, J.S.; Ladkani, D.; Filippi, M. Effects of seasons on magnetic resonance imagingmeasured disease activity in patients with multiple sclerosis. *Ann. Neurol.* **2001**, *49*, 415–416. [CrossRef] [PubMed]
111. Killestein, J.; Rep, M.H.; Meilof, J.F.; Adèr, H.J.; Uitdehaag, B.M.; Barkhof, F.; van Lier, R.A.; Polman, C.H. Seasonal variation in immune measurements and MRI markers of disease activity in, M.S. *Neurology* **2002**, *58*, 1077–1080. [CrossRef] [PubMed]
112. Smolders, J.; Menheere, P.; Kessels, A.; Damoiseaux, J.; Hupperts, R. Association of vitamin D metabolite levels with relapse rate and disability in multiple sclerosis. *Mult. Scler. J.* **2008**, *14*, 1220–1224. [CrossRef] [PubMed]
113. Weinstock-Guttman, B.; Zivadinov, R.; Qu, J.; Cookfair, D.; Bang, E.; Bergsland, N.; Hussein, S.; Cherneva, M.; Willis, L.; et al. Vitamin D metabolites are associated with clinical and MRI outcomes in multiple sclerosis patients. *J. Neurol. Neurosurg. Psychiatry* **2011**, *82*, 189–195. [CrossRef] [PubMed]
114. Koven, N.; Cadden, M.; Murali, S.; Ross, M. Vitamin D and long-term memory in multiple sclerosis. *Cognit. Behav. Neurol.* **2013**, *26*, 155–160. [CrossRef] [PubMed]
115. Kimball, S.M.; Ursell, M.R.; O'Connor, P.; Vieth, R. Safety of vitamin D3 in adults with multiple sclerosis. *Am. J. Clin. Nutr.* **2007**, *86*, 645–651. [CrossRef] [PubMed]

116. Soilu-Hanninen, M.; Aivo, J.; Lindstro¨m, B.; Elovaara, I.; Sumelahti, M.L.; Färkkilä, M.; Tienari, P.; Atula, S.; Sarasoja, T.; Herrala, L.; et al. A randomised, double blind, placebo controlled trial with vitamin D3as an add on treatment to interferon b-1b in patients with multiple sclerosis. *J. Neurol. Neurosurg. Psychiatry* **2012**, *83*, 565–571. [CrossRef] [PubMed]
117. Etemadifar, M.; Janghorbani, M. Efficacy of high-dose vitamin D3 supplementation in vitamin D deficient pregnant women with multiple sclerosis: Preliminary findings of a randomized-controlled trial. *Iran. J. Neurol.* **2015**, *14*, 67–73. [PubMed]
118. Smolders, J.; Hupperts, R.M.M.; Vieth, R.; Grimaldi, L.M.; Holmoy, T.; Killestein, J.; Rieckmann, P.; Schluep, M.; Vieth, R.; Hostalek, U.; et al. High dose cholecalciferol (vitamin D3) oil as add-on therapy in subjects with relapsing-remitting multiple sclerosis (RRMS) receiving subcutaneous interferon s-1a (scIFNs-1a). *ECTRIMS Online Libr.* **2016**, *16*, 147013.
119. Camu, W. Cholecalciferol supplementation in relapsing multiple sclerosis patients treated with subcutaneous interferon beta-1a: A randomized controlled trial. *Neurology* **2017**, *88* (Suppl. 16), S44.004.
120. Darwish, H.; Haddad, R.; Osman, S.; Ghassan, S.; Yamout, B.; Tamim, H.; Khoury, S. Effect of vitamin D replacement on cognition in multiple sclerosis patients. *Sci. Rep.* **2017**, *7*, 45926. [CrossRef] [PubMed]
121. Solomon, A.J.; Whitham, R.H. Multiple Sclerosis and Vitamin D: A Review and Recommendations. *Curr. Neurol. Neurosci. Rep.* **2010**, *10*, 389–396. [CrossRef] [PubMed]
122. Shoemaker, T.J.; Mowry, E.M. A review of vitamin D supplementation as disease-modifying therapy. *Mult. Scler.* **2018**, *24*, 6–11. [CrossRef] [PubMed]
123. Mozaffarian, D.; Benjamin, E.J.; Go, A.S.; Arnett, D.K.; Blaha, M.J.; Cushman, M.; Das, S.R.; de Ferranti, S.; Després, J.P.; Fullerton, H.J.; et al. Heart Disease and Stroke Statistics-2016 Update: A Report from the American Heart Association. *Circulation* **2016**, *133*, e38–e360. [CrossRef] [PubMed]
124. Sadovnick, A.D. Genetic background of multiple sclerosis. *Autoimmun. Rev.* **2012**, *11*, 163–166. [CrossRef] [PubMed]
125. Daubail, B.; Jacquin, A.; Guilland, J.-C.; Hervieu, M.; Osseby, G.-V.; Rouaud, O.; Giroud, M.; Béjot, Y. Serum 25-hydroxyvitamin D predicts severity and prognosis in stroke patients. *Eur. J. Neurol.* **2013**, *20*, 57–61. [CrossRef] [PubMed]
126. Judd, S.E.; Morgan, C.J.; Panwar, B.; Howard, V.J.; Wadley, V.G.; Jenny, N.S.; Kissela, B.M.; Gutiérrez, O.M. Vitamin D deficiency and incident stroke risk in community-living black and white adults. *Int. J. Stroke* **2016**, *11*, 93–102. [CrossRef] [PubMed]
127. Vianello, E.; Dozio, E.; Barassi, A.; Tacchini, L.; Lamont, J.; Trimarchi, S.; Marrocco-Trischitta, M.M.; Romanelli, M.C. Vitamin D Deficiency Is Associated with Increased Osteocalcin Levels in Acute Aortic Dissection: A Pilot Study on Elderly Patients. *Hindawi Mediat. Inflamm.* **2017**, 6412531. [CrossRef] [PubMed]
128. Kato, S. The function of vitamin D receptor in vitamin D action. *J. Biochem.* **2000**, *127*, 717–722. [CrossRef] [PubMed]
129. Borges, A.C.; Feres, T.; Vianna, L.M.; Therezinha, B.P. Effect of cholecalciferol treatment on the relaxant responses of spontaneously hypertensive rat arteries to acetylcholine. *Hypertension* **1999**, *34*, 897–901. [CrossRef] [PubMed]
130. Sanket, S.; Madireddi, J.; Stanley, W.; Sura, P.; Prabhu, M. Relation between Vitamin D Deficiency and Severity of Chronic Obstructive Pulmonary Disease-A Case Control Study. *J. Clin. Diagn. Res.* **2016**, *10*, OC16–OC19. [CrossRef] [PubMed]
131. Manouchehri, N.; Vakil-Asadollahi, M.; Zandifar, A.; Rasmani, F.; Saadatnia, M. Vitamin D Status in Small Vessel and Large Vessel Ischemic Stroke Patients: A Case–control Study. *Adv. Biomed. Res.* **2017**, *6*, 146. [PubMed]
132. Qiu, H.; Wang, M.; Mi, D.; Zhao, J.; Tu, W.; Liu, Q. Vitamin D Status and the Risk of Recurrent Stroke and Mortality in Ischemic Stroke Patients: Data from a 24-Month Follow-Up Study in China. *J. Nutr. Health Aging* **2017**, *21*, 766–771. [CrossRef] [PubMed]
133. Daubail, B.; Jacquin, A.; Guilland, J.-C.; Khoumri, C.; Aboa-Eboulé, C.; Giroud, M.; Béjot, Y. Association between serum concentration of vitamin D and 1-year mortality in stroke patients. *Cerebrovasc. Dis.* **2014**, *37*, 364–367. [CrossRef] [PubMed]
134. Alfieri, D.F.; Lehmann, M.F.; Oliveira, S.R.; Flauzino, T.; Delongui, F.; de Araújo, M.C.; Dichi, I.; Delfino, V.D.; Mezzaroba, L.; Simão, A.N.; et al. Vitamin D deficiency is associated with acute ischemic stroke, C-reactive protein, and short-term outcome. *Metab. Brain Dis.* **2017**, *32*, 493–502. [CrossRef] [PubMed]

135. Kim, K.; Cho, K.H.; Im, S.H.; Choi, J.; Yu, J.; Kim, M. Decrement of Serum Vitamin D Level After Stroke. *Ann. Rehabil. Med.* **2017**, *41*, 944–950. [CrossRef] [PubMed]
136. Artaza, J.N.; Mehrotra, R.; Norris, K.C. Vitamin D and the cardiovascular system. *Clin. J. Am. Soc. Nephrol.* **2009**, *4*, 1515–1522. [CrossRef] [PubMed]
137. Cannell, J.J.; Grant, W.B.; Holick, M.F. Vitamin D and inflammation. *Dermatoendocrinology* **2014**, *6*, e983401. [CrossRef] [PubMed]
138. Cohen-Lahav, M.; Shany, S.; Tobvin, D.; Chaimovitz, C.; Douvdevani, A. Vitamin D decreases NFkappaB activity by increasing IkappaBalpha levels. *Nephrol. Dial. Transplant.* **2006**, *21*, 889–897. [CrossRef] [PubMed]
139. Liu, X.; Nelson, A.; Wang, X.; Farid, M.; Gunji, Y.; Ikari, J.; Iwasawa, S.; Basma, H.; Feghali-Bostwick, C.; Rennard, S.I. Vitamin D modulates prostaglandin E2 synthesis and degradation in human lung fibroblasts. *Am. J. Respir. Cell Mol. Biol.* **2014**, *50*, 40–50. [PubMed]
140. Penna, G.; Roncari, A.; Amuchastegui, S.; Daniel, K.C.; Berti, E.; Colonna, M.; Adorini, L. Expression of the inhibitory receptor ILT3 on dendritic cells is dispensable for induction of CD4 + Foxp3 + regulatory T cells by 1,25-dihydroxyvitamin D3. *Blood* **2005**, *106*, 3490–3497. [CrossRef] [PubMed]
141. Tarcin, O.; Yavuz, D.G.; Ozben, B.; Telli, A.; Ogunc, A.V.; Yuksel, M.; Toprak, A.; Yazici, D.; Sancak, S.; Deyneli, O.; et al. Effect of Vitamin D Deficiency and Replacement on Endothelial Function in Asymptomatic Subjects. *J. Clin. Endocrinol. Metab.* **2009**, *94*, 4023–4030. [CrossRef] [PubMed]
142. Marniemi, J.; Alanen, E.; Impivaara, O.; Seppänen, R.; Hakala, P.; Rajala, T.; Rönnemaa, T. Dietary and serum vitamins and minerals as predictors of myocardial infarction and stroke in elderly subjects. *Nutr. Metab. Cardiovasc. Dis.* **2005**, *15*, 188–197. [CrossRef] [PubMed]
143. Sun, Q.; Pan, A.; Hu, F.B.; Manson, J.E.; Rexrode, K.M. 25-Hydroxyvitamin D Levels and the Risk of Stroke: A Prospective Study and Meta-analysis. *Stroke* **2012**, *43*, 1470–1477. [CrossRef] [PubMed]
144. Cirillo, P.; Golino, P.; Calabro, P.; Calì, G.; Ragni, M.; De Rosa, S.; Cimmino, G.; Pacileo, M.; De Palma, R.; Forte, L.; et al. C-reactive protein induces tissue factor expression and promotes smooth muscle and endothelial cell proliferation. *Cardiovasc. Res.* **2005**, *68*, 47–55. [CrossRef] [PubMed]
145. Chen, C.; Nan, B.; Lin, P.; Yao, Q. C-reactive protein increases plasminogen activator inhibitor-1 expression in human endothelial cells. *Thromb. Res.* **2008**, *122*, 125–133. [CrossRef] [PubMed]
146. Hattori, Y.; Matsumura, K.K.; Kasai, K. Vascular smooth muscle cell activation by C-reactive protein. *Cardiovasc. Res.* **2003**, *58*, 186–195. [CrossRef]
147. Pilz, S.; Tomarchitz, A.; Drechsler, C.; Zittermann, A.; Dekker, J.M.; März, W. Vitamin [8]D supplementation: A promising approach for the prevention and treatment of strokes. *Curr. Drug Targets* **2011**, *12*, 88–96. [CrossRef] [PubMed]
148. Park, K.Y.; Chung, P.W.; Kim, Y.B.; Moon, H.S.; Suh, B.C.; Won, Y.S.; Kim, J.M.; Youn, Y.C.; Kwon, O.S. Serum vitamin [9]D status as a predictor of prognosis in patients with acute ischemic stroke. *Cerebrovasc. Dis.* **2015**, *40*, 73–80. [CrossRef] [PubMed]
149. Ladeby, R.; Wirenfeldt, M.; Garcia-Ovejero, D.; Fenger, C.; Dissing-Olesen, L.; Dalmau, I.; Finsen, B. Microglial cell population dynamics in the injured adult central nervous system. *Brain Res. Brain Res. Rev.* **2005**, *48*, 196–206. [CrossRef] [PubMed]
150. Wei, Z.; Kuang, J. Research Article: Vitamin D deficiency in relation to the poor functional outcomes in nondiabetic patients with ischemic stroke. *Biosci. Rep.* **2018**, *38*, BSR20171509. [CrossRef] [PubMed]
151. Bjelakovic, G.; Gluud, L.L.; Nikolova, D.; Whitfield, K.; Wetterslev, J.; Simonetti, R.G.; Bjelakovic, M.; Gluud, C. Vitamin D supplementation for prevention of mortality in adults. *Cochrane Database Syst. Rev.* **2011**, *7*, CD007470.
152. Gupta, A.; Prabhakar, S.; Modi, M.; Bhadada, S.K.; Kalaivani, M.; Lal, V.; Khurana, D. Effect of Vitamin D and calcium supplementation on ischaemic stroke outcome: A randomised controlled open-label trial. *Int. J. Clin. Pract.* **2016**, *70*, 764–770. [CrossRef] [PubMed]
153. Manson, J.E. Vitamin D and the heart: Why we need large-scale clinical trials. *Cleve Clin. J. Med.* **2010**, *77*, 903–910. [CrossRef] [PubMed]
154. LeBoff, M.S.; Yue, A.Y.; Copeland, T.; Cook, N.R.; Buring, J.E.; Manson, J.E. VITAL-Bone Health: Rationale and design of two ancillary studies evaluating the effects of vitamin D and/or omega-3 fatty acid supplements on incident fractures and bone health outcomes in the VITamin D and OmegA-3 TriaL (VITAL). *Contemp. Clin. Trials* **2015**, *41*, 259–268. [CrossRef] [PubMed]

155. Shaffer, J.A.; Edmondson, D.; Wasson, L.T.; Falzon, L.; Homma, K.; Ezeokoli, N.; Li, P.; Davidson, K.W. Vitamin D supplementation for depressive symptoms: A systematic review and meta-analysis of randomized controlled trials. *Psychosom. Med.* **2014**, *76*, 190–196. [CrossRef] [PubMed]
156. Karran, E.; Mercken, M.; Strooper, B.D. The amyloid cascade hypothesis for Alzheimer's disease: An appraisal for the development of therapeutics. *Nat. Rev. Drug Discov.* **2011**, *10*, 698–712. [CrossRef] [PubMed]
157. Roher, A.E.; Lowenson, J.D.; Clarke, S.; Woods, A.S.; Cotter, R.J.; Gowing, E.; Ball, M.J. Beta amyloid (1–42) is a major component of cerebrovascular amyloid deposits: Implications for the pathology of Alzheimer's disease. *Proc. Natl. Acad. Sci. USA* **1993**, *90*, 10836–10840. [CrossRef] [PubMed]
158. Choi, S.H.; Kim, Y.H.; Hebisch, M.; Sliwinski, C.; Lee, S.; D'Avanzo, C.; Chen, H.; Hooli, B.; Asselin, C.; Muffat, J.; et al. A three dimensional human neural cell culture model of Alzheimer's disease. *Nature* **2014**, *515*, 274–278. [CrossRef] [PubMed]
159. Lahiri, D.K.; Maloney, B. The LEARn (Latent early life associated regulation) model integrates environmental risk factors and the developmental basis of Alzheimer's disease, and proposes remedial steps. *Exp. Gerontol.* **2010**, *45*, 291–296. [CrossRef] [PubMed]
160. Banerjee, A.; Khemka, V.K.; Gaungly, A.; Roy, D.; Gauguly, U.; Chakrabarti, S. Vitamin D and Alzheimer's Disease: Neurocognition to therapeutics. *Int. J. Alzheimers Dis.* **2015**, *2015*. [CrossRef] [PubMed]
161. Gezen, A.K.D.; Dursun, B.; Bilgic, B.; Hanağasi, H.; Ertan, T.; Gürvit, H.; Emre, M.; Eker, E.; Ulutin, T.; Uysal, O.; et al. Vitamin D receptor gene haplotype is associated with late-onset Alzheimer's Disease. *Tohoku J. Exp. Med.* **2012**, *228*, 189–196. [CrossRef]
162. Dursun, E.; Gezen Ak, D.; Ylmazer, S. A new mechanism for amyloid Beta induction of iNOS: Vitamin D-VDR pathwy disruption. *J. Alzheimers Dis.* **2013**, *36*, 459–474. [CrossRef] [PubMed]
163. Brewer, L.D.; Thibault, V.; Chen, K.C.; Langub, M.C.; Landfield, P.W.; Porter, N.M. Vitamin D hormone confers neuroprotection in parallel with downregulation of L-type calcium channel expression in hippocampal neurons. *J. Neurosci.* **2001**, *21*, 98–108. [CrossRef] [PubMed]
164. Thibault, O.; Landfield, P.W. Increase in single L-type calcium channels in hippocampal neurons during aging. *Science* **1996**, *272*, 1017–1020. [CrossRef] [PubMed]
165. Porter, N.M.; Thibault, O.; Thibault, V.; Chen, K.C.; Landfield, P.W. Calcium-channel density and hippocampal cell death with age in long-term culture. *J. Neurosci.* **1997**, *17*, 5629–5639. [CrossRef] [PubMed]
166. Gezen-Ak, D.; Dursun, E.; Yilmazer, S. Vitamin D inquiry in hippocampal neurons: Consequences of vitamin D-VDR pathway disruption on calcium channel and the vitamin D requirement. *Neurol. Sci.* **2013**, *34*, 1453–1458. [CrossRef] [PubMed]
167. Wang, L.; Har, K.; Van Baaren, J.M.; Price, J.C.; Beecham, G.W.; Gallins, P.J.; Whitehead, P.L.; Wang, G.; Lu, C.; Slifer, M.A.; et al. Vitamin D receptor and AD: A genetic and functional study. *Neurobiol. Aging* **2012**, *33*, 1844.e1–1844.e9. [CrossRef] [PubMed]
168. Kuningans, M.; Mooijart, S.P.; Jolles, J.; Slagboom, P.E.; Westendorp, R.G.; van Heemst, D. VDR genes variants associate with cognitive functions and depressive symptom in old age. *Neurobiol. Aging* **2009**, *30*, 466–473. [CrossRef] [PubMed]
169. Buell, J.S.; Dawson-Hughes, B.; Scott, T.M.; Weiner, D.E.; Dallal, G.E.; Qui, W.Q.; Bergethon, P.; Rosenberg, I.H.; Folstein, M.F.; Patz, S.; et al. 25-Hydroxyvitamin D, dementia and cerebrovascular pathology in elders receiving home services. *Neurology* **2010**, *74*, 18–26. [CrossRef] [PubMed]
170. Grimm, M.O.W.; Lehmann, J.; Mett, J.; Zimmer, V.C.; Grösgen, S.; Stahlmann, C.P.; Hundsdörfer, B.; Haupenthal, V.J.; Rothhaar, T.L.; Herr, C.; et al. Impact of vitamin D on amyloid precursor protein processing and amyloid beta peptide degradation in Alzheimer's Disease. *Neurodegen. Dis.* **2014**, *13*, 75–81. [CrossRef] [PubMed]
171. Miziwicki, M.T.; Menegaz, D.; Zhang, J.; Barrientos-Durán, A.; Tse, S.; Cashman, J.R.; Griffin, P.R.; Fiala, M. Genomic and nongenomic signaling induced by 1 alpha 25 OH2 vitamin D3 promotes the recovery of amyloid phagocytosis by Alzheimer's disease macrophages. *J. Alzheimers Dis.* **2012**, *29*, 51–62. [CrossRef] [PubMed]
172. Taniura, H.; Ito, M.; Sanada, N.; Kuramoto, N.; Ohno, Y.; Nakamichi, N.; Yoneda, Y. Chronic vitamin d3 treatment protects against neurotoxicity by glutamate in association with upregulation of vitamin D receptor mRNA expression in cultured rat cortical neurons. *J. Neurosci. Res.* **2006**, *83*, 1179–1189. [CrossRef] [PubMed]

173. Garcion, E.; Sindij, L.; Leblondel, G.; Brachet, P.; Darcy, F. 1–25 dihydroxyvitamin D3 regulates the synthesis of gamma glutamyl transpeptidase and gluthatione levels in rat primary astrocytes. *J. Neurochem.* **1999**, *73*, 859–866. [CrossRef] [PubMed]
174. Briones, T.L.; Darwish, H. Decrease in age related tau hyperphosphorylation and cognitive improvement following vitamin D supplementation are associated with modulation of brain energy metabolism and redox state. *Neuroscience* **2014**, *262*, 143–155. [CrossRef] [PubMed]
175. Thomas, M.K.; Lloyd-Jones, D.M.; Thadani, R.I.; Shaw, A.C.; Deraska, D.J.; Kitch, B.T.; Vamvakas, E.C.; Dick, I.M.; Prince, R.L.; Finkelstein, J.S. Hypovitaminosis D in medical inpatients. *N. Engl. J. Med.* **1998**, *338*, 777–783. [CrossRef] [PubMed]
176. Gloth, F.M.; Gundberg, C.M.; Hollis, B.W.; Haddad, J.G.; Tobin, J.D. Vitamin D deficiency in homebound elderly persons. *JAMA* **1995**, *274*, 1683–1686. [CrossRef] [PubMed]
177. Moon, J.H.; Lim, S.; Han, J.W.; Kim, K.M.; Choi, S.H.; Kim, K.W.; Jang, H.C. Serum 25-hydroxyvitamin D level and the risk of mild cognitive impairment and dementia: The Korean Longitudinal Study on Health and Aging (KloSHA). *Clin. Endocrinol.* **2015**, *83*, 36–42. [CrossRef] [PubMed]
178. Khachaturian, Z.S. The role of calcium regulation in brain aging: Reexamination of a hypothesis. *Aging* **1989**, *1*, 17–34. [CrossRef] [PubMed]
179. Annweiler, C.; Montero-Odasso, M.; Llewellyn, D.J.; Richard Devantoy, S.; Duque, G.; Beauchet, O. Meta-analysis of memory and executive dysfunctions in relation to vitamin D. *J. Alzheimers Dis.* **2013**, *37*, 147–171. [CrossRef] [PubMed]
180. Annweiler, C.; Rolland, Y.; Schott, A.M.; Blain, H.; Vellas, B.; Herrmann, F.R.; Beauchet, O. Higher vitamin D dietary intake is associated with lower risk of AD: A 7-year follow-up. *J. Gerontol. Ser. A Biol. Sci. Med. Sci.* **2012**, *67*, 1205–1211. [CrossRef] [PubMed]
181. Fiala, M.; Miziwiki, M.T. Neuroprotective and immune effects of active forms of vitamin D3 and docosahexaenoic acid in AD patients. *Funct. Foods Health Dis.* **2011**, *1*, 545–554.
182. Annweiler, C.; Herrmann, F.R.; Fantino, B.; Brugg, B.; Beauchet, O. Effectiveness of the combination of memantine plus vitamin D on cognition in patients with AD: A pre–post pilot study. *Cognit. Behav. Neurol.* **2012**, *25*, 121–127. [CrossRef] [PubMed]
183. Stein, M.S.; Schere, S.C.; Ladd, K.S.; Harrison, L.C. A randomized controlled trial of high dose vitamin D2 followed by intranasal insulin in, A.D. *J. Alzheimers Dis.* **2011**, *26*, 477–484. [CrossRef] [PubMed]
184. Przybelski, R.; Agrawal, S.; Krueger, D.; Engelke, J.A.; Walbrun, F.; Binkley, N. Rapid correction of low vitamin D status in nursing home residents. *Osteoporos. Int.* **2008**, *19*, 1621–1628. [CrossRef] [PubMed]
185. LaPrincess, C.B.; Michos, E.D.; Reis, J.P. Vitamin D in atherosclerosis, vascular disease, and endothelial function. *Curr. Drug Targets* **2011**, *12*, 54–60.
186. Prabhakar, P.; Chandra, S.R.; Supriya, M.; Issac, T.G.; Prasad, C.; Christopher, R. Vitamin D status and vascular dementia due to cerebral small vessel disease in the elderly Asian Indian population. *J. Neurol. Sci.* **2015**, *359*, 108–111. [CrossRef] [PubMed]
187. Alagiakrishnan, K.; Hsueh, J.; Zhang, E.; Khan, K.; Senthilselvan, A. Small vessel disease/white matter disease of the brain and its association with osteoporosis. *J. Clin. Med. Res.* **2015**, *7*, 297–302. [CrossRef] [PubMed]
188. Chung, P.W.; Park, K.Y.; Lim, J.M.; Shin, D.W.; Park, M.S.; Chung, Y.J.; Ha, S.Y.; Ahn, S.W.; Shin, H.W.; Kim, Y.B.; et al. 25-Hydroxyvitmain D status is associated with chronic cerebral small vessel disease. *Stroke* **2015**, *46*, 248–251. [CrossRef] [PubMed]
189. Mancuso, P.; Rahman, A.; Hershey, S.D.; Dandu, L.; Nibbelink, K.A.; Simpson, R.U. 1,25-Dihydroxyvitamin-D3 treatment reduces cardiac hypertrophy and left ventricular diameter in spontaneously hypertensive heart failure-prone (cp/+) rats independent of changes in serum leptin. *J. Cardiovasc. Pharmacol.* **2008**, *51*, 559–564. [CrossRef] [PubMed]
190. Bodyak, N.; Ayus, J.C.; Achinger, S.; Shivalingappa, V.; Ke, Q.; Chen, Y.S.; Debra, L.R.; Isaac, S.; Hector, T.; Paul, E.K.; et al. Activated vitamin D attenuates left ventricular abnormalities induced by dietary sodium in DAHL salt-sensitive animals. *Proc. Natl. Acad. Sci. USA* **2007**, *104*, 16810–16815. [CrossRef] [PubMed]
191. Wang, T.J.; Pencina, M.J.; Booth, S.L.; Jacques, P.F.; Ingelsson, E.; Lanier, K.; Benjamin, E.J.; D'Agostino, R.B.; Wolf, M.; Vasan, R.S. Vitamin D deficiency and risk of cardiovascular disease. *Circulation* **2008**, *117*, 503–511. [CrossRef] [PubMed]

192. Zittermann, A.; Schleithoff, S.S.; Tenderich, G.; Berthold, H.K.; Körfer, R.; Stehle, P. Low vitamin D status a contributing factor in the pathogensis of congestive heart failure? *J. Am. Coll. Cardiol.* **2003**, *41*, 105–112. [CrossRef]
193. Somjen, D.; Weisman, Y.; Kohen, F.; Gayer, B.; Limor, R.; Sharon, O.; Jaccard, N.; Knoll, E.; Stern, N. 25-hydroxyvitamin D3–1alpha-hydroxylase is expressed in human vascular smooth muscle cells and is upregulated by parathyroid hormone and estrogenic compounds. *Circulation* **2005**, *111*, 1666–1671. [CrossRef] [PubMed]
194. Danielsson, C.; Nayeri, S.; Wiesinger, H.; Thieroff-Ekerdt, R.; Carlberg, C. Potent gene regulatory and antiproliferative activities of 20-methyl analogues of 1,25 dihydroxyvitamin D3. *J. Cell. Biochem.* **1996**, *63*, 199–206. [CrossRef]
195. Eyles, D.W.; Burne, T.H.J.; McGrath, J.J. Vitamin D effects on brain development, adult brain function and the links between low levels of vitamin D and neuropsychiatric disease. *Front. Neuroendocrinol.* **2013**, *34*, 47–64. [CrossRef] [PubMed]
196. Almeras, L.; Eyles, D.; Benech, P.; Laffite, D.; Villard, C.; Patatian, A.; Boucraut, J.; Mackay-Sim, A.; McGrath, J.; Féron, F. Developmental vitamin D deficiency alters brain protein expression in the adult rat: Implications for neuropsychiatric disorders. *Proteomics* **2007**, *7*, 769–780. [CrossRef] [PubMed]
197. Sutherland, M.K.; Somerville, M.J.; Yoong, L.K.K.; Bergeron, C.; Haussler, M.R.; Crapper McLachlan, D.R. Reduction of vitamin D hormone receptor mRNA levels in Alzheimer as compared to Huntington hippocampus: Correlation with calbindin-28k mRNA levels. *Mol. Brain Res.* **1992**, *3*, 239–250. [CrossRef]
198. Moretti, R.; Furlanis, G.; Caruso, P.; Signori, R.; Gazzin, S.; Tiribelli, C. Vitamin D in the Small Vessel disease. *Curr. Neurobiol.* **2017**, *8*, 112–124.
199. Li, Y.C.; Kong, J.; Wei, M.; Chen, Z.F.; Liu, S.Q.; Cao, L.P. 1,25 Dihydroxyvitamin D(3) is a negative endocrine regulator of the renin-angiotensin system. *J. Clin. Investig.* **2002**, *110*, 229–238. [CrossRef] [PubMed]
200. Buell, J.S.; Dawson-Hughes, B. Vitamin D and neurocognitive dysfunction: Preventing "D"ecline. *Mol. Asp. Med.* **2008**, *29*, 415–422. [CrossRef] [PubMed]
201. De Silva, T.M.; Miller, A.A. Cerebral small vessel disease: Targeting oxydative stress as a novel therapeutic strategy. *Front. Pharmacol.* **2016**. [CrossRef] [PubMed]
202. Miller, A.A.; Drummond, G.R.; De Silva, T.M.; Mast, A.E.; Hickey, H.; Williams, J.P.; Broughton, B.R.; Sobey, C.G. NADPH oxidase activity is higher in cerebral versus systemic arteries of four animal species: Role of Nox2. *Am. J. Physiol. Heart Circ. Physiol.* **2009**, *296*, 220–225. [CrossRef] [PubMed]
203. Kong, X.F.; Zhi, X.H.; Pei, Y.L.; Jackson, D.M.; Holick, M.F. Molecular cloning, characterization, and promoter analysis of the human 25-hydroxyvitamin D3-1aplha.hydroxyalse gene. *Proc. Natl. Acad. Sci. USA* **1999**, *96*, 6988–6993. [CrossRef] [PubMed]
204. Timms, P.M.; Mannan, N.; Hitman, G.A.; Noonan, K.; Mills, P.G.; Syndercombe-Court, D.; Aganna, E.; Price, C.P.; Boucher, B.J. Circualtion MMMP9, vitamin D, and variation in the TIMP-1 response with VDR genotype: Mechanism for inflammatory damage in chronic disorders. *QJM* **2002**, *95*, 787–796. [CrossRef] [PubMed]
205. Raymond, M.A.; Desrmeaux, A.; Labelle, A.; Soulez, M.; Soluez, G.; Langelier, Y.; Pshezhetsky, A.V.; Hébert, M.J. Endothelial stress induces the release of vitamin D binding protein, a novel growth factor. *Biochem. Biophys. Res. Commun.* **2005**, *338*, 1374–1382. [CrossRef] [PubMed]
206. Nakagawa, K.; Sasaki, Y.; Kato, S.; Kubodera, N.; Okano, T. 22-oxa-1-alpha,25 dyhydroxyvitamin D3 inhibits metastastasis and angiogenesis in lung cancer. *Carcinogensesis* **2005**, *26*, 1044–1054. [CrossRef] [PubMed]
207. Zittermnann, A.; Koerfer, R. Protective and toxic effects of vitamin D on vascular calcification: Clinical implications. *Mol. Asp. Med.* **2008**, *29*, 423–432. [CrossRef] [PubMed]
208. Andress, D.I. Non classical aspects of differential vitamin D receptor activation. *Drugs* **2007**, *67*, 1999–2012. [CrossRef] [PubMed]
209. Williamson, J.B.; Lewis, G.F.; Nyenhuis, D.L.; Stebbins, G.T.; Murphy, C.; Handelman, M.; Harden, E.; Harden, E.; Heilman, K.M.; Gorelick, P.B.; Porges, S.W. The effects of cerebral white matter changes on cardiovascular responses to cognitive and physical activity in a stroke population. *Psychophysiology* **2012**, *49*, 1618–1628. [CrossRef] [PubMed]
210. Laurent, S.; Katsahian, S.; Fassot, C.; Tropeano, A.I.; Gautier, I.; Laloux, B.; Boutouyrie, P. Aortic stiffness is an independent predictor of fatal stroke in essential hypertension. *Stroke* **2003**, *34*, 1203–1206. [CrossRef] [PubMed]

211. Baumbach, G.L.; Heistad, D.D. Adaptive changes in cerebral blood vessels during chronic hypertension. *J. Hypertens.* **1991**, *9*, 987–991. [CrossRef] [PubMed]
212. Huneau, C.; Benali, H.; Chabriat, H. Investigating human neurovascular coupling using functional neuroimaging: A critical review of dynamic models. *Front. Neurosci.* **2015**, *9*, 467. [CrossRef] [PubMed]
213. Phillips, A.A.; Chan, F.H.N.; Zheng, M.M.Z.; Krassioukov, A.V.; Ainslie, P.N. Neurovascular coupling in human: Physiology, methodological advances and clinical implications. *JCBFM* **2016**, *36*, 647–664. [CrossRef] [PubMed]
214. Kitazono, T.; Faraci, F.M.; Tagchi, H.; Heistad, D.D. Role of potassium channels in cerebral blood vessels. *Stroke* **1995**, *26*, 1713–1723. [CrossRef] [PubMed]
215. Nelson, M.T.; Patlak, J.B.; Worley, J.F.; Standen, N.B. Calcium channels, potassium channels, and voltage dependence of arterial smooth muscle tone. *Am. J. Physiol.* **1990**, *259*, 3–18. [CrossRef] [PubMed]
216. Bolotina, V.; Gericke, M.; Bregoestovski, P. Kinetic differences between calcium activate potassium channels in smooth muscle isolated from normal and atherosclerotic human aorta. *Proc. R. Soc. Lond. B Biol. Sci.* **1991**, *244*, 51–55. [CrossRef] [PubMed]
217. Cui, X.; Pelekanos, M.; Liu, P.Y.; Burne, T.H.J.; McGrath, J.J.; Eyles, D.W. The vitamin D receptor in dopamine neurons; its presence in human substantia nigra and its ontogenesis in rat midbrain. *Neuroscience* **2013**, *236*, 77–87. [CrossRef] [PubMed]
218. Abou Raya, S.; Helmii, M.; Abou Raya, A. Bone and mineral metabolism in older adults with Parkinson's disease. *Age Ageing* **2009**, *38*, 675–680. [CrossRef] [PubMed]
219. Lu'o'ng, K.; Nguyen, L. Role of vitamin D in Parkinson's Disease. *Int. Sch. Res. Netw.* **2012**, *2012*, 124289.
220. Fiszer, U.; Mix, E.; Fredrikson, S.; Kostulas, V.; Link, H. Parkinson's disease and immunological abnormalities increase of HLA-DR expression on monocytes in cerebrospinal fluid and of CD45ro+ T cells in peripheral blood. *Acta Neurol. Scand.* **1994**, *90*, 160–166. [CrossRef] [PubMed]
221. McGeer, P.L.; Itagaki, S.; Boyes, B.E.; McGeer, E.G. Reactive microglia are positive for HLA-DR in the substantia nigra of PD and AD' disease brain. *Neurology* **1988**, *38*, 1285–12919. [CrossRef] [PubMed]
222. Tokuda, N.; Levy, R.B. 1,25 Dihydroxyvitamin D3 stimulates phagocytosis but suppresses HLA-DR and CD13 antigen expression in human mononuclear phagocytes. *Proc. Soc. Exp. Biol. Med.* **1996**, *211*, 244–250. [CrossRef] [PubMed]
223. Tone, T.; Eto, K.; Katsuoka, K.; Nishioka, K.; Nishiyama, S. Suppression of gamma interferon induced HLA-DR antigen expression on normal and transformed keratocytes by 1,25 $(OH)_2$ vitamin D3. *Jpn. J. Dermatol.* **1991**, *101*, 519–525.
224. Stefanovic, M.; Topic, E.; Khanna, V.K.; Shukla, R.; PArmar, D. Association of polymorphism in cytochrome P450 2D6 and N-Acetyltransferase-2 with Parkinson's disease. *Dis. Mark.* **2010**, *28*, 87–93.
225. Singh, S.; Singh, K.; Patel, D.K.; Singh, C.; Nath, C.; Singh, V.K.; Singh, R.K.; Singh, M.P. The expression of cyp2d33, an ortholog of human cyp2D6 in mouse striatum and its modulation in 1-MPTP induced PD phenotype and nicotine-mediated neuroprotection. *Rejuv. Res.* **2009**, *12*, 185–197. [CrossRef] [PubMed]
226. Shojaee, S.; Sina, F.; Bnihossein, S.; Kazemi, M.H.; Kalhor, R.; Shahidi, G.A.; Fakhrai-Rad, H.; Ronaghi, M.; Elahi, E. Genome-wide linkage analysis of a parkinsonian pyramidal syndrome pedigree by 500 K SNP arrays. *Am. J. Hum. Genet.* **2008**, *82*, 1375–1384. [CrossRef] [PubMed]
227. Wilhelmsen, K.; Mirel, D.; Marder, K.; Bernstein, M.; Naini, A.; Leal, S.M.; Cote, L.J.; Tang, M.X.; Freyer, G.; Graziano, J.; et al. Is there a genetic susceptibility locus for PD on chromosome 22q13? *Ann. Neurol.* **1997**, *41*, 813–817. [CrossRef] [PubMed]
228. Stagi, S.; Lapi, E.; Gambiner, E.; Manoni, C.; Genuardi, M.; Colarusso, G.; Conti, C.; Chiarelli, F.; de Martino, M.; Azzari, C. Bone density and metabolism in subjects with microdeletion of chromosome 22q11. *Eur. J. Endocr.* **2010**, *163*, 329–337. [CrossRef] [PubMed]
229. Ryu, H.; Lee, J.; Zamam, K.; Kubilis, J.; Ferrante, R.J.; Ross, B.D.; Neve, R.; Ratan, R.R. Sp1 and Sp3 are oxidative stress-inducible, anti-death transcription factors in cortical neurons. *J. Neurosci.* **2003**, *23*, 3597–3606. [CrossRef] [PubMed]
230. Wang, J.; BAnnon, M.J. Sp1 and Sp3 activate transcription of the human dopamine transporter gene. *J. Neurochem.* **2005**, *93*, 474–482. [CrossRef] [PubMed]
231. Yajima, S.; Lee, S.H.; Minowa, T.; Mouradian, M.M. Sp family transcription factors regulate expression of rat D2 dopamine receptor gene. *DNA Cell Biol.* **1998**, *17*, 471–479. [CrossRef] [PubMed]

232. Choi, J.M.; Hong, J.H.; Chae, M.J.; Ngyuen, P.H.; Kang, H.S.; Ma, H.I.; Kim, Y.J. Analysis of mutations and the association between polymorphisms in the cerebral dopamine neurotrophic factor (CDNF) gene and, P.D. *Neurosci. Lett.* **2011**, *493*, 97–101. [CrossRef] [PubMed]
233. Baranano, D.; Snyder, S.H. Neural roles for heme oxygenase: Contrasts to nitric oxide synthase. *Proc. Natl. Acad. Sci. USA* **2001**, *98*, 10996–11002. [CrossRef] [PubMed]
234. Mateo, I.; Infante, J.; Sanchez-Juan, P.; García-Gorostiaga, I.; Rodríguez-Rodríguez, E.; Vázquez-Higuera, J.L.; Berciano, J.; Combarros, O. Serum heme oxygenase-1 levels are increased in PD but not in, A.D. *Acta Neurol. Scand.* **2010**, *121*, 136–138. [CrossRef] [PubMed]
235. Castellani, R.; Smith, M.A.; Richey, P.L.; Perry, G. Glycoxidation and oxidative stress in PD and diffuse Lewy body disease. *Brain Res.* **1996**, *737*, 195–200. [CrossRef]
236. Oermann, E.; Bidmon, H.J.; Witte, O.W.; Zilles, K. Effects of 1 alpha, 25 dihydroxyvitamin D3 on the expression of HO1 and GFAP in glial cells of the photothrombotically lesioned cerebral cortex. *J. Chem. Neuroanat.* **2004**, *28*, 225–238. [CrossRef] [PubMed]
237. Soos, J.; Engelhardt, I.; Siklos, L.; Havas, L.; Majtenyi, K. The expression of PARP, NF-κB and parvalbumin is increased in, O.D. *Neuroreport* **2004**, *15*, 1715–1718. [CrossRef] [PubMed]
238. Mabley, J.G.; Wallace, R.; Pacher, P.; Murphy, K.; Szabo, C. Inhibition of PARP polymerase by the active form of vitamin D. *Int. J. Mol. Med.* **2007**, *19*, 947–952. [PubMed]
239. Suzuki, M.; Yoshioka, M.; Hashimoto, M.; Murakami, M.; Noya, M.; Takahashi, D.; Urashima, M. Randomized, double-blind, placebo-controlled trial of vitamin D supplement in Parkinson's disease. *Am. J. Clin. Nutr.* **2013**, *97*, 1004–1013. [CrossRef] [PubMed]
240. Ohmura, K.; Kato, M.; Watanabe, T.; Oku, K.; Bohgaki, T.; Horita, T.; Yasuda, S.; Ito, Y.M.; Sato, N.; Atsumi, T. Effect of combined treatment with bisphosphonate and vitamin D on atherosclerosis in patients with systemic lupus erythematosus: A propensity scorebased analysis. *Arthrit. Res. Ther.* **2018**, *20*, 72. [CrossRef] [PubMed]
241. Aydoğan, N.H.; Özel, İ.; İltar, S.; Kara, T.; Özmeriç, A.; Alemdaroğlu, K.B. The effect of vitamin D and bisphosphonate on fracture healing: An experimental study. *J. Clin. Orthop. Trauma* **2016**, *7*, 90–94. [CrossRef] [PubMed]
242. Kang, Y.M.; Hong, S.H.; Yang, J.H.; Oh, J.C.; Park, J.O.; Lee, B.H.; Lee, S.Y.; Kim, H.S.; Lee, H.M.; Moon, S.H. Pamidronate down-regulates tumor necrosis factor-alpha induced matrix metalloproteinases expression in human intervertebral disc cells. *J. Bone Metab.* **2016**, *23*, 165–173. [CrossRef] [PubMed]
243. Kennel, K.A.; Drake, M.T.; Hurley, D.L. Vitamin D Deficiency in Adults: When to Test and How to Treat. *Mayo Clin. Proc.* **2010**, *85*, 752–758. [CrossRef] [PubMed]

9

Extra-Skeletal Effects of Vitamin D

Rose Marino and Madhusmita Misra *

Pediatric Endocrine Unit, Massachusetts General Hospital and Harvard Medical School, Boston, MA 02114, USA
* Correspondence: mmisra@mgh.harvard.edu

Abstract: The vitamin D receptor is expressed in multiple cells of the body (other than osteoblasts), including beta cells and cells involved in immune modulation (such as mononuclear cells, and activated T and B lymphocytes), and most organs in the body including the brain, heart, skin, gonads, prostate, breast, and gut. Consequently, the extra-skeletal impact of vitamin D deficiency has been an active area of research. While epidemiological and case-control studies have often suggested a link between vitamin D deficiency and conditions such as type 1 and type 2 diabetes, connective tissue disorders, inflammatory bowel disorders, chronic hepatitis, food allergies, asthma and respiratory infections, and cancer, interventional studies for the most part have failed to confirm a causative link. This review examines available evidence to date for the extra-skeletal effects of vitamin D deficiency, with a focus on randomized controlled trials and meta-analyses.

Keywords: vitamin D; type 1 diabetes; type 2 diabetes; metabolic syndrome; autoimmune; children; cancer

---

1. Introduction

While the skeletal effects of vitamin D are well recognized and described extensively in the literature [1–3], its extra-skeletal effects have been subject to some controversy with conflicting data reported, particularly for case-control or epidemiologic vs. prospective and interventional studies. This review aims to summarize and synthesize data regarding many extra-skeletal effects of vitamin D. Given the extensive literature reported in this area over the last two decades, we have discussed key papers that illustrate variations in data reported from the various kinds of studies, with a focus on randomized controlled trials (RCTs) and meta-analyses of existing studies.

Vitamin D_3 (cholecalciferol) is synthesized primarily in the skin on exposure to ultraviolet radiation, while vitamin D_2 (ergocalciferol) is derived from plant sources. 7-dehydrocholesterol (provitamin D; present in the stratum basale and stratum spinosum of the epidermis), is converted to previtamin D on exposure to ultraviolet radiation-B (UV-B), which is then isomerized to vitamin D. Vitamin D passes into dermal capillaries and is carried by vitamin D binding protein (DBP) to the liver, where microsomal vitamin D 25-hydroxylase catalyzes its conversion to 25-hydroxy vitamin D [25(OH)D], the storage form of vitamin D. 25(OH)D is what is reported when we ask for levels of vitamin D, and most assays report both 25(OH)D_2 and 25(OH)D_3. While controversy persists around the normative range for 25(OH)D levels, the Institute of Medicine has indicated that a 25(OH)D level at or above 20 ng/mL (50 nmol/L) is likely sufficient to optimize its skeletal effects [4]. Normative ranges for its possible extra-skeletal effects remain to be determined. Vitamin D supplements may contain either vitamin D_2 or D_3, or alfacalcidiol (1-hydroxycholecalciferol). Overall, data suggest that vitamin D_3 may be more effective in raising 25(OH)D levels than vitamin D_2 (reviewed in [5]).

25(OH)D is transported to the kidney by DBP, where cytochromal 25-hydroxyvitamin D 1-α hydroxylase catalyzes its conversion to 1,25 dihydroxy vitamin D [1,25(OH)$_2$D], the active form of vitamin D. The vitamin D receptor (VDR) is expressed in multiple cells including the osteoblasts, mononuclear cells, activated T and B lymphocytes and beta cells, and most organs in the body including the brain, heart, skin, gonads, prostate, breast, and gut. How vitamin D deficiency affects disease states in these multiple organ systems has been an active area of research. Repletion of vitamin D stores to mitigate and improve disease processes has been attempted in certain conditions, although there is a paucity of data to direct clear treatment protocols, especially in the pediatric population.

2. Immune and Anti-Inflammatory Effects

There is evidence that vitamin D modulates B and T lymphocyte function [6–9], and vitamin D deficiency has been associated with conditions such as multiple sclerosis, type 1 diabetes (T1D), rheumatoid arthritis, systemic lupus erythematosus, dermatomyositis, inflammatory bowel disease, hepatitis, asthma and respiratory infections.

2.1. Type 1 Diabetes

Data regarding associations of 25(OH)D levels or vitamin D sufficiency/insufficiency/deficiency status are conflicting with some [10,11], but not all [12–14], studies reporting an association between low vitamin D status and occurrence of T1D. Pancreatic beta cells have VDRs and express 1-α hydroxylase (encoded by *CYP27B1*) [15], and the human insulin gene promoter has a vitamin D response element [16]. Further, vitamin D plays a role in T-cell regulatory responses and may protect beta cells from immune attack [17]. In addition, T1D patients are reported to have lower 25(OH)D levels compared to age matched controls [11,18,19]. Cooper et al. [20] linked the genetic determinants of circulating 25(OH)D (*DHCR7* and *CYP2R1*, which encode 7-dehydrocholesterol reductase and 25-hydroxylase) and vitamin D signaling in T cells (*CYP27B1*) with risk of T1D, while others (including a meta-analysis of nine studies with 1053 patients and 1017 controls) have linked specific polymorphisms of the VDR gene with risk for T1D [21]. Another study linked T-cell proliferation with DBP, and reported higher levels and frequencies of serum anti-DBP antibodies in patients with T1D vs. controls. This study postulated that DBP (expressed in α-cells of pancreatic islets) may be an autoantigen in T1D [22]. Further, lower maternal third trimester DBP levels and cord blood DBP levels have been associated with risk of T1D in offspring [23,24]. Further investigation into the role of CYP27B1 in immune cells such as monocytes, macrophages and T-cells is needed to better understand the role of vitamin D in the pathogenesis and perhaps prevention of T1D. Under this umbrella of research, prospective studies of vitamin D supplementation have attempted to elucidate causality of T1D and use of vitamin D as a potential therapy.

Interventional studies: Table 1 describes details of some representative studies of vitamin D supplementation in T1D. a beneficial effect of cholecalciferol supplementation on regulatory T-cells (T-regs) has been reported, with an increase in T-reg percentage [25] and suppressive capacity [26], and reduced progression to undetectable C-peptide. Consistent with these findings, a meta-analysis of five observational studies reported a protective effect of vitamin D supplementation in early childhood against development of T1D with a dose response effect [27], while another reported that such supplementation may have prevented 27% of the predicted T1D cases in England and Wales in 2012 [28]. Similarly, a beneficial impact has been reported with respect to fasting C-peptide with lower daily insulin doses [29], peripheral vascular resistance and inflammatory renal markers [30]. However, many other studies have not demonstrated a beneficial effect of vitamin D supplementation in preventing or improving the course of T1D. Importantly, the prospective Environmental Determinants of Diabetes in the Young (TEDDY) Study demonstrated no benefit of maternal vitamin D supplementation during pregnancy on the risk of islet autoimmunity in the offspring [31]. Other studies have failed to demonstrate a beneficial impact on beta cell function [32], HbA1C levels [25,33,34] or insulin requirement [25,34]. While the reason for these conflicting results is unclear, one may speculate that differences in study design, sample size and vitamin D dosing may contribute. Overall, randomized controlled studies investigating vitamin D replacement in preventing T1D or treating at diagnosis to prolong endogenous insulin secretion are few. Vitamin D replacement is necessary in those deficient for optimal bone health. However, current data do not provide definitive evidence that supplementation will improve the inflammatory state in a clinically significant manner.

Table 1. Summary of studies of vitamin D administration in type 1 and type 2 diabetes.

Reference	Type of Study	Intervention	Participants	Results (Intervention)
Type 1 Diabetes				
Studies examining effects on immune modulation				
[25]	18-month randomized controlled trial (RCT)	2000 IUs vitamin D_3 daily or placebo	38 participants; 35 completers; 7–30 years old	Increase in regulatory T-cell (T-reg) percentage; lower cumulative incidence of progression to undetectable C-peptide; no difference in HbA1C, insulin requirement or BMI
[26]	12-month RCT	70 IUs/kg/day vitamin D_3 vs. placebo	29 Participants; >6 years old; <3 months duration of T1D	Increase in suppressive capacity of T-regs
Studies of prevention of islet autoimmunity or T1D				
[27]	Meta-analysis of four case-control and one cohort study	Vitamin D supplementation (variable doses)	Infants	Four case control studies: risk of T1D decreased; similar findings in cohort study; some evidence of a dose-response effect
[28]	Population impact number of eliminating a risk factor (PIN-ER-*t*) Statistical method	Vitamin D supplementation (variable doses)	Babies born in 2012	For a population of 729,674 babies born in England and Wales in 2012, 374 cases of T1D (out of 1357 total predicted cases) could be prevented over 18 years if all were supplemented with vitamin D
[31]	Cohort study; assessment every 3 months between 3–48 months, and then every 6 months	Maternal vitamin D supplementation during pregnancy (based on recall); cumulative intake of vitamin D supplements and n-3 FAs analyzed	8676 children with increased genetic risk for T1D in Finland, Germany, Sweden and the US	Vitamin D supplementation during pregnancy was not associated with risk for development of islet autoantibodies (any/none and cumulative intake)
Studies examining course or complications of T1D				
[29]	6-month RCT	0.25 mcg twice daily of alfacalcidol vs. placebo	61 participants; 54 completers; 8–15 years old; <8 weeks duration of T1D	Higher fasting C-peptide; lower daily insulin dose
[30]	12–24 weeks single arm intervention study	1000–2000 IUs of vitamin D_3 daily	271 adolescents with T1D with 25(OH)D <15 ng/mL	Improved endothelial function; decreased urinary inflammatory cytokines/chemokines; no change in systolic or diastolic blood pressure, lipids, HbA1C and albumin/creatinine ratio
[32]	2-year RCT	0.25 mcg daily of calcitriol or placebo	34 participants 11–35 years old with recent onset T1D and high basal C-peptide	No effect on beta cell function
[33]	Single dose single arm intervention study	Vitamin D_3: 100,000 IUs for those 2–10 years old; 160,000 IUs for those >10 years	40 children <19 years with T1D and vitamin D deficiency (<20 ng/mL) included in ITT analysis	No difference in HbA1C levels at 3 months or at 1 year
[34]	6-month RCT	Vitamin D_3 60,000 IUs once a month for 6 months	52 children with T1D 1–18 years old	Higher mean C-peptide level; no difference in HbA1C or insulin requirement

Table 1. *Cont.*

Reference	Type of Study	Intervention	Participants	Results (Intervention)
			Obesity, Prediabetes or Type 2 Diabetes	
			Adults	
[35]	Single arm intervention study	Vitamin D_3 two doses of 100,000 IUs at 2-week intervals	33 adults with vitamin D deficiency (25(OH)D < 20 ng/mL) and without T2D	No change in mean blood glucose or insulin, or insulin sensitivity (assessed using an OGTT)
[36]	6-month RCT	Vitamin D_3 4000 IUs daily or placebo	82 insulin resistant, vitamin D deficient (25(OH)D < 20 ng/mL) South Asian women in New Zealand without T2D	HOMA-IR improved when 25(OH)D level rose to >32 ng/mL; no differences in insulin secretion, CRP, BMI or lipid levels
[37]	6-month intervention study	Vitamin D_3 20,000 IUs or placebo given twice weekly over 6 months	104 adults with vitamin D deficiency; 94 completers	No difference in insulin secretion, insulin sensitivity (using a hyperglycemic clamp) or lipids
[38]	4-month RCT	Vitamin D_3 2500 IUs or placebo daily	114 post-menopausal women with 25(OH)D between 10–60 ng/mL	No improvement in blood pressure, endothelial function, arterial stiffness, inflammation and CRP
[39]	16-week RCT	Vitamin D_3 supplementation 200 IUs or placebo daily	165 healthy women 18–35 years	No change in lipids; modest change in systolic and diastolic blood pressure
[40]	5-year RCT	Vitamin D_3 20,000 IUs/week or placebo; followed every 6 months	556 adults 25–80 years old with prediabetes; 503 completers	25(OH)D increased from ~24 ng/mL to 48 ng/mL with supplementation; no effect on progression to T2D, measures of glucose metabolism, serum lipids or blood pressure in the group as a whole, or in those with vitamin D deficiency
[41]	Pooled meta-analysis of 28 RCTs	Vitamin D_3 supplementation, variable doses	Adults at risk for T2D (no T2D)	No effect on controlling fasting plasma glucose levels, improving insulin resistance, or preventing T2D; stratified analysis suggested a possible beneficial effect in those without obesity, those with prediabetes, when 25(OH)D levels were ≥20 ng/mL, and when the supplemental dose was >2000 IUs per day and given without calcium supplementation
[42]	RCT	Vitamin D_3 4000 IUs or placebo regardless of vitamin D status	2423 adult participants meeting criteria for prediabetes (2382 randomized)	No differences in baseline 25(OH)D; supplemented group had 25(OH)D levels about twice that in the placebo group; no difference in progression to T2D (9.4 vs. 10.7 events per 100 person-years respectively at a median follow-up of 2.5 years)
			Children	
[43]	6-month RCT	Vitamin D_3 4000 IUs daily or placebo	35 adolescents with obesity 9–19 years old	Improved HOMA-IR and QUICKI (but not fasting glucose, HbA1C, CRP, IL-6 or TNF-alpha) in those who received vitamin D
[44]	1-year open label parallel arm prospective study	Vitamin D_3 5000 IUs weekly for 8 weeks vs. no intervention	70 indigenous Argentinean children vs. 20 non-supplemented children	Improved HDL

Table 1. *Cont.*

Reference	Type of Study	Intervention	Participants	Results (Intervention)
[45]	12-week RCT	Vitamin D_3 300,000 IUs weekly or placebo	50 children with obesity 10–16 years old	Improved serum insulin and HOMA-IR with no effect on lipids, fasting blood sugar or blood pressure
[46]	Retrospective study	Vitamin D supplementation	43 children 3–18 years old with T2D for >12 months and a diagnosis of vitamin D deficiency (25(OH)D < 20 ng/mL)	Decrease in BMI-SDS, HbA1C and ALT in supplemented group
[47]	12-week RCT	Vitamin D_3 2000 IUs daily or placebo	58 adolescents with obesity 12–18 years old	No change in fasting glucose, insulin, HOMA-IR, lipids or CRP
[48]	12-week RCT	Vitamin D_3 two doses (400 IU/day and 2000 IU/day) for 12 weeks	51 Caucasian adolescents with obesity 12–18 years old; 46 completers	No change in 25(OH)D levels in the in 400 IU/day group and a modest increase in the 2000 IU/day group. No change in fasting HOMA-IR, insulin, glucose or lipid levels post-supplementation
[49]	2-year prospective study	Vitamin D_3 100,00 IUs/year to both groups	104 children in Group a (treated in 2014) and 86 in Group B (treated in 2013)	Changes in 25(OH)D levels were significantly associated with lower LDL-C and Apo-B levels.
[50]	3-month open label, prospective study	Vitamin D_3 100,000 IUs monthly for 3 months	19 children with obesity and vitamin D deficiency 13–18 years old	No change in endothelial function, fasting lipids, glucose, insulin and CRP values
[51]	12-week RCT	Vitamin D_3 at either 0, 400, 1000, 2000 or 4000 IU/day for 12 weeks	323 early pubertal children At baseline, 15% had 25(OH)D levels that were insufficient <25 ng/mL, 6% had levels <16 ng/mL and 1% had levels lower than 12 ng/mL	At baseline, 25(OH)D levels were inversely associated with insulin and HOMA-IR. However, glucose, insulin and insulin resistance increased over 12 weeks in all dosage groups
[52]	12-week RCT	Vitamin D_3 50,000 IUs per week vs. placebo	29 African American children with obesity 13–17 years old	No impact on insulin secretion or sensitivity

2.2. Multiple Sclerosis

The risk for multiple sclerosis (MS) is higher in people living above 35° latitudes than those who live below this latitude [53] (although effects were attenuated over time in this study), and studies have reported an association between risk for MS and lower sunlight exposure [54–59], vitamin D intake [60] and serum 25(OH)D levels [61–64]. Increased sun exposure in children has been linked to a lower risk of MS in studies out of Tasmania [57], twin studies where only one monozygotic twin developed MS [55], a study from Cuba, Martinique and Sicily [54], as well as studies in adults from Iran [58] and Sweden [59]. Other studies have linked the reduced risk of MS following sun exposure to the melanocortin 1 receptor genotype [56]. Further, polymorphisms in genes that impact 25(OH)D levels have been linked to risk of relapse in children with MS [65].

Munger et al. reported an inverse relationship between serum 25(OH)D and the risk of MS [61], and that before onset, MS risk decreases by 40% for every 20 ng/mL increase in 25(OH)D levels. In another study, women (but not men) with MS had lower 25(OH)D levels than controls 11 years after disease onset [62], with a 19% reduction in the odds for MS for every 4 ng/mL increase in winter 25(OH)D concentrations. Similar lower 25(OH)D in patients with MS versus controls has been reported in other studies for winter [63] or summer levels [64].

Data suggest that vitamin D sufficient states in the mother and infant may protect against MS [66]. Increased first trimester exposure to UVR reduced MS risk in the child in a dose dependent fashion [67]. Higher MS rates in children born in the summer or spring, and lower rates in those born in the fall may be related to maternal vitamin D insufficiency [68,69]. In the Nurses Health Study, women born to mothers with high vitamin D intake during pregnancy had a reduced risk of MS [70].

Interventional Studies: protective effects of vitamin D supplementation have been demonstrated against MS in a few studies [60]. The Nurses Health Study reported that women taking at least 400 IU of vitamin D supplements daily were at lower risk compared to those not on supplements [60,71]. a meta-analysis of 12 RCTs that included 950 adult patients with MS reported non-significant trends in improvement in annualized relapse rate Expanded Disability Status Scale scores and MRI findings in those who received vitamin D supplementation, although higher vitamin D doses (2850–10,400 IUs) performed significantly worse compared to lower doses (800–1000 IUs) [72]. One RCT did report an improvement in MRI lesions when vitamin D_3 was employed as add-on treatment to interferon beta-1b in patients with MS [73]. Data are lacking for effects of vitamin D supplementation in children with MS.

Overall, although case-control and epidemiological studies suggest that people with lower 25(OH)D levels may be at higher risk for MS, confounding factors, such as the association of higher latitudes (also a risk factor for MS) with lower 25(OH)D levels need to be considered. Interventional studies examining the preventive effect of vitamin D supplementation on the risk for developing MS are lacking. Existing RCTs in adult patients with established MS are not convincing for a significant role for vitamin D supplementation in reducing MS outcomes, although trends for a positive effect have been reported, particularly with low dose supplementation. Data to date indicate deleterious effects of high dose vitamin D supplementation on MS outcomes. RCTs assessing the impact of vitamin D supplementation on MS outcomes in children are lacking.

2.3. Rheumatoid Arthritis

One meta-analysis of 15 studies (including 1143 rheumatoid arthritis (RA) patients and 963 controls) confirmed lower 25(OH)D levels and a higher prevalence of vitamin D deficiency in patients compared with controls (55% vs. 33%) [74]. Similarly, a meta-analysis of three cohort studies that included 215,757 participants and 874 incident cases of RA reported that individuals in the highest quartile for vitamin D intake had a 24% lower risk of developing RA compared to those in the lowest quartile [75]. In addition, inverse associations of 25(OH)D levels with disease activity scores in RA patients have been reported [74,76–79]. Further, specific VDR polymorphisms have been demonstrated to contribute significantly to RA risk [80,81].

Interventional Studies: consistent with the findings from epidemiologic studies, protective effects of vitamin D supplementation have been demonstrated against RA in some studies [82]. Chandrashekara and Patted reported a reduction in disease severity scores following vitamin D replacement (60,000 IU of vitamin D weekly for six weeks followed by 60,000 IU monthly) over three months in RA patients who were vitamin D deficient (25(OH)D levels <20 ng/mL) and had persistent disease activity [83]. However, a meta-analysis that included five RCTs in patients with RA reported borderline significance for reduction in disease recurrence, but not for disease activity [84]. Calcitriol enhances inhibition of T cell activation by abatacept (CTLA-4-Ig), a CD28-ligand blocker to which patients with RA respond with variable efficacy [85], suggesting that vitamin D or calcitriol may be used as an adjunct therapy to improve efficacy of abatacept in RA patients. Overall, these data suggest that lower 25(OH)D levels may predict susceptibility to RA and its severity, but it is not clear that vitamin D supplementation reduces the risk of developing RA or its disease activity/severity. Further, data in children with RA are currently lacking.

2.4. *Systemic Lupus Erythematosus (SLE) and Juvenile Dermatomyositis*

Many studies have reported inverse associations of 25(OH)D levels with the occurrence and severity of SLE and dermatomyosits in adults and children [86–92]. In children, greater disease severity of SLE is reported in those with 25(OH)D levels <20 ng/mL [88].

Interventional Studies: in contrast to other autoimmune conditions, several interventional studies have reported an improvement in markers of severity of disease following vitamin D supplementation in patients with SLE. One study in adolescents and adults with juvenile onset SLE reported an improvement in disease severity scores and fatigue in those randomized to 50,000 IU per week of vitamin D supplementation compared to placebo over 6 months [93]. Similar findings are reported in studies of adults with SLE. a reduction in inflammatory and hemostatic markers, and disease activity was reported in those randomized to 2000 IU of vitamin D daily compared to placebo for 12 months [94]. Further, a meta-analysis of three RCTs of vitamin D supplementation in patients with SLE reported a significant reduction in anti-dsDNA positivity with supplementation [84]. Another study reported an increase of T-regs and a decrease of effector Th1 and Th17 cells, memory B cells and anti-DNA antibodies in adults with SLE given 100,000 IU of vitamin D weekly for 4 weeks followed by 100,000 IU monthly for 6 months [95]. No flares were observed over the study duration [95].

Overall, these data suggest that low 25(OH)D levels are concerning for greater risk of developing SLE and increased severity of the condition, and a possible beneficial effect of vitamin D supplementation on disease severity, particularly when levels are low. However, more RCTs, including in children, are necessary to confirm these data. Of note, symptoms of SLE can worsen after UV radiation exposure which will otherwise increase the vitamin D status of the individual [96]. Thus, excessive sun exposure to improve 25(OH)D levels in patients with SLE may worsen symptoms of the disease.

2.5. *Psoriasis*

Keratinocytes express the vitamin D receptor (VDR), and vitamin D inhibits the growth of keratinocytes, stimulates them to differentiate, and helps maintain the cutaneous barrier integrity [97]. This has led to the use of topical vitamin D analogs to treat psoriasis [98]. However, no VDR genotype (other than the Taql polymorphsm in Caucasians) has been linked to an increased risk for psoriasis [99,100]. In addition, there is no correlation between the change in 25(OH)D post phototherapy and change in severity of symptoms of psoriasis [101,102].

Interventional Studies: a 6-month RCT of 60,000 IUs of vitamin D vs. placebo given every 2 weeks to 45 patients with psoriasis showed an increase in 25(OH)D levels in the active group associated with a reduction in the Psoriasis Area and Severity Index (PASI) [103]. Topical vitamin D analogs (calcipotriene/calcipotriol/maxacalcitol) given with topical betamethasone have also been shown to be effective in improving plaque psoriasis [104–106] by disrupting the IL-36 and IL-23/IL-17 positive feedback loop, key factors in the pathogenesis of psoriasis.

Overall, while studies suggest an association between 25(OH)D levels and psoriasis, causation is yet to be established. Additionally, RCTs to date are promising for an impact of vitamin D on psoriasis severity, but studies are small, and more and larger RCTs are necessary to confirm these preliminary findings. Data in children are lacking.

2.6. *Inflammatory Bowel Disease (IBD)*

Protective effects of vitamin D supplementation have been demonstrated against IBD [107]. Vitamin D deficient and vitamin D receptor (*Vdr*) null mice are at high risk of IBD [108], with more severe disease and more spontaneous recurrences. Further, polymorphisms in the *Vdr* gene (TaqI) may confer susceptibility to IBD [109]. a meta-analysis of VDR genotyping in relation to IBD reported that ApaI polymorphism may increase the risk of Crohn's disease, whereas the TaqI polymorphism may decrease the risk of ulcerative colitis, especially in Caucasians [110]. a connection has been proposed between seasonal vitamin D status and risk for both Crohn's disease and ulcerative colitis [111,112], with an association between vitamin D deficiency and more complicated disease course. a recent meta-analysis reported lower 25(OH)D levels in patients with both Crohn's disease and ulcerative colitis than controls, a two-fold risk of vitamin D deficiency in those with IBD, and greater severity of Crohn's disease in those with vitamin D deficiency [113,114]. However, these studies are associative and confounded by the fact that malabsorption (particularly in Crohn's disease) may contribute to lower 25(OH)D levels, with more severe disease being associated with more malabsorption.

Interventional studies: there are few randomized controlled trials that have examined the impact of vitamin D supplementation on disease occurrence or severity. One randomized controlled trial of 400 vs. 2000 IU of vitamin D supplementation in children and adolescents with IBD did report that the higher dose of vitamin D led to lower levels of pro-inflammatory markers [115]. Vitamin D has also been shown to exert marked anti-inflammatory effects on peripheral and intestinal CD4+ and CD8+ T cells of patients with inflammatory bowel disorders in vitro, and inhibit production of TH1 and TH17 cytokines in patients with Crohn's disease in vivo [116].

Overall, while data to date suggest that vitamin D deficiency may impact disease course in patients with inflammatory bowel disorders, we are in need of robust RCTs that will help determine whether vitamin D supplementation is indeed efficacious in reducing disease severity in these patients, including in children.

2.7. *Food Allergies*

Although associations of low 25(OH)D levels with a risk of atopy, asthma and food allergies have been reported [117], recent birth cohort studies demonstrate no association of 25(OH)D levels (including antenatal vitamin D exposure) with the incidence of food allergy [118,119]. One meta-analysis of more than 5000 children did not find a significant association between vitamin D status and food allergy [120].

Interventional Studies: data for the role of vitamin D supplementation in preventing food allergies is inconsistent, and large trials are necessary to determine the role if any of vitamin D in reducing the risk for food allergies [121]. One RCT of 400 vs. 1200 IUs of vitamin D supplementation in 975 infants from the age of 2 weeks found no impact of higher-dose vitamin D supplementation on allergic sensitization or allergic diseases (food or aeroallergen) at 12-months of age [122]. Overall, current data do not support a role of vitamin D status in impacting the risk for food allergies in children, and non-interventional studies may be confounded by variables such as associated malabsorption.

2.8. *Chronic Hepatitis B and C*

Certain vitamin D receptor gene (*VDR* a/a) polymorphisms have been linked to greater severity of hepatitis B infection and a higher viral load [123]. In addition, polymorphisms in the T/T allele of exon 9 of the *VDR* gene (but not intron 8 polymorphisms) are associated with occult hepatitis B infection [124]. Further, a meta-analysis of seven studies involving 814 patients with chronic hepatitis B and 696 controls showed lower 25(OH)D levels in patients with chronic hepatitis B associated with higher viral loads [125]. Petta et al. [126] reported that lower 25(OH)D levels in chronic hepatitis C infection were related to decreased CYP27A1 expression, female gender, necrosis and inflammation, severe fibrosis and poor viral response to interferon based therapy. Of note, polymorphisms in the VDR gene have been associated with development of hepatocellular carcinoma in patients with hepatitis C [127].

Interventional Studies: in in vitro studies, 25(OH)D has been shown to inhibit hepatitis C virus production by suppressing apolipoprotein expression [128]. In 42 patients with recurrent hepatitis C infections treated with INF-α and ribavirin for 48 weeks, vitamin D deficiency was associated with an unfavorable response to antiviral medication, and 15 patients given oral vitamin D supplements had a better and more sustained response to antiviral treatment [129]. One short 6-week RCT of vitamin D supplementation vs. placebo in 54 patients with chronic hepatitis C with vitamin D deficiency demonstrated improved serum markers of hepatic fibrogenesis upon correction of 25(OH)D levels [130].

Overall, data suggest deleterious effects of vitamin D deficiency on the course of chronic hepatitis B and C infections, with some studies suggesting a possible role (and mechanism) for vitamin D supplementation in improving outcomes in these patients. However, we are in need of larger RCTs and of longer duration to effectively confirm these findings, and data in children are lacking.

2.9. Asthma and Respiratory Infections

Several studies have reported an association between vitamin D deficiency (25(OH)D < 20 ng/mL) and increased airway inflammation, decreased lung function, increased exacerbations, and poor prognosis in patients with asthma (reviewed in [131]).

Interventional Studies: a literature review of RCTs of vitamin D supplementation in children older than 2 years found a possible effect of vitamin D supplementation in improving bronchial asthma exacerbation [132,133], but no effect on the severity of asthma [132]. a subsequent meta-analysis that included 435 children (seven trials) and 658 adults (two trials) similarly reported a reduction in asthma exacerbations requiring systemic corticosteroids and the risk for an exacerbation requiring an emergency department visit or hospitalization in those who received vitamin D supplementation, but not on measures of severity (% predicted forced expiratory volume in one second or Asthma Control test Scores [134]. The improvement in asthma exacerbation has been attributed to a decrease in respiratory infections [12].

RCTs of vitamin D supplementation (300–1200 IUs per day) vs. placebo report a potential effect of vitamin D in reducing the risk for influenza infections during the winter months [135], although a subsequent analysis reported that benefits observed in the first month of supplementation were lost in the second month, and overall there was no difference among groups for influenza prevalence over the entire season [136]. a meta-analysis of 25 RCTs using vitamin D supplementation of any duration in individuals 0–95 years old demonstrated that vitamin D reduced the risk for acute respiratory infections overall, with the greatest benefit in those with low 25(OH)D levels (<10 ng/mL), and those receiving daily or weekly vitamin D supplementation vs. bolus doses [137,138]. Effects may be less robust in those 1–5 years old [139], and a dose effect has not been demonstrated [140].

Overall, these data suggest that vitamin D may have an effect in reducing the risk for respiratory infections in children, with more pronounced effects after 5 years of age, and in those that are vitamin D deficient. This effect may explain the reduced risk of asthma exacerbations in children with vitamin D supplementation (although asthma severity does not appear to improve with vitamin D). The mechanism underlying the effect on respiratory infections needs to be determined, but may involve the impact of vitamin D on inflammatory pathways.

3. Metabolic Syndrome and Type 2 Diabetes Mellitus

Although, VDR polymorphisms are unlikely to play a major role in obesity-related phenotypes, as reported in a population of Caucasian adults [141], vitamin D deficiency has been associated with obesity in both pediatric and adult populations. The prevalence of vitamin D deficiency is about 50% in children with obesity [142,143], and attributable to decreased sun exposure secondary to low activity level, poor nutrition with decreased consumption of vitamin D containing foods such as milk, as well as storage in adipose tissue [142]. With the increased prevalence of obesity in children there has also been concern of increased prevalence of type 2 DM (T2D), dyslipidemia and hypertension, the metabolic syndrome [1]. The role vitamin D plays in contributing to these disorders has been of interest given the above association and implications for potential treatment. Exactly which aspects of the metabolic syndrome are associated with vitamin D deficiency have not been definitively delineated as studies show varied results. Olson et al. found a negative correlation between 25(OH)D levels and HOMA-IR (homeostasis model assessment of insulin resistance) and weaker but significant inverse correlations with 2-h glucose levels in an oral glucose tolerance test (OGTT). There was no correlation with HbA1C, systolic blood pressure (SBP) or diastolic blood pressure (DBP) [142]. In another study vitamin D deficiency in children with obesity was associated with higher BMI and SBP, and decreased HDL-C [143]. After adjusting for BMI in Native American children, 25(OH)D levels were inversely associated with log transformed fasting 2-h glucose, fasting insulin, HOMA-IR, triglyceride and CRP levels, and SBP and DBP. There was a positive correlation with HDL but no correlation with total or LDL cholesterol [144]. Studies have postulated that adipokines such as adiponectin and resistin may be involved in the pathogenesis of insulin resistance and vitamin D deficiency. a study of 125 children and adolescents with obesity showed a trend toward lower 25(OH)D levels being associated with low adiponectin levels and higher insulin resistance even after adjusting for body mass, though there was no correlation between 25(OH)D levels and resistin [145].

Conversely, Poomthavorn et al. [146] found no correlation between vitamin D deficiency and abnormal glucose homeostasis in 150 children and adolescents with obesity living in Thailand. In fact, the five children identified with T2D in this study were all vitamin D sufficient. They also found the same degree of vitamin D deficiency in 29 healthy children without obesity [146]. Similarly, Bril et al. found no relationship between lower 25(OH)D levels and insulin resistance (using an euglycemic insulin clamp), liver fat accumulation or steatohepatitis when adult patients with the latter were matched for BMI and total adiposity with controls [147]. More recently, in a study of 215 children with T1D and 326 children with T2D vs. youth of similar age without diabetes from the 2005–2006 NHANES Survey, the prevalence of vitamin D deficiency or insufficiency did not differ in children with vs. those without diabetes [14]. Additionally, although latitude and the winter months have been associated with a higher risk of hypertension, recent studies suggest that the effect of ultraviolet light on blood pressure is likely mediated via nitric oxide synthesis and not through vitamin D production [148]. Limitations of pediatric studies include the fact that these associative studies often do not include controls matched for measures of adiposity, or use euglycemic clamps to assess insulin resistance. In addition, sample sizes are small and length of studies short. Associations of vitamin D deficiency with worsening insulin resistance or other aspects of the metabolic syndrome are yet to be proven.

Interventional studies in adults and adolescents are described in detail in Table 1 and are summarized here.

Interventional Studies in Adults with Obesity, Prediabetes and T2D: the contribution of vitamin D to the metabolic phenotype of obesity is of interest given implications for treatment. If these associations have a biological basis, repleting vitamin D should improve the phenotype. How this should be done, to what level of replacement, and the actual efficacy have been the basis of several studies. Vitamin D administration in adults has had mixed results for progression to T2D and cardio-metabolic outcomes. Among short-term studies with small numbers of participants, most have reported no changes in insulin sensitivity [35], insulin secretion [36,37], CRP [36,38], BMI [36], lipids [36,37,39], blood pressure, endothelial function, and arterial stiffness [38] following vitamin D administration, while a few have reported an improvement in insulin sensitivity [36] and blood pressure [39]. Among larger and longer-term studies, a five-year interventional study in 556 adults 25–80 years old at risk for developing T2D, reported no impact of vitamin D administration on progression to T2D, measures of glucose metabolism, serum lipids or blood pressure [40]. a subsequent pooled meta-analysis of 23 RCTs similarly found no effect of vitamin D supplementation in controlling fasting plasma glucose levels, improving insulin resistance, or preventing T2D; however, stratified analysis suggested a possible beneficial effect in those without obesity, those with prediabetes, when 25(OH)D levels were at least 20 ng/mL, and when the supplemental dose was >2000 IUs per day and given without calcium supplementation [41]. Yet, an RCT in adult participants meeting criteria for prediabetes (but not diabetes) reported no difference between groups for onset of diabetes over the study duration [42].

Interventional Studies in Children with Obesity, Prediabetes and T2D: similar to the adult literature, the pediatric literature includes conflicting data regarding effects of vitamin D supplementation [43–52] (Table 1). a retrospective study of vitamin D supplementation in 43 children 3–18 years old with T2D reported a decrease in BMI-SDS and HbA1C in those supplemented with vitamin D [46]. A few prospective studies in adolescents with obesity have similarly reported improved HOMA-IR and QUICKI (but not in fasting glucose, HbA1C, CRP, inflammatory markers, blood pressure) [43,45] following vitamin D administration, and an association of reductions in Apo-B and LDL-C, and increases in HDL with increases in 25(OH)D levels after supplementation [44,49]. However, most prospective interventional studies in children with obesity have failed to demonstrate a beneficial effect of vitamin D administration on fasting lipids, glucose, insulin and CRP values [47,48,50,51], and insulin secretion or sensitivity [52], and dose response studies have similarly not been able to demonstrate an effect of increasing vitamin D doses on fasting glucose, insulin and insulin resistance [48,51] or lipid levels [48].

Overall data indicate that there is an association between obesity and vitamin D deficiency (likely related to sequestration of vitamin D in adipose depots). However, the biological effect of vitamin D deficiency on insulin resistance, hypertension, hyperlipidemia and progression to T2D is likely small. Data are conflicting regarding associations of vitamin D deficiency with components of the metabolic syndrome, as well as a treatment effect. Some differences may be attributable to the type of study, sample size, and dose of vitamin D used (Table 1). Larger and longer-term prospective studies are needed to definitively determine causality.

4. Cancer

In cell culture studies, 25(OH)D concentrations of >30 ng/mL prevent unregulated cell growth [149–151]. There are very little data for the role of vitamin D in preventing or ameliorating the course of cancer in children, although low 25(OH)vitamin D levels may contribute to poor bone health in children with hematological and other malignancies [152–154]. Much of the data for the impact of vitamin D in preventing or reducing the morbidity of cancer comes from studies in adults, particularly in the context of breast, colorectal and prostate cancer. This section briefly reviews existing literature for these three kinds of cancer.

In breast cancer cell lines, vitamin D signaling inhibits expression of a tumor progression gene (Id1), and ablation of VDR expression causes increased tumor growth and development of metastases [155]. This pathway is inhibited in murine models of breast cancer associated with vitamin D deficiency, and epidemiological studies in humans suggest associations of vitamin D deficiency and the risk of breast, prostate and colon cancer [156–158]. However, data are conflicting regarding the impact of vitamin D receptor genotype and cancer risk at this time [159]. One study reported that *VDR* single nucleotide polymorphisms and haplotypes may determine how inflammatory markers change in breast cancer survivors with vitamin D deficiency, following vitamin D supplementation [160].

In general, vitamin D deficiency is associated with increased risk of progression and mortality in breast cancers [161–163]. Of note, these data have been questioned in that meta-analyses indicate that while case control studies suggest a reduction in breast cancer risk in those with higher 25(OH)D levels, this is not evident in prospective studies [163,164]. Data suggest that weight and alcohol intake may modify associations between vitamin D intake and breast cancer risk [165]. Of note, the Women's Health Initiative demonstrated no reduction in risk for breast cancer in women receiving 400 IU vitamin D_3 and 1000 mg of calcium vs. placebo [166]. However, a decreased risk was noted in postmenopausal women on hormone replacement therapy from daily vitamin D and calcium supplements [167], and another study reported improved breast cancer survival in patients after surgery of invasive breast cancer in de novo vitamin D users [168]. One recent 12-month RCT of 20,000 IUs of vitamin D vs. placebo in 208 premenopausal women at high risk for breast cancer found no effect of vitamin D supplementation in reducing breast cancer risk (assessed using mammographic density) [169]. Similarly, an RCT of 2000 IUs of vitamin D and omega-3 fatty acids (1 g daily) (2×2 factorial design) in women 55 and older and men 50 and older found no effect of vitamin D supplementation in lowering the incidence of invasive cancer compared to placebo [170].

Meta-analyses have reported inverse associations of 25(OH)D levels and vitamin D intake with the incidence and recurrence of colorectal adenoma [171–174]. One meta-analysis suggested a 10%–20% reduction in risk of incidence or recurrence of colorectal adenomas with every 20 ng/mL increase in 25(OH)D levels [171]. Another meta-analysis suggested a 26% reduction in risk with every 10 ng/mL increase in 25(OH)D levels [175,176]. However, a large Mendelian randomization study that included 10,725 colorectal cancer cases and 30,794 controls found no evidence for a causal relationship between circulating 25(OH)D and colorectal cancer risk. These authors suggested that circulating vitamin D may be a biomarker of colorectal cancer, rather than a causative factor [177]. Thus far, data for a role of VDR polymorphisms in mediating the risk of colorectal adenomas are conflicting, with no associations reported in more recent studies [176,178].

Some studies have suggested that vitamin D with or without calcium supplementation promotes colorectal epithelial cell differentiation, reduces proliferation, and promotes apoptosis, and is thus chemopreventive against colorectal neoplasms [179]. Further, a higher expression of CYP24A1, which reduces local 1,25-D (3) availability and thus its antiproliferative effect, has been demonstrated in colorectal adenocarcinomas, associated with increased expression of the proliferation marker Ki-67 [180]. Despite these data and consistent with the Mendelian randomization study, randomized controlled trials and meta-analyses do not support a role of vitamin D supplementation in preventing these cancers [161,181,182] or relapses [183–185]. Baron et al. disappointingly reported that daily supplementation with vitamin D_3 (1000 IU), calcium (1200 mg), or both after removal of colorectal adenomas did not reduce the risk of recurrence over a 3–5 year period [184]. Similarly, Urashima et al. reported no improvement in relapse free survival in patients with digestive tract cancers (48% were colorectal cancers) randomized to 2000 IUs of vitamin D vs. placebo (AMATERASU RCT) [185]. However, in the SUNSHINE trial (a phase 2 RCT in which 139 patients with advanced or metastatic colorectal cancer were randomized to chemotherapy plus high-dose vitamin D_3 supplementation (8000 IUs daily for one month followed by 4000 IUs daily vs. chemotherapy plus standard-dose vitamin D_3 (400 IUs daily)) the higher vitamin D dose was associated with a multivariable hazard ratio of 0.64 for progression-free survival or death that was statistically significant [186].

Sun exposure may delay the onset of prostate cancer [157] while serum 25(OH)D levels of at least 20 ng/mL appear to reduce the risk for prostate cancer by 50% [187]. However, data for associations of vitamin D deficiency with incidence of prostate cancer are weaker than those for colon cancer, and data for associations with progression are inconsistent [161,188].

Overall, at this time, data do not support a significant role of vitamin D supplementation in preventing or changing the course of breast, colorectal or prostate cancer.

5. Conclusions

In conclusion, vitamin D may have biological effects well beyond the skeleton. While it is important to maintain adequate 25(OH)D levels for optimal bone health, this may have benefits in a variety of different organ systems. However, interventional studies to prevent or ameliorate disease processes attributable to vitamin D deficiency in large populations have been disappointing thus far for the most part. More investigation is needed to determine optimal dosing and serum levels to effect positive biological outcomes.

Author Contributions: R.M. and M.M. contributed equally to the concept of this manuscript, the required literature review, and the writing of this manuscript. Both authors approved the submitted version of the manuscript.

References

1. Misra, M.; Pacaud, D.; Petryk, A.; Collett-Solberg, P.F.; Kappy, M. Vitamin D deficiency in children and its management: Review of current knowledge and recommendations. *Pediatrics* **2008**, *122*, 398–417. [CrossRef] [PubMed]
2. Holick, M.F.; Binkley, N.C.; Bischoff-Ferrari, H.A.; Gordon, C.M.; Hanley, D.A.; Heaney, R.P.; Murad, M.H.; Weaver, C.M. Guidelines for preventing and treating vitamin D deficiency and insufficiency revisited. *J. Clin. Endocrinol. Metab.* **2012**, *97*, 1153–1158. [CrossRef] [PubMed]
3. Holick, M.F.; Binkley, N.C.; Bischoff-Ferrari, H.A.; Gordon, C.M.; Hanley, D.A.; Heaney, R.P.; Murad, M.H.; Weaver, C.M. Evaluation, treatment, and prevention of vitamin D deficiency: An Endocrine Society clinical practice guideline. *J. Clin. Endocrinol. Metab.* **2011**, *96*, 1911–1930. [CrossRef] [PubMed]
4. Ross, A.C.; Manson, J.E.; Abrams, S.A.; Aloia, J.F.; Brannon, P.M.; Clinton, S.K.; Durazo-Arvizu, R.A.; Gallagher, J.C.; Gallo, R.L.; Jones, G.; et al. The 2011 report on dietary reference intakes for calcium and vitamin D from the Institute of Medicine: What clinicians need to know. *J. Clin. Endocrinol. Metab.* **2011**, *96*, 53–58. [CrossRef] [PubMed]
5. Guo, J.; Lovegrove, J.A.; Givens, D.I. 25(OH)D_3-enriched or fortified foods are more efficient at tackling inadequate vitamin D status than vitamin D_3. *Proc. Nutr. Soc.* **2018**, *77*, 282–291. [CrossRef] [PubMed]
6. Tsoukas, C.D.; Provvedini, D.M.; Manolagas, S.C. 1,25-dihydroxyvitamin D_3: A novel immunoregulatory hormone. *Science* **1984**, *224*, 1438–1440. [CrossRef] [PubMed]
7. Bhalla, A.K.; Amento, E.P.; Clemens, T.L.; Holick, M.F.; Krane, S.M. Specific high-affinity receptors for 1,25-dihydroxyvitamin D_3 in human peripheral blood mononuclear cells: Presence in monocytes and induction in T lymphocytes following activation. *J. Clin. Endocrinol. Metab.* **1983**, *57*, 1308–1310. [CrossRef] [PubMed]
8. Drozdenko, G.; Scheel, T.; Heine, G.; Baumgrass, R.; Worm, M. Impaired T cell activation and cytokine production by calcitriol-primed human B cells. *Clin. Exp. Immunol.* **2014**, *178*, 364–372. [CrossRef] [PubMed]
9. Milliken, S.V.; Wassall, H.; Lewis, B.J.; Logie, J.; Barker, R.N.; Macdonald, H.; Vickers, M.A.; Ormerod, A.D. Effects of ultraviolet light on human serum 25-hydroxyvitamin D and systemic immune function. *J. Allergy Clin. Immunol.* **2012**, *129*, 1554–1561. [CrossRef]
10. Al-Zubeidi, H.; Leon-Chi, L.; Newfield, R.S. Low vitamin D level in pediatric patients with new onset type 1 diabetes is common, especially if in ketoacidosis. *Pediatr. Diabetes* **2016**, *17*, 592–598. [CrossRef]
11. Savastio, S.; Cadario, F.; Genoni, G.; Bellomo, G.; Bagnati, M.; Secco, G.; Picchi, R.; Giglione, E.; Bona, G. Vitamin D Deficiency and Glycemic Status in Children and Adolescents with Type 1 Diabetes Mellitus. *PLoS ONE* **2016**, *11*, e0162554. [CrossRef] [PubMed]
12. Makinen, M.; Mykkanen, J.; Koskinen, M.; Simell, V.; Veijola, R.; Hyoty, H.; Ilonen, J.; Knip, M.; Simell, O.; Toppari, J. Serum 25-Hydroxyvitamin D Concentrations in Children Progressing to Autoimmunity and Clinical Type 1 Diabetes. *J. Clin. Endocrinol. Metab.* **2016**, *101*, 723–729. [CrossRef] [PubMed]
13. Granfors, M.; Augustin, H.; Ludvigsson, J.; Brekke, H.K. No association between use of multivitamin supplement containing vitamin D during pregnancy and risk of Type 1 Diabetes in the child. *Pediatr. Diabetes* **2016**, *17*, 525–530. [CrossRef] [PubMed]
14. Wood, J.R.; Connor, C.G.; Cheng, P.; Ruedy, K.J.; Tamborlane, W.V.; Klingensmith, G.; Schatz, D.; Gregg, B.; Cengiz, E.; Willi, S.; et al. Vitamin D status in youth with type 1 and type 2 diabetes enrolled in the Pediatric Diabetes Consortium (PDC) is not worse than in youth without diabetes. *Pediatr. Diabetes* **2016**, *17*, 584–591. [CrossRef] [PubMed]
15. Bland, R.; Markovic, D.; Hills, C.E.; Hughes, S.V.; Chan, S.L.; Squires, P.E.; Hewison, M. Expression of 25-hydroxyvitamin D_3-1alpha-hydroxylase in pancreatic islets. *J. Steroid Biochem. Mol. Biol.* **2004**, *89*, 121–125. [CrossRef] [PubMed]
16. Maestro, B.; Davila, N.; Carranza, M.C.; Calle, C. Identification of a Vitamin D response element in the human insulin receptor gene promoter. *J. Steroid Biochem. Mol. Biol.* **2003**, *84*, 223–230. [CrossRef]
17. El-Fakhri, N.; McDevitt, H.; Shaikh, M.G.; Halsey, C.; Ahmed, S.F. Vitamin D and its effects on glucose homeostasis, cardiovascular function and immune function. *Horm. Res. Paediatr.* **2014**, *81*, 363–378. [CrossRef]
18. Bae, K.N.; Nam, H.K.; Rhie, Y.J.; Song, D.J.; Lee, K.H. Low levels of 25-hydroxyvitamin D in children and adolescents with type 1 diabetes mellitus: A single center experience. *Ann. Pediatr. Endocrinol. Metab.* **2018**, *23*, 21–27. [CrossRef]

19. Federico, G.; Genoni, A.; Puggioni, A.; Saba, A.; Gallo, D.; Randazzo, E.; Salvatoni, A.; Toniolo, A. Vitamin D status, enterovirus infection, and type 1 diabetes in Italian children/adolescents. *Pediatr. Diabetes* **2018**, *19*, 923–929. [CrossRef]
20. Cooper, J.D.; Smyth, D.J.; Walker, N.M.; Stevens, H.; Burren, O.S.; Wallace, C.; Greissl, C.; Ramos-Lopez, E.; Hypponen, E.; Dunger, D.B.; et al. Inherited variation in vitamin D genes is associated with predisposition to autoimmune disease type 1 diabetes. *Diabetes* **2011**, *60*, 1624–1631. [CrossRef]
21. Sahin, O.A.; Goksen, D.; Ozpinar, A.; Serdar, M.; Onay, H. Association of vitamin D receptor polymorphisms and type 1 diabetes susceptibility in children: A meta-analysis. *Endocr. Connect.* **2017**, *6*, 159–171. [CrossRef] [PubMed]
22. Kodama, K.; Zhao, Z.; Toda, K.; Yip, L.; Fuhlbrigge, R.; Miao, D.; Fathman, C.G.; Yamada, S.; Butte, A.J.; Yu, L. Expression-Based Genome-Wide Association Study Links Vitamin D-Binding Protein with Autoantigenicity in Type 1 Diabetes. *Diabetes* **2016**, *65*, 1341–1349. [CrossRef] [PubMed]
23. Sorensen, I.M.; Joner, G.; Jenum, P.A.; Eskild, A.; Brunborg, C.; Torjesen, P.A.; Stene, L.C. Vitamin D-binding protein and 25-hydroxyvitamin D during pregnancy in mothers whose children later developed type 1 diabetes. *Diabetes Metab. Res. Rev.* **2016**, *32*, 883–890. [CrossRef] [PubMed]
24. Tapia, G.; Marild, K.; Dahl, S.R.; Lund-Blix, N.A.; Viken, M.K.; Lie, B.A.; Njolstad, P.R.; Joner, G.; Skrivarhaug, T.; Cohen, A.S.; et al. Maternal and Newborn Vitamin D-Binding Protein, Vitamin D Levels, Vitamin D Receptor Genotype, and Childhood Type 1 Diabetes. *Diabetes Care* **2019**, *42*, 553–559. [CrossRef] [PubMed]
25. Gabbay, M.A.; Sato, M.N.; Finazzo, C.; Duarte, A.J.; Dib, S.A. Effect of cholecalciferol as adjunctive therapy with insulin on protective immunologic profile and decline of residual beta-cell function in new-onset type 1 diabetes mellitus. *Arch. Pediatr. Adolesc. Med.* **2012**, *166*, 601–607. [CrossRef]
26. Treiber, G.; Prietl, B.; Frohlich-Reiterer, E.; Lechner, E.; Ribitsch, A.; Fritsch, M.; Rami-Merhar, B.; Steigleder-Schweiger, C.; Graninger, W.; Borkenstein, M.; et al. Cholecalciferol supplementation improves suppressive capacity of regulatory T-cells in young patients with new-onset type 1 diabetes mellitus—A randomized clinical trial. *Clin. Immunol.* **2015**, *161*, 217–224. [CrossRef] [PubMed]
27. Zipitis, C.S.; Akobeng, A.K. Vitamin D supplementation in early childhood and risk of type 1 diabetes: A systematic review and meta-analysis. *Arch. Dis. Child.* **2008**, *93*, 512–517. [CrossRef] [PubMed]
28. Zipitis, C.S.; Mughal, Z.M.; Clayton, P.E. Assessing the population impact of low rates of vitamin D supplementation on type 1 diabetes using a new statistical method. *JRSM Open* **2016**, *7*. [CrossRef] [PubMed]
29. Ataie-Jafari, A.; Loke, S.C.; Rahmat, A.B.; Larijani, B.; Abbasi, F.; Leow, M.K.; Yassin, Z. a randomized placebo-controlled trial of alphacalcidol on the preservation of beta cell function in children with recent onset type 1 diabetes. *Clin. Nutr.* **2013**, *32*, 911–917. [CrossRef]
30. Deda, L.; Yeshayahu, Y.; Sud, S.; Cuerden, M.; Cherney, D.Z.; Sochett, E.B.; Mahmud, F.H. Improvements in peripheral vascular function with vitamin D treatment in deficient adolescents with type 1 diabetes. *Pediatr. Diabetes* **2018**, *19*, 457–463. [CrossRef] [PubMed]
31. Silvis, K.; Aronsson, C.A.; Liu, X.; Uusitalo, U.; Yang, J.; Tamura, R.; Lernmark, A.; Rewers, M.; Hagopian, W.; She, J.X.; et al. Maternal dietary supplement use and development of islet autoimmunity in the offspring: TEDDY study. *Pediatr. Diabetes* **2019**, *20*, 86–92. [CrossRef] [PubMed]
32. Bizzarri, C.; Pitocco, D.; Napoli, N.; Di Stasio, E.; Maggi, D.; Manfrini, S.; Suraci, C.; Cavallo, M.G.; Cappa, M.; Ghirlanda, G.; et al. No protective effect of calcitriol on beta-cell function in recent-onset type 1 diabetes: The IMDIAB XIII trial. *Diabetes Care* **2010**, *33*, 1962–1963. [CrossRef] [PubMed]
33. Perchard, R.; Magee, L.; Whatmore, A.; Ivison, F.; Murray, P.; Stevens, A.; Mughal, M.Z.; Ehtisham, S.; Campbell, J.; Ainsworth, S.; et al. a pilot interventional study to evaluate the impact of cholecalciferol treatment on HbA1c in type 1 diabetes (T1D). *Endocr. Connect.* **2017**, *6*, 225–231. [CrossRef] [PubMed]
34. Sharma, S.; Biswal, N.; Bethou, A.; Rajappa, M.; Kumar, S.; Vinayagam, V. Does Vitamin D Supplementation Improve Glycaemic Control in Children with Type 1 Diabetes Mellitus?—A Randomized Controlled Trial. *J. Clin. Diagn. Res.* **2017**, *11*, SC15. [CrossRef] [PubMed]
35. Tai, K.; Need, A.G.; Horowitz, M.; Chapman, I.M. Glucose tolerance and vitamin D: Effects of treating vitamin D deficiency. *Nutrition* **2008**, *24*, 950–956. [CrossRef] [PubMed]
36. Von Hurst, P.R.; Stonehouse, W.; Coad, J. Vitamin D supplementation reduces insulin resistance in South Asian women living in New Zealand who are insulin resistant and vitamin D deficient—A randomised, placebo-controlled trial. *Br. J. Nutr.* **2010**, *103*, 549–555. [CrossRef] [PubMed]

37. Grimnes, G.; Figenschau, Y.; Almas, B.; Jorde, R. Vitamin D insulin secretion, sensitivity, and lipids: Results from a case-control study and a randomized controlled trial using hyperglycemic clamp technique. *Diabetes* **2011**, *60*, 2748–2757. [CrossRef]
38. Gepner, A.D.; Ramamurthy, R.; Krueger, D.C.; Korcarz, C.E.; Binkley, N.; Stein, J.H. a prospective randomized controlled trial of the effects of vitamin D supplementation on cardiovascular disease risk. *PLoS ONE* **2012**, *7*, e36617. [CrossRef]
39. Toxqui, L.; Blanco-Rojo, R.; Wright, I.; Perez-Granados, A.M.; Vaquero, M.P. Changes in blood pressure and lipid levels in young women consuming a vitamin D-fortified skimmed milk: A randomised controlled trial. *Nutrients* **2013**, *5*, 4966–4977. [CrossRef]
40. Jorde, R.; Sollid, S.T.; Svartberg, J.; Schirmer, H.; Joakimsen, R.M.; Njolstad, I.; Fuskevag, O.M.; Figenschau, Y.; Hutchinson, M.Y. Vitamin D 20,000 IU per Week for Five Years Does Not Prevent Progression from Prediabetes to Diabetes. *J. Clin. Endocrinol. Metab.* **2016**, *101*, 1647–1655. [CrossRef]
41. He, S.; Yu, S.; Zhou, Z.; Wang, C.; Wu, Y.; Li, W. Effect of vitamin D supplementation on fasting plasma glucose, insulin resistance and prevention of type 2 diabetes mellitus in non-diabetics: A systematic review and meta-analysis. *Biomed. Rep.* **2018**, *8*, 475–484. [CrossRef] [PubMed]
42. Pittas, A.G.; Dawson-Hughes, B.; Sheehan, P.; Ware, J.H.; Knowler, W.C.; Aroda, V.R.; Brodsky, I.; Ceglia, L.; Chadha, C.; Chatterjee, R.; et al. Vitamin D Supplementation and Prevention of Type 2 Diabetes. *N. Engl. J. Med.* **2019**. [CrossRef] [PubMed]
43. Belenchia, A.M.; Tosh, A.K.; Hillman, L.S.; Peterson, C.A. Correcting vitamin D insufficiency improves insulin sensitivity in obese adolescents: A randomized controlled trial. *Am. J. Clin. Nutr.* **2013**, *97*, 774–781. [CrossRef] [PubMed]
44. Hirschler, V.; Maccallini, G.; Sanchez, M.; Claudio, G.; Molinari, C.; Figueroa, M.; Arnada, C.; Hidalgo, M. Improvement of Apolipoprotein B in Argentine Indigenous School Children after Vitamin D Supplementation. *Cardiovasc. Hematol. Agents Med. Chem.* **2015**, *13*, 137–145. [CrossRef] [PubMed]
45. Kelishadi, R.; Salek, S.; Salek, M.; Hashemipour, M.; Movahedian, M. Effects of vitamin D supplementation on insulin resistance and cardiometabolic risk factors in children with metabolic syndrome: A triple-masked controlled trial. *J. Pediatr.* **2014**, *90*, 28–34. [CrossRef] [PubMed]
46. Nwosu, B.U.; Maranda, L. The effects of vitamin D supplementation on hepatic dysfunction, vitamin D status, and glycemic control in children and adolescents with vitamin D deficiency and either type 1 or type 2 diabetes mellitus. *PLoS ONE* **2014**, *9*, e99646. [CrossRef] [PubMed]
47. Nader, N.S.; Aguirre Castaneda, R.; Wallace, J.; Singh, R.; Weaver, A.; Kumar, S. Effect of vitamin D_3 supplementation on serum 25(OH)D, lipids and markers of insulin resistance in obese adolescents: A prospective, randomized, placebo-controlled pilot trial. *Horm. Res. Paediatr.* **2014**, *82*, 107–112. [CrossRef] [PubMed]
48. Javed, A.; Vella, A.; Balagopal, P.B.; Fischer, P.R.; Weaver, A.L.; Piccinini, F.; Dalla Man, C.; Cobelli, C.; Giesler, P.D.; Laugen, J.M.; et al. Cholecalciferol supplementation does not influence beta-cell function and insulin action in obese adolescents: A prospective double-blind randomized trial. *J. Nutr.* **2015**, *145*, 284–290. [CrossRef] [PubMed]
49. Hirschler, V.; Maccallini, G.; Sanchez, M.S.; Castano, L.; Molinari, C. Improvement in high-density lipoprotein cholesterol levels in argentine Indian school children after vitamin D supplementation. *Horm. Res. Paediatr.* **2013**, *80*, 335–342. [CrossRef] [PubMed]
50. Javed, A.; Kullo, I.J.; Balagopal, P.B.; Kumar, S. Effect of vitamin D_3 treatment on endothelial function in obese adolescents. *Pediatr. Obes.* **2016**, *11*, 279–284. [CrossRef] [PubMed]
51. Ferira, A.J.; Laing, E.M.; Hausman, D.B.; Hall, D.B.; McCabe, G.P.; Martin, B.R.; Hill Gallant, K.M.; Warden, S.J.; Weaver, C.M.; Peacock, M.; et al. Vitamin D Supplementation Does Not Impact Insulin Resistance in Black and White Children. *J. Clin. Endocrinol. Metab.* **2016**, *101*, 1710–1718. [CrossRef] [PubMed]
52. Sethuraman, U.; Zidan, M.A.; Hanks, L.; Bagheri, M.; Ashraf, A. Impact of vitamin D treatment on 25 hydroxy vitamin D levels and insulin homeostasis in obese African American adolescents in a randomized trial. *J. Clin. Transl. Endocrinol.* **2018**, *12*, 13–19. [CrossRef] [PubMed]
53. Hernan, M.A.; Olek, M.J.; Ascherio, A. Geographic variation of MS incidence in two prospective studies of US women. *Neurology* **1999**, *53*, 1711–1718. [CrossRef] [PubMed]

54. Dalmay, F.; Bhalla, D.; Nicoletti, A.; Cabrera-Gomez, J.A.; Cabre, P.; Ruiz, F.; Druet-Cabanac, M.; Dumas, M.; Preux, P.M. Multiple sclerosis and solar exposure before the age of 15 years: Case-control study in Cuba, Martinique and Sicily. *Mult. Scler.* **2010**, *16*, 899–908. [CrossRef] [PubMed]
55. Islam, T.; Gauderman, W.J.; Cozen, W.; Mack, T.M. Childhood sun exposure influences risk of multiple sclerosis in monozygotic twins. *Neurology* **2007**, *69*, 381–388. [CrossRef] [PubMed]
56. Dwyer, T.; van der Mei, I.; Ponsonby, A.L.; Taylor, B.V.; Stankovich, J.; McKay, J.D.; Thomson, R.J.; Polanowski, A.M.; Dickinson, J.L. Melanocortin 1 receptor genotype, past environmental sun exposure, and risk of multiple sclerosis. *Neurology* **2008**, *71*, 583–589. [CrossRef] [PubMed]
57. van der Mei, I.A.; Ponsonby, A.L.; Dwyer, T.; Blizzard, L.; Simmons, R.; Taylor, B.V.; Butzkueven, H.; Kilpatrick, T. Past exposure to sun, skin phenotype, and risk of multiple sclerosis: Case-control study. *BMJ* **2003**, *327*, 316. [CrossRef]
58. Alonso, A.; Cook, S.D.; Maghzi, A.H.; Divani, A.A. a case-control study of risk factors for multiple sclerosis in Iran. *Mult. Scler.* **2011**, *17*, 550–555. [CrossRef]
59. Baarnhielm, M.; Hedstrom, A.K.; Kockum, I.; Sundqvist, E.; Gustafsson, S.A.; Hillert, J.; Olsson, T.; Alfredsson, L. Sunlight is associated with decreased multiple sclerosis risk: No interaction with human leukocyte antigen-DRB1*15. *Eur. J. Neurol.* **2012**, *19*, 955–962. [CrossRef]
60. Munger, K.L.; Zhang, S.M.; O'Reilly, E.; Hernan, M.A.; Olek, M.J.; Willett, W.C.; Ascherio, A. Vitamin D intake and incidence of multiple sclerosis. *Neurology* **2004**, *62*, 60–65. [CrossRef]
61. Munger, K.L.; Levin, L.I.; Hollis, B.W.; Howard, N.S.; Ascherio, A. Serum 25-hydroxyvitamin D levels and risk of multiple sclerosis. *JAMA* **2006**, *296*, 2832–2838. [CrossRef]
62. Kragt, J.; van Amerongen, B.; Killestein, J.; Dijkstra, C.; Uitdehaag, B.; Polman, C.; Lips, P. Higher levels of 25-hydroxyvitamin D are associated with a lower incidence of multiple sclerosis only in women. *Mult. Scler.* **2009**, *15*, 9–15. [CrossRef]
63. Shaygannejad, V.; Golabchi, K.; Haghighi, S.; Dehghan, H.; Moshayedi, A. a Comparative Study of 25 (OH) Vitamin D Serum Levels in Patients with Multiple Sclerosis and Control Group in Isfahan, Iran. *Int. J. Prev. Med.* **2010**, *1*, 195–201.
64. Soilu-Hanninen, M.; Airas, L.; Mononen, I.; Heikkila, A.; Viljanen, M.; Hanninen, A. 25-Hydroxyvitamin D levels in serum at the onset of multiple sclerosis. *Mult. Scler.* **2005**, *11*, 266–271. [CrossRef]
65. Graves, J.S.; Barcellos, L.F.; Krupp, L.; Belman, A.; Shao, X.; Quach, H.; Hart, J.; Chitnis, T.; Weinstock-Guttman, B.; Aaen, G.; et al. Vitamin D genes influence MS relapses in children. *Mult. Scler.* **2019**. [CrossRef]
66. Willer, C.J.; Dyment, D.A.; Sadovnick, A.D.; Rothwell, P.M.; Murray, T.J.; Ebers, G.C. Timing of birth and risk of multiple sclerosis: Population based study. *BMJ* **2005**, *330*, 120. [CrossRef]
67. Staples, J.; Ponsonby, A.L.; Lim, L. Low maternal exposure to ultraviolet radiation in pregnancy, month of birth, and risk of multiple sclerosis in offspring: Longitudinal analysis. *BMJ* **2010**, *340*, c1640.
68. Torkildsen, O.; Grytten, N.; Aarseth, J.; Myhr, K.M.; Kampman, M.T. Month of birth as a risk factor for multiple sclerosis: An update. *Acta Neurol. Scand. Suppl.* **2012**, *126*, 58–62. [CrossRef]
69. Disanto, G.; Morahan, J.M.; Ramagopalan, S.V. Multiple sclerosis: Risk factors and their interactions. *CNS Neurol. Disord. Drug Targets* **2012**, *11*, 545–555. [CrossRef]
70. Mirzaei, F.; Michels, K.B.; Munger, K.; O'Reilly, E.; Chitnis, T.; Forman, M.R.; Giovannucci, E.; Rosner, B.; Ascherio, A. Gestational vitamin D and the risk of multiple sclerosis in offspring. *Ann. Neurol.* **2011**, *70*, 30–40. [CrossRef]
71. McKay, K.A.; Jahanfar, S.; Duggan, T.; Tkachuk, S.; Tremlett, H. Factors associated with onset, relapses or progression in multiple sclerosis: A systematic review. *Neurotoxicology* **2016**, *61*, 189–212. [CrossRef]
72. McLaughlin, L.; Clarke, L.; Khalilidehkordi, E.; Butzkueven, H.; Taylor, B.; Broadley, S.A. Vitamin D for the treatment of multiple sclerosis: A meta-analysis. *J. Neurol.* **2018**, *265*, 2893–2905. [CrossRef]
73. Soilu-Hanninen, M.; Aivo, J.; Lindstrom, B.M.; Elovaara, I.; Sumelahti, M.L.; Farkkila, M.; Tienari, P.; Atula, S.; Sarasoja, T.; Herrala, L.; et al. a randomised, double blind, placebo controlled trial with vitamin D_3 as an add on treatment to interferon beta-1b in patients with multiple sclerosis. *J. Neurol. Neurosurg. Psychiatry* **2012**, *83*, 565–571. [CrossRef]
74. Lee, Y.H.; Bae, S.C. Vitamin D level in rheumatoid arthritis and its correlation with the disease activity: A meta-analysis. *Clin. Exp. Rheumatol.* **2016**, *34*, 827–833.
75. Son, K.M.; Song, S.H.; Lim, S.K.; Seo, Y.I.; Kim, H.A. Characteristics of patients with rheumatoid arthritis in clinical remission: The many aspects of DAS28 remission. *Clin. Exp. Rheumatol.* **2012**, *30*, 947–950.

76. Song, G.G.; Bae, S.C.; Lee, Y.H. Association between vitamin D intake and the risk of rheumatoid arthritis: A meta-analysis. *Clin. Rheumatol.* **2012**, *31*, 1733–1739. [CrossRef]
77. Lin, J.; Liu, J.; Davies, M.L.; Chen, W. Serum Vitamin D Level and Rheumatoid Arthritis Disease Activity: Review and Meta-Analysis. *PLoS ONE* **2016**, *11*, e0146351. [CrossRef]
78. Wang, Y.; Zhang, F.; Wang, S.; Shang, X.; Luo, S.; Zhou, H.; Shi, H.; Cai, L. Serum Vitamin D Level is Inversely Associated with Anti-Cyclic Citrullinated Peptide Antibody Level and Disease Activity in Rheumatoid Arthritis Patients. *Arch. Rheumatol.* **2016**, *31*, 64–70. [CrossRef]
79. Zakeri, Z.; Sandoughi, M.; Mashhadi, M.A.; Raeesi, V.; Shahbakhsh, S. Serum vitamin D level and disease activity in patients with recent onset rheumatoid arthritis. *Int. J. Rheum. Dis.* **2016**, *19*, 343–347. [CrossRef]
80. Tizaoui, K.; Hamzaoui, K. Association between VDR polymorphisms and rheumatoid arthritis disease: Systematic review and updated meta-analysis of case-control studies. *Immunobiology* **2015**, *220*, 807–816. [CrossRef]
81. Song, G.G.; Bae, S.C.; Lee, Y.H. Vitamin D receptor FokI, BsmI, and TaqI polymorphisms and susceptibility to rheumatoid arthritis: A meta-analysis. *Z. Rheumatol.* **2016**, *75*, 322–329. [CrossRef]
82. Merlino, L.A.; Curtis, J.; Mikuls, T.R.; Cerhan, J.R.; Criswell, L.A.; Saag, K.G. Vitamin D intake is inversely associated with rheumatoid arthritis: Results from the Iowa Women's Health Study. *Arthritis Rheum.* **2004**, *50*, 72–77. [CrossRef]
83. Chandrashekara, S.; Patted, A. Role of vitamin D supplementation in improving disease activity in rheumatoid arthritis: An exploratory study. *Int. J. Rheum. Dis.* **2015**, *20*, 825–831. [CrossRef]
84. Franco, A.S.; Freitas, T.Q.; Bernardo, W.M.; Pereira, R.M.R. Vitamin D supplementation and disease activity in patients with immune-mediated rheumatic diseases: A systematic review and meta-analysis. *Medicine* **2017**, *96*, e7024. [CrossRef] [PubMed]
85. Gardner, D.H.; Jeffery, L.E.; Soskic, B.; Briggs, Z.; Hou, T.Z.; Raza, K.; Sansom, D.M. 1,25$(OH)_2D_3$ Promotes the Efficacy of CD28 Costimulation Blockade by Abatacept. *J. Immunol.* **2015**, *195*, 2657–2665. [CrossRef]
86. Amital, H.; Szekanecz, Z.; Szucs, G.; Danko, K.; Nagy, E.; Csepany, T.; Kiss, E.; Rovensky, J.; Tuchynova, A.; Kozakova, D.; et al. Serum concentrations of 25-OH vitamin D in patients with systemic lupus erythematosus (SLE) are inversely related to disease activity: Is it time to routinely supplement patients with SLE with vitamin D? *Ann. Rheum. Dis.* **2010**, *69*, 1155–1157. [CrossRef]
87. Robinson, A.B.; Thierry-Palmer, M.; Gibson, K.L.; Rabinovich, C.E. Disease activity, proteinuria, and vitamin D status in children with systemic lupus erythematosus and juvenile dermatomyositis. *J. Pediatr.* **2012**, *160*, 297–302. [CrossRef]
88. Wright, T.B.; Shults, J.; Leonard, M.B.; Zemel, B.S.; Burnham, J.M. Hypovitaminosis D is associated with greater body mass index and disease activity in pediatric systemic lupus erythematosus. *J. Pediatr.* **2009**, *155*, 260–265. [CrossRef]
89. Kamen, D.; Aranow, C. Vitamin D in systemic lupus erythematosus. *Curr. Opin. Rheumatol.* **2008**, *20*, 532–537. [CrossRef]
90. AlSaleem, A.; AlE'ed, A.; AlSaghier, A.; Al-Mayouf, S.M. Vitamin D status in children with systemic lupus erythematosus and its association with clinical and laboratory parameters. *Clin. Rheumatol.* **2015**, *34*, 81–84. [CrossRef]
91. Borba, V.Z.; Vieira, J.G.; Kasamatsu, T.; Radominski, S.C.; Sato, E.I.; Lazaretti-Castro, M. Vitamin D deficiency in patients with active systemic lupus erythematosus. *Osteoporos. Int.* **2009**, *20*, 427–433. [CrossRef] [PubMed]
92. Schneider, L.; Dos Santos, A.S.; Santos, M.; da Silva Chakr, R.M.; Monticielo, O.A. Vitamin D and systemic lupus erythematosus: State of the art. *Clin. Rheumatol.* **2014**, *33*, 1033–1038. [CrossRef] [PubMed]
93. Lima, G.L.; Paupitz, J.; Aikawa, N.E.; Takayama, L.; Bonfa, E.; Pereira, R.M. Vitamin D Supplementation in Adolescents and Young Adults with Juvenile Systemic Lupus Erythematosus for Improvement in Disease Activity and Fatigue Scores: A Randomized, Double-Blind, Placebo-Controlled Trial. *Arthritis Care Res.* **2016**, *68*, 91–98. [CrossRef] [PubMed]
94. Abou-Raya, A.; Abou-Raya, S.; Helmii, M. The effect of vitamin D supplementation on inflammatory and hemostatic markers and disease activity in patients with systemic lupus erythematosus: A randomized placebo-controlled trial. *J. Rheumatol.* **2013**, *40*, 265–272. [CrossRef] [PubMed]

95. Terrier, B.; Derian, N.; Schoindre, Y.; Chaara, W.; Geri, G.; Zahr, N.; Mariampillai, K.; Rosenzwajg, M.; Carpentier, W.; Musset, L.; et al. Restoration of regulatory and effector T cell balance and B cell homeostasis in systemic lupus erythematosus patients through vitamin D supplementation. *Arthritis Res. Ther.* **2012**, *14*, R221. [CrossRef] [PubMed]
96. Shoenfeld, Y.; Giacomelli, R.; Azrielant, S.; Berardicurti, O.; Reynolds, J.A.; Bruce, I.N. Vitamin D and systemic lupus erythematosus—The hype and the hope. *Autoimmun. Rev.* **2018**, *17*, 19–23. [CrossRef] [PubMed]
97. Smith, E.L.; Walworth, N.C.; Holick, M.F. Effect of 1 alpha,25-dihydroxyvitamin D_3 on the morphologic and biochemical differentiation of cultured human epidermal keratinocytes grown in serum-free conditions. *J. Investig. Dermatol.* **1986**, *86*, 709–714. [CrossRef] [PubMed]
98. Smith, E.L.; Pincus, S.H.; Donovan, L.; Holick, M.F. a novel approach for the evaluation and treatment of psoriasis. Oral or topical use of 1,25-dihydroxyvitamin D_3 can be a safe and effective therapy for psoriasis. *J. Am. Acad. Dermatol.* **1988**, *19*, 516–528. [CrossRef]
99. Stefanic, M.; Rucevic, I.; Barisic-Drusko, V. Meta-analysis of vitamin D receptor polymorphisms and psoriasis risk. *Int. J. Dermatol.* **2013**, *52*, 705–710. [CrossRef]
100. Lee, Y.H. Vitamin D receptor ApaI, TaqI, BsmI, and FokI polymorphisms and psoriasis susceptibility: An updated meta-analysis. *Clin. Exp. Dermatol.* **2019**, *44*, 498–505. [CrossRef]
101. Saleky, S.; Bulur, I.; Saracoglu, Z.N. Narrowband UVB treatment increases serum 25-hydroxyvitamin D levels in patients with chronic plaque psoriasis. *Cutis* **2017**, *99*, 431–435. [PubMed]
102. Gupta, A.; Arora, T.C.; Jindal, A.; Bhadoria, A.S. Efficacy of narrowband ultraviolet B phototherapy and levels of serum vitamin D_3 in psoriasis: A prospective study. *Indian Dermatol. Online J.* **2016**, *7*, 87–92. [CrossRef] [PubMed]
103. Disphanurat, W.; Viarasilpa, W.; Chakkavittumrong, P.; Pongcharoen, P. The Clinical Effect of Oral Vitamin D_2 Supplementation on Psoriasis: A Double-Blind, Randomized, Placebo-Controlled Study. *Dermatol. Res. Pract.* **2019**, *2019*. [CrossRef] [PubMed]
104. Del Rosso, J.Q.; Kircik, L.H. The Effect of Calcipotriene-Betamethasone Dipropionate Aerosol Foam versus Vehicle on Target Lesions in Moderate Severity Plaque Psoriasis: Focus on Elbows and Knees. *J. Drugs Dermatol.* **2019**, *18*, 358–361. [PubMed]
105. German, B.; Wei, R.; Hener, P.; Martins, C.; Ye, T.; Gottwick, C.; Yang, J.; Seneschal, J.; Boniface, K.; Li, M. Disrupting the IL-36 and IL-23/IL-17 loop underlies the efficacy of calcipotriol and corticosteroid therapy for psoriasis. *JCI Insight.* **2019**, *4*. [CrossRef] [PubMed]
106. Hau, C.S.; Shimizu, T.; Tada, Y.; Kamata, M.; Takeoka, S.; Shibata, S.; Mitsui, A.; Asano, Y.; Sugaya, M.; Kadono, T.; et al. The vitamin D_3 analog, maxacalcitol, reduces psoriasiform skin inflammation by inducing regulatory T cells and downregulating IL-23 and IL-17 production. *J. Dermatol. Sci.* **2018**, *92*, 117–126. [CrossRef] [PubMed]
107. Cantorna, M.T.; Munsick, C.; Bemiss, C.; Mahon, B.D. 1,25-Dihydroxycholecalciferol prevents and ameliorates symptoms of experimental murine inflammatory bowel disease. *J. Nutr.* **2000**, *130*, 2648–2652. [CrossRef]
108. Bouillon, R.; Carmeliet, G.; Verlinden, L.; van Etten, E.; Verstuyf, A.; Luderer, H.F.; Lieben, L.; Mathieu, C.; Demay, M. Vitamin D and human health: Lessons from vitamin D receptor null mice. *Endocr. Rev.* **2008**, *29*, 726–776. [CrossRef]
109. Simmons, J.D.; Mullighan, C.; Welsh, K.I.; Jewell, D.P. Vitamin D receptor gene polymorphism: Association with Crohn's disease susceptibility. *Gut* **2000**, *47*, 211–214. [CrossRef]
110. Wang, L.; Wang, Z.T.; Hu, J.J.; Fan, R.; Zhou, J.; Zhong, J. Polymorphisms of the vitamin D receptor gene and the risk of inflammatory bowel disease: A meta-analysis. *Genet. Mol. Res.* **2014**, *13*, 2598–2610. [CrossRef]
111. Peyrin-Biroulet, L.; Oussalah, A.; Boucekkine, T.; Bigard, M.A. TNF antagonists in the treatment of inflammatory bowel disease: Results of a survey of gastroenterologists in the French region of Lorraine. *Gastroenterol. Clin. Biol.* **2009**, *33*, 23–30. [CrossRef] [PubMed]
112. Janssen, C.E.; Globig, A.M.; Busse Grawitz, A.; Bettinger, D.; Hasselblatt, P. Seasonal variability of vitamin D status in patients with inflammatory bowel disease—A retrospective cohort study. *PLoS ONE* **2019**, *14*, e0217238. [CrossRef] [PubMed]
113. Lu, C.; Yang, J.; Yu, W.; Li, D.; Xiang, Z.; Lin, Y.; Yu, C. Association between 25(OH)D Level, Ultraviolet Exposure, Geographical Location, and Inflammatory Bowel Disease Activity: A Systematic Review and Meta-Analysis. *PLoS ONE* **2015**, *10*, e0132036. [CrossRef] [PubMed]

114. Del Pinto, R.; Pietropaoli, D.; Chandar, A.K.; Ferri, C.; Cominelli, F. Association between Inflammatory Bowel Disease and Vitamin D Deficiency: A Systematic Review and Meta-analysis. *Inflamm. Bowel Dis.* **2015**, *21*, 2708–2717. [CrossRef] [PubMed]
115. Pappa, H.M.; Mitchell, P.D.; Jiang, H.; Kassiff, S.; Filip-Dhima, R.; DiFabio, D.; Quinn, N.; Lawton, R.C.; Bronzwaer, M.E.; Koenen, M.; et al. Maintenance of optimal vitamin D status in children and adolescents with inflammatory bowel disease: A randomized clinical trial comparing two regimens. *J. Clin. Endocrinol. Metab.* **2014**, *99*, 3408–3417. [CrossRef]
116. Schardey, J.; Globig, A.M.; Janssen, C.; Hofmann, M.; Manegold, P.; Thimme, R.; Hasselblatt, P. Vitamin D inhibits pro-inflammatory T cell function in patients with inflammatory bowel disease. *J. Crohn's Colitis* **2019**. [CrossRef] [PubMed]
117. Guo, H.; Zheng, Y.; Cai, X.; Yang, H.; Zhang, Y.; Hao, L.; Jin, Y.; Yang, G. Correlation between serum vitamin D status and immunological changes in children affected by gastrointestinal food allergy. *Allergol. Immunopathol.* **2018**, *46*, 39–44. [CrossRef]
118. Hennessy, A.; Hourihane, J.O.; Malvisi, L.; Irvine, A.D.; Kenny, L.C.; Murray, D.M.; Kiely, M.E. Antenatal vitamin D exposure and childhood eczema, food allergy, asthma and allergic rhinitis at 2 and 5 years of age in the atopic disease-specific Cork BASELINE Birth Cohort Study. *Allergy* **2018**, *73*, 2182–2191. [CrossRef]
119. Molloy, J.; Koplin, J.J.; Allen, K.J.; Tang, M.L.K.; Collier, F.; Carlin, J.B.; Saffery, R.; Burgner, D.; Ranganathan, S.; Dwyer, T.; et al. Vitamin D insufficiency in the first 6 months of infancy and challenge-proven IgE-mediated food allergy at 1 year of age: A case-cohort study. *Allergy* **2017**, *72*, 1222–1231. [CrossRef]
120. Willits, E.K.; Wang, Z.; Jin, J.; Patel, B.; Motosue, M.; Bhagia, A.; Almasri, J.; Erwin, P.J.; Kumar, S.; Joshi, A.Y. Vitamin D and food allergies in children: A systematic review and meta-analysis. *Allergy Asthma Proc.* **2017**, *38*, 21–28. [CrossRef]
121. Peroni, D.G.; Boner, A.L. Food allergy: The perspectives of prevention using vitamin, D. *Curr. Opin. Allergy Clin. Immunol.* **2013**, *13*, 287–292. [CrossRef] [PubMed]
122. Rosendahl, J.; Pelkonen, A.S.; Helve, O.; Hauta-Alus, H.; Holmlund-Suila, E.; Valkama, S.; Enlund-Cerullo, M.; Viljakainen, H.; Hytinantti, T.; Makitie, O.; et al. High-Dose Vitamin D Supplementation Does Not Prevent Allergic Sensitization of Infants. *J. Pediatr.* **2019**, *209*, 139–145.e1. [CrossRef] [PubMed]
123. Suneetha, P.V.; Sarin, S.K.; Goyal, A.; Kumar, G.T.; Shukla, D.K.; Hissar, S. Association between vitamin D receptor, CCR5, TNF-alpha and TNF-beta gene polymorphisms and HBV infection and severity of liver disease. *J. Hepatol.* **2006**, *44*, 856–863. [CrossRef] [PubMed]
124. Nosratabadi, R.; Arababadi, M.K.; Salehabad, V.A.; Shamsizadeh, A.; Mahmoodi, M.; Sayadi, A.R.; Kennedy, D. Polymorphisms within exon 9 but not intron 8 of the vitamin D receptor are associated with the nephropathic complication of type-2 diabetes. *Int. J. Immunogenet.* **2010**, *37*, 493–497. [CrossRef] [PubMed]
125. Hu, Y.C.; Wang, W.W.; Jiang, W.Y.; Li, C.Q.; Guo, J.C.; Xun, Y.H. Low vitamin D levels are associated with high viral loads in patients with chronic hepatitis B: A systematic review and meta-analysis. *BMC Gastroenterol.* **2019**, *19*, 84. [CrossRef] [PubMed]
126. Petta, S.; Camma, C.; Scazzone, C.; Tripodo, C.; Di Marco, V.; Bono, A.; Cabibi, D.; Licata, G.; Porcasi, R.; Marchesini, G.; et al. Low vitamin D serum level is related to severe fibrosis and low responsiveness to interferon-based therapy in genotype 1 chronic hepatitis, C. *Hepatology* **2010**, *51*, 1158–1167. [CrossRef]
127. Barooah, P.; Saikia, S.; Bharadwaj, R.; Sarmah, P.; Bhattacharyya, M.; Goswami, B.; Medhi, S. Role of VDR, GC, and CYP2R1 Polymorphisms in the Development of Hepatocellular Carcinoma in Hepatitis C Virus-Infected Patients. *Genet. Test. Mol. Biomark.* **2019**, *23*, 325–331. [CrossRef]
128. Murayama, A.; Saitoh, H.; Takeuchi, A.; Yamada, N.; Matsumura, T.; Shiina, M.; Muramatsu, M.; Wakita, T.; Imawari, M.; Kato, T. Vitamin D derivatives inhibit hepatitis C virus production through the suppression of apolipoprotein. *Antivir. Res.* **2018**, *160*, 55–63. [CrossRef]
129. Bitetto, D.; Fabris, C.; Fornasiere, E.; Pipan, C.; Fumolo, E.; Cussigh, A.; Bignulin, S.; Cmet, S.; Fontanini, E.; Falleti, E.; et al. Vitamin D supplementation improves response to antiviral treatment for recurrent hepatitis C. *Transpl. Int.* **2011**, *24*, 43–50. [CrossRef]
130. Komolmit, P.; Kimtrakool, S.; Suksawatamnuay, S.; Thanapirom, K.; Chattrasophon, K.; Thaimai, P.; Chirathaworn, C.; Poovorawan, Y. Vitamin D supplementation improves serum markers associated with hepatic fibrogenesis in chronic hepatitis C patients: A randomized, double-blind, placebo-controlled study. *Sci. Rep.* **2017**, *7*, 8905. [CrossRef]

131. Hall, S.C.; Agrawal, D.K. Vitamin D and Bronchial Asthma: An Overview of Data from the Past 5 Years. *Clin. Ther.* **2017**, *39*, 917–929. [CrossRef]
132. Reinehr, T.; Schnabel, D.; Wabitsch, M.; Bechtold-Dalla Pozza, S.; Buhrer, C.; Heidtmann, B.; Jochum, F.; Kauth, T.; Korner, A.; Mihatsch, W.; et al. Vitamin D supplementation after the second year of life: Joint position of the Committee on Nutrition, German Society for Pediatric and Adolescent Medicine (DGKJ e.V.), and the German Society for Pediatric Endocrinology and Diabetology (DGKED e.V.). *Mol. Cell. Pediatr.* **2019**, *6*, 3. [CrossRef] [PubMed]
133. Jolliffe, D.A.; Greenberg, L.; Hooper, R.L.; Griffiths, C.J.; Camargo, C.A., Jr.; Kerley, C.P.; Jensen, M.E.; Mauger, D.; Stelmach, I.; Urashima, M.; et al. Vitamin D supplementation to prevent asthma exacerbations: A systematic review and meta-analysis of individual participant data. *Lancet Respir. Med.* **2017**, *5*, 881–890. [CrossRef]
134. Martineau, A.R.; Cates, C.J.; Urashima, M.; Jensen, M.; Griffiths, A.P.; Nurmatov, U.; Sheikh, A.; Griffiths, C.J. Vitamin D for the management of asthma. *Cochrane Database Syst. Rev.* **2016**, *9*, CD011511. [CrossRef] [PubMed]
135. Urashima, M.; Segawa, T.; Okazaki, M.; Kurihara, M.; Wada, Y.; Ida, H. Randomized trial of vitamin D supplementation to prevent seasonal influenza a in schoolchildren. *Am. J. Clin. Nutr.* **2010**, *91*, 1255–1260. [CrossRef] [PubMed]
136. Urashima, M.; Mezawa, H.; Noya, M.; Camargo, C.A., Jr. Effects of vitamin D supplements on influenza a illness during the 2009 H1N1 pandemic: A randomized controlled trial. *Food Funct.* **2014**, *5*, 2365–2370. [CrossRef] [PubMed]
137. Martineau, A.R.; Jolliffe, D.A.; Hooper, R.L.; Greenberg, L.; Aloia, J.F.; Bergman, P.; Dubnov-Raz, G.; Esposito, S.; Ganmaa, D.; Ginde, A.A.; et al. Vitamin D supplementation to prevent acute respiratory tract infections: Systematic review and meta-analysis of individual participant data. *BMJ* **2017**, *356*, i6583. [CrossRef] [PubMed]
138. Martineau, A.R.; Jolliffe, D.A.; Greenberg, L.; Aloia, J.F.; Bergman, P.; Dubnov-Raz, G.; Esposito, S.; Ganmaa, D.; Ginde, A.A.; Goodall, E.C.; et al. Vitamin D supplementation to prevent acute respiratory infections: Individual participant data meta-analysis. *Health Technol. Assess.* **2019**, *23*, 1–44. [CrossRef] [PubMed]
139. Yakoob, M.Y.; Salam, R.A.; Khan, F.R.; Bhutta, Z.A. Vitamin D supplementation for preventing infections in children under five years of age. *Cochrane Database Syst. Rev.* **2016**, *11*, CD008824. [CrossRef]
140. Aglipay, M.; Birken, C.S.; Parkin, P.C.; Loeb, M.B.; Thorpe, K.; Chen, Y.; Laupacis, A.; Mamdani, M.; Macarthur, C.; Hoch, J.S.; et al. Effect of High-Dose vs Standard-Dose Wintertime Vitamin D Supplementation on Viral Upper Respiratory Tract Infections in Young Healthy Children. *JAMA* **2017**, *318*, 245–254. [CrossRef]
141. Correa-Rodriguez, M.; Carrillo-Avila, J.A.; Schmidt-RioValle, J.; Gonzalez-Jimenez, E.; Vargas, S.; Martin, J.; Rueda-Medina, B. Genetic association analysis of vitamin D receptor gene polymorphisms and obesity-related phenotypes. *Gene* **2018**, *640*, 51–56. [CrossRef]
142. Olson, M.L.; Maalouf, N.M.; Oden, J.D.; White, P.C.; Hutchison, M.R. Vitamin D deficiency in obese children and its relationship to glucose homeostasis. *J. Clin. Endocrinol. Metab.* **2012**, *97*, 279–285. [CrossRef]
143. Smotkin-Tangorra, M.; Purushothaman, R.; Gupta, A.; Nejati, G.; Anhalt, H.; Ten, S. Prevalence of vitamin D insufficiency in obese children and adolescents. *J. Pediatr. Endocrinol. Metab.* **2007**, *20*, 817–823. [CrossRef] [PubMed]
144. Nsiah-Kumi, P.A.; Erickson, J.M.; Beals, J.L.; Ogle, E.A.; Whiting, M.; Brushbreaker, C.; Borgeson, C.D.; Qiu, F.; Yu, F.; Larsen, J.L. Vitamin D insufficiency is associated with diabetes risk in Native American children. *Clin. Pediatr.* **2012**, *51*, 146–153. [CrossRef] [PubMed]
145. Roth, C.L.; Elfers, C.; Kratz, M.; Hoofnagle, A.N. Vitamin d deficiency in obese children and its relationship to insulin resistance and adipokines. *J. Obes.* **2011**, *2011*, 495101. [CrossRef] [PubMed]
146. Poomthavorn, P.; Saowan, S.; Mahachoklertwattana, P.; Chailurkit, L.; Khlairit, P. Vitamin D status and glucose homeostasis in obese children and adolescents living in the tropics. *Int. J. Obes.* **2012**, *36*, 491–495. [CrossRef] [PubMed]
147. Bril, F.; Maximos, M.; Portillo-Sanchez, P.; Biernacki, D.; Lomonaco, R.; Subbarayan, S.; Correa, M.; Lo, M.; Suman, A.; Cusi, K. Relationship of vitamin D with insulin resistance and disease severity in non-alcoholic steatohepatitis. *J. Hepatol.* **2015**, *62*, 405–411. [CrossRef]

148. Liu, D.; Fernandez, B.O.; Hamilton, A.; Lang, N.N.; Gallagher, J.M.C.; Newby, D.E.; Feelisch, M.; Weller, R.B. UVA irradiation of human skin vasodilates arterial vasculature and lowers blood pressure independently of nitric oxide synthase. *J. Investig. Dermatol.* **2014**, *134*, 1839–1846. [CrossRef]
149. Tangpricha, V.; Flanagan, J.N.; Whitlatch, L.W.; Tseng, C.C.; Chen, T.C.; Holt, P.R.; Lipkin, M.S.; Holick, M.F. 25-hydroxyvitamin D-1alpha-hydroxylase in normal and malignant colon tissue. *Lancet* **2001**, *357*, 1673–1674. [CrossRef]
150. Mawer, E.B.; Hayes, M.E.; Heys, S.E.; Davies, M.; White, A.; Stewart, M.F.; Smith, G.N. Constitutive synthesis of 1,25-dihydroxyvitamin D_3 by a human small cell lung cancer cell line. *J. Clin. Endocrinol. Metab.* **1994**, *79*, 554–560. [PubMed]
151. Cross, H.S.; Bareis, P.; Hofer, H.; Bischof, M.G.; Bajna, E.; Kriwanek, S.; Bonner, E.; Peterlik, M. 25-Hydroxyvitamin D(3)-1alpha-hydroxylase and vitamin D receptor gene expression in human colonic mucosa is elevated during early cancerogenesis. *Steroids* **2001**, *66*, 287–292. [CrossRef]
152. Fouda, A.; Kandil, S.; Boujettif, K.; Fayea, N. Hypovitamininosis D in Childhood Cancer Survivors: Importance of Vitamin D Supplementation and Measurement Over Different Points of Time. *J. Pediatr. Hematol. Oncol.* **2018**, *40*, e83–e90. [CrossRef] [PubMed]
153. Demirsoy, U.; Sarper, N.; Aylan Gelen, S.; Zengin, E.; Kum, T.; Demir, H. The Association of Oral Vitamin D and Calcium Supplementation with Bone Mineral Density in Pediatric Acute Lymphoblastic Leukemia Patients. *J. Pediatr. Hematol. Oncol.* **2017**, *39*, 287–292. [CrossRef] [PubMed]
154. Genc, D.B.; Vural, S.; Yagar, G. The Incidence of and Factors Associated with Vitamin D Deficiency in Newly Diagnosed Children with Cancer. *Nutr. Cancer* **2016**, *68*, 756–761. [CrossRef] [PubMed]
155. Williams, J.D.; Aggarwal, A.; Swami, S.; Krishnan, A.V.; Ji, L.; Albertelli, M.A.; Feldman, B.J. Tumor Autonomous Effects of Vitamin D Deficiency Promote Breast Cancer Metastasis. *Endocrinology* **2016**, *157*, 1341–1347. [CrossRef] [PubMed]
156. Grant, W.B. An ecologic study of dietary and solar ultraviolet-B links to breast carcinoma mortality rates. *Cancer* **2002**, *94*, 272–281. [CrossRef] [PubMed]
157. Bodiwala, D.; Luscombe, C.J.; French, M.E.; Liu, S.; Saxby, M.F.; Jones, P.W.; Ramachandran, S.; Fryer, A.A.; Strange, R.C. Susceptibility to prostate cancer: Studies on interactions between UVR exposure and skin type. *Carcinogenesis* **2003**, *24*, 711–717. [CrossRef] [PubMed]
158. Pritchard, R.S.; Baron, J.A.; de Verdier, M.G. Dietary calcium, vitamin, D.; and the risk of colorectal cancer in Stockholm, Sweden. *Cancer Epidemiol. Biomark. Prev.* **1996**, *5*, 897–900.
159. Gandini, S.; Gnagnarella, P.; Serrano, D.; Pasquali, E.; Raimondi, S. Vitamin D receptor polymorphisms and cancer. *Adv. Exp. Med. Biol.* **2014**, *810*, 69–105.
160. Kazemian, E.; Akbari, M.E.; Moradi, N.; Gharibzadeh, S.; Mondul, A.M.; Jamshidi-Naeini, Y.; Khademolmele, M.; Zarins, K.R.; Ghodoosi, N.; Amouzegar, A.; et al. Vitamin D Receptor Genetic Variation and Cancer Biomarkers among Breast Cancer Patients Supplemented with Vitamin D_3: A Single-Arm Non-Randomized Before and After Trial. *Nutrients* **2019**, *11*, 1264. [CrossRef]
161. Jacobs, E.T.; Kohler, L.N.; Kunihiro, A.G.; Jurutka, P.W. Vitamin D and Colorectal, Breast, and Prostate Cancers: A Review of the Epidemiological Evidence. *J. Cancer* **2016**, *7*, 232–240. [CrossRef] [PubMed]
162. Yin, L.; Grandi, N.; Raum, E.; Haug, U.; Arndt, V.; Brenner, H. Meta-analysis: Serum vitamin D and breast cancer risk. *Eur. J. Cancer* **2010**, *46*, 2196–2205. [CrossRef] [PubMed]
163. Kim, Y.; Je, Y. Vitamin D intake, blood 25(OH)D levels, and breast cancer risk or mortality: A meta-analysis. *Br. J. Cancer* **2014**, *110*, 2772–2784. [CrossRef] [PubMed]
164. Gandini, S.; Boniol, M.; Haukka, J.; Byrnes, G.; Cox, B.; Sneyd, M.J.; Mullie, P.; Autier, P. Meta-analysis of observational studies of serum 25-hydroxyvitamin D levels and colorectal, breast and prostate cancer and colorectal adenoma. *Int. J. Cancer* **2011**, *128*, 1414–1424. [CrossRef] [PubMed]
165. Deschasaux, M.; Souberbielle, J.C.; Latino-Martel, P.; Sutton, A.; Charnaux, N.; Druesne-Pecollo, N.; Galan, P.; Hercberg, S.; Le Clerc, S.; Kesse-Guyot, E.; et al. Weight Status and Alcohol Intake Modify the Association between Vitamin D and Breast Cancer Risk. *J. Nutr.* **2016**, *146*, 576–585. [CrossRef]
166. Chlebowski, R.T.; Johnson, K.C.; Kooperberg, C.; Pettinger, M.; Wactawski-Wende, J.; Rohan, T.; Rossouw, J.; Lane, D.; O'Sullivan, M.J.; Yasmeen, S.; et al. Calcium plus vitamin D supplementation and the risk of breast cancer. *J. Natl. Cancer Inst.* **2008**, *100*, 1581–1591. [CrossRef]

167. Cadeau, C.; Fournier, A.; Mesrine, S.; Clavel-Chapelon, F.; Fagherazzi, G.; Boutron-Ruault, M.C. Interaction between current vitamin D supplementation and menopausal hormone therapy use on breast cancer risk: Evidence from the E3N cohort. *Am. J. Clin. Nutr.* **2015**, *102*, 966–973. [CrossRef]
168. Madden, J.M.; Murphy, L.; Zgaga, L.; Bennett, K. De novo vitamin D supplement use post-diagnosis is associated with breast cancer survival. *Breast Cancer Res. Treat.* **2018**, *172*, 179–190. [CrossRef]
169. Crew, K.D.; Anderson, G.L.; Hershman, D.L.; Terry, M.B.; Tehranifar, P.; Lew, D.L.; Yee, M.; Brown, E.A.; Kairouz, S.S.; Kuwajerwala, N.; et al. Randomized Double-Blind Placebo-Controlled Biomarker Modulation Study of Vitamin D in Premenopausal Women at High Risk for Breast Cancer (SWOG S0812). *Cancer Prev. Res.* **2019**. [CrossRef]
170. Manson, J.E.; Cook, N.R.; Lee, I.M.; Christen, W.; Bassuk, S.S.; Mora, S.; Gibson, H.; Gordon, D.; Copeland, T.; D'Agostino, D.; et al. Vitamin D Supplements and Prevention of Cancer and Cardiovascular Disease. *N. Engl. J. Med.* **2019**, *380*, 33–44. [CrossRef]
171. Yin, L.; Grandi, N.; Raum, E.; Haug, U.; Arndt, V.; Brenner, H. Meta-analysis: Serum vitamin D and colorectal adenoma risk. *Prev. Med.* **2011**, *53*, 10–16. [CrossRef] [PubMed]
172. Wei, M.Y.; Garland, C.F.; Gorham, E.D.; Mohr, S.B.; Giovannucci, E. Vitamin D and prevention of colorectal adenoma: A meta-analysis. *Cancer Epidemiol. Biomark. Prev.* **2008**, *17*, 2958–2969. [CrossRef] [PubMed]
173. Jacobs, E.T.; Hibler, E.A.; Lance, P.; Sardo, C.L.; Jurutka, P.W. Association between circulating concentrations of 25(OH)D and colorectal adenoma: A pooled analysis. *Int. J. Cancer* **2013**, *133*, 2980–2988. [CrossRef] [PubMed]
174. Garland, C.F.; Gorham, E.D. Dose-response of serum 25-hydroxyvitamin D in association with risk of colorectal cancer: A meta-analysis. *J. Steroid Biochem. Mol. Biol.* **2017**, *168*, 1–8. [CrossRef] [PubMed]
175. Ma, Y.; Zhang, P.; Wang, F.; Yang, J.; Liu, Z.; Qin, H. Association between vitamin D and risk of colorectal cancer: A systematic review of prospective studies. *J. Clin. Oncol.* **2011**, *29*, 3775–3782. [CrossRef] [PubMed]
176. Sheng, S.; Chen, Y.; Shen, Z. Correlation between polymorphism of vitamin D receptor TaqI and susceptibility to colorectal cancer: A meta-analysis. *Medicine* **2017**, *96*, e7242. [CrossRef] [PubMed]
177. He, Y.; Timofeeva, M.; Farrington, S.M.; Vaughan-Shaw, P.; Svinti, V.; Walker, M.; Zgaga, L.; Meng, X.; Li, X.; Spiliopoulou, A.; et al. Exploring causality in the association between circulating 25-hydroxyvitamin D and colorectal cancer risk: A large Mendelian randomisation study. *BMC Med.* **2018**, *16*, 142. [CrossRef]
178. Grau, M.V.; Baron, J.A.; Sandler, R.S.; Haile, R.W.; Beach, M.L.; Church, T.R.; Heber, D. Vitamin D calcium supplementation, and colorectal adenomas: Results of a randomized trial. *J. Natl. Cancer Inst.* **2003**, *95*, 1765–1771. [CrossRef]
179. Gao, Y.; Um, C.Y.; Fedirko, V.; Rutherford, R.E.; Seabrook, M.E.; Barry, E.L.; Baron, J.A.; Bostick, R.M. Effects of supplemental vitamin D and calcium on markers of proliferation, differentiation, and apoptosis in the normal colorectal mucosa of colorectal adenoma patients. *PLoS ONE* **2018**, *13*, e0208762. [CrossRef]
180. Horvath, H.C.; Lakatos, P.; Kosa, J.P.; Bacsi, K.; Borka, K.; Bises, G.; Nittke, T.; Hershberger, P.A.; Speer, G.; Kallay, E. The candidate oncogene CYP24A1: A potential biomarker for colorectal tumorigenesis. *J. Histochem. Cytochem.* **2010**, *58*, 277–285. [CrossRef]
181. Wactawski-Wende, J.; Kotchen, J.M.; Anderson, G.L.; Assaf, A.R.; Brunner, R.L.; O'Sullivan, M.J.; Margolis, K.L.; Ockene, J.K.; Phillips, L.; Pottern, L.; et al. Calcium plus vitamin D supplementation and the risk of colorectal cancer. *N. Engl. J. Med.* **2006**, *354*, 684–696. [CrossRef] [PubMed]
182. Autier, P.; Mullie, P.; Macacu, A.; Dragomir, M.; Boniol, M.; Coppens, K.; Pizot, C. Effect of vitamin D supplementation on non-skeletal disorders: A systematic review of meta-analyses and randomised trials. *Lancet Diabetes Endocrinol.* **2017**, *5*, 986–1004. [CrossRef]
183. Calderwood, A.H.; Baron, J.A.; Mott, L.A.; Ahnen, D.J.; Bostick, R.M.; Figueiredo, J.C.; Passarelli, M.N.; Rees, J.R.; Robertson, D.J.; Barry, E.L. No Evidence for Posttreatment Effects of Vitamin D and Calcium Supplementation on Risk of Colorectal Adenomas in a Randomized Trial. *Cancer Prev. Res.* **2019**, *12*, 295–304. [CrossRef] [PubMed]
184. Baron, J.A.; Barry, E.L.; Ivanova, A. Calcium and Vitamin D for the Prevention of Colorectal Adenomas. *N. Engl. J. Med.* **2016**, *374*, 791–792. [CrossRef] [PubMed]
185. Urashima, M.; Ohdaira, H.; Akutsu, T.; Okada, S.; Yoshida, M.; Kitajima, M.; Suzuki, Y. Effect of Vitamin D Supplementation on Relapse-Free Survival among Patients with Digestive Tract Cancers: The AMATERASU Randomized Clinical Trial. *JAMA* **2019**, *321*, 1361–1369. [CrossRef] [PubMed]

186. Ng, K.; Nimeiri, H.S.; McCleary, N.J.; Abrams, T.A.; Yurgelun, M.B.; Cleary, J.M.; Rubinson, D.A.; Schrag, D.; Miksad, R.; Bullock, A.J.; et al. Effect of High-Dose vs Standard-Dose Vitamin D_3 Supplementation on Progression-Free Survival among Patients with Advanced or Metastatic Colorectal Cancer: The SUNSHINE Randomized Clinical Trial. *JAMA* **2019**, *321*, 1370–1379. [CrossRef] [PubMed]
187. Tuohimaa, P.; Tenkanen, L.; Ahonen, M.; Lumme, S.; Jellum, E.; Hallmans, G.; Stattin, P.; Harvei, S.; Hakulinen, T.; Luostarinen, T.; et al. Both high and low levels of blood vitamin D are associated with a higher prostate cancer risk: A longitudinal, nested case-control study in the Nordic countries. *Int. J. Cancer* **2004**, *108*, 104–108. [CrossRef] [PubMed]
188. Petrou, S.; Mamais, I.; Lavranos, G.; Tzanetakou, P.T.; Chrysostomou, S. Effect of Vitamin D Supplementation in Prostate Cancer: A Systematic Review of Randomized Control Trials. *Int. J. Vitam. Nutr. Res.* **2018**, *88*, 100–112. [CrossRef] [PubMed]

10

Relationship between 1,25-Dihydroxyvitamin D and Body Composition in Middle-Aged Sedentary Adults: The FIT-AGEING Study

Alejandro De-la-O [1,*], Lucas Jurado-Fasoli [1], Manuel J. Castillo [1], Luis Gracia-Marco [2], Ángel Gutierrez [1,†] and Francisco J. Amaro-Gahete [1,2,*,†]

1 EFFECTS 262 Research Group, Department of Physiology, Faculty of Medicine, University of Granada, 18071 Granada, Spain; juradofasoli@ugr.es (L.J.-F.); gutierre@ugr.es (Á.G.); mcgarzon@ugr.es (M.J.C.)

2 PROFITH "PROmoting FITness and Health Through Physical Activity" Research Group, Sport and Health University Research Institute (iMUDS), Department of Physical Education and Sports, Faculty of Sport Sciences, University of Granada, 18071 Granada, Spain; lgracia@ugr.es

* Correspondence: delao@ugr.es (A.D.-l.-O.); amarof@ugr.es (F.J.A.-G.);

† These authors contributed equally to this work.

Abstract: Vitamin D deficiency is a worldwide health problem that, in addition to its well-known negative effects on musculoskeletal health, has been related to a wide range of acute and chronic age-related diseases. However, little is known about the association of body composition with the active, hormonal form of vitamin D, 1,25-dihydroxyvitamin D plasma levels (1,25(OH)$_2$D). Therefore, the aim of this study was to investigate the association of 1,25(OH)$_2$D with body composition including lean and fat body mass as well as bone mineral density (BMD) in middle-aged sedentary adults. A total of 73 (39 women) middle-aged sedentary adults (53.7 ± 5.1 years old) participated in the current study. We measured weight and height, and we used dual energy X-ray absorptiometry to measure lean body mass, fat body mass and BMD. Body mass index (BMI), lean mass index (LMI), and fat mass index (FMI) were calculated. 1,25(OH)$_2$D was measured using a DiaSorin Liaison®immunochemiluminometric analyzer. The results showed a negative association of 1,25(OH)$_2$D with BMI, LMI and BMD ($\beta = -0.274$, $R^2 = 0.075$, $p = 0.019$; $\beta = -0.268$, $R^2 = 0.072$, $p = 0.022$; and $\beta = -0.325$, $R^2 = 0.105$, $p = 0.005$, respectively), which persisted after controlling for age and sex. No significant differences in 1,25(OH)$_2$D across body weight status were observed after controlling for the same covariates. In summary, our results suggest that 1,25(OH)$_2$D could be negatively associated with BMI, LMI and BMD whereas no association was found with FMI in middle-aged sedentary adults.

Keywords: vitamin D; calcitriol; body mass index; lean mass; fat mass; bone mineral density

1. Introduction

As the world´s population ages, the prevalence of chronic diseases increases, particularly over the last decades, becoming one of the great challenges that society faces [1,2]. Abnormalities in body composition such as a decrease of lean body mass and/or bone mineral density (BMD) or an increment in fat body mass are powerful predictors of morbidity and mortality risk as well as overall quality of life [3]. Epidemiologic studies indicate that these body composition changes are closely related to obesity, sarcopenia and/or osteoporosis in the elderly population [3,4]. However, these chronic diseases are progressive and initiate at a younger age [5,6]. Their high prevalence and concomitant health risk make them a particularly relevant worldwide public health problem and a social and economic burden [7–9].

Vitamin D is a fat-soluble vitamin essential for normal homeostasis of calcium and phosphorus, as well as for bone health [10] and preventing falls [11] and fractures [12]. Globally, vitamin D deficiency has been considered as a major public health problem affecting not only musculoskeletal health but also a wide range of several age-related chronic diseases [13]. 25-hydroxyvitamin D (25(OH)D) is the most commonly used biomarker when evaluating the relationship of vitamin D status with health-related outcomes [14–17]. However, 25(OH)D is thought to be largely inactive since it requires to be metabolized in the kidney by the enzyme 25-hydroxyvitamin D-1α-hydroxylase to be active. Therefore, 1,25-dihydroxyvitamin D (1,25$(OH)_2$D), also known as calcitriol, is responsible for most, if not all, of its biological effects [18,19]. The association between 1,25$(OH)_2$D and body composition parameters has been hard to establish for several reasons: (i) previously there was not a reliable and sensitive assay for calcitriol [20,21] and (ii) 25(OH)D has a higher concentration and longer half-life than 1,25$(OH)_2$D, thus requiring less sample volume for reliable measurements [22].

Consequently, epidemiological data are scarce, and a review of the scientific literature found no large studies examining the relationship between 1,25$(OH)_2$D and body composition outcomes. There is some evidence of the existence of an inverse association of 1,25$(OH)_2$D with body mass index (BMI) and fat body mass [23,24], however these data are conflicting with other studies [25–28]. In contrast, data are scarce on the potential relationship between 1,25$(OH)_2$D and lean body mass. Two recent studies found a significant association between low 1,25$(OH)_2$D and low lean body mass [29,30], which is highly dependent on the individual's age [29]. Similarly, controversial findings have been discovered regarding the role of 1,25$(OH)_2$D in bone health. Previous cross-sectional studies have reported an inverse association between 1,25$(OH)_2$D and BMD [31–33], whereas other studies found that 1,25$(OH)_2$D was unrelated to bone mineral content [34], bone loss [33,35] or hip fracture risk [36,37].

There are limited data on the study of body composition parameters in relation to 1,25$(OH)_2$D status in middle-aged adults. Thus, understanding whether 1,25$(OH)_2$D is associated with body composition parameters in this population is of clinical interest since, as previously established, the interventions to delay or reverse body composition related diseases are preferable when individuals are still relatively young and healthy [38,39].

Therefore, the aim of this study was to investigate the association of 1,25$(OH)_2$D with body composition including lean and fat body mass as well as BMD in middle-aged sedentary adults.

2. Materials and Methods

2.1. Study Design and Participants

The present cross-sectional study was conducted under the framework of the FIT-AGEING study (clinicaltrial.gov: ID: NCT03334357) [40]. The Ethics Committee on Human Research of the Regional Government of Andalucía approved the rationale, design, and methodology of the study [0838-N-2017] and all participants signed written informed consent in accordance with the Declaration of Helsinki (last revision guidelines, 2013).

Seventy-three middle-aged sedentary adults were recruited via electronic media, social networks and leaflets. The inclusion criteria were as follows: (i) to be sedentary (i.e., less than 20 min of physical activity on less than 3 days/week), (ii) not to have had greater body weight changes than 3 kg in the past 3 months, (iii) to be aged between 45 and 65 years old, (iv) not to be a smoker, (v) to be taking no long-term medication, (vi) not to be pregnant and (vii) not to suffer from any chronic cardiometabolic disease.

All tests were performed during September–October 2016/17 at the Sport and Health University Research Institute (iMUDS, Granada, Spain) and at the "Campus de la Salud" Hospital (Granada, Spain).

2.2. Anthropometric Parameters and Body Composition Assessment

A pre-validated Seca model 799 scale and stadiometer (Seca, Hamburg, Germany) was used to measure body weight and height with light clothing and without shoes. BMI was subsequently calculated as weight (kg)/height (m^2). Body composition outcomes were determined by a dual-energy X-ray absorptiometry scanner (Discovery Wi, Hologic, Inc., Bedford, MA, USA) obtaining lean body mass in kg, fat body mass in kg, and BMD in g/cm^2. A spine phantom quality check scan was conducted on each study day. A whole-body scan was performed considering all manufacturer´s guidelines (i.e., the positioning of participants, the analysis of results and the quality controls among others). The APEX 4.0.2. software was used to draw an automatic delineation of anatomic regions. The lean mass index (LMI) was calculated as lean body mass (kg)/body height (m^2). Similarly, we calculated the fat mass index (FMI) as fat body mass (kg)/body height (m^2). Fat mass was also expressed as a percentage of the total body mass. The participants were categorized into three groups on the basis of BMI levels: (i) normal weight (BMI $\geq$ 18.5 and <25 kg/m^2), (ii) overweight (BMI $\geq$ 25 and <30 kg/m^2), and (iii) obese (BMI $\geq$ 30 kg/m^2).

2.3. *Dietary Intake Assessment*

We performed a total of three 24-hour dietary recalls collected on non-consecutive days (one weekend day included). This validated method is able to determine the energy intake to within 8–10% of the current energy intake [41]. The interviews were meal sequence-based, in which a detailed description of the food consumed by the participants was recorded. The 24-hour dietary recalls were collected by an experimented and qualified research dietitian (L.J.-F.), using a photograph guide to improve the quality of the information provided on portion sizes of food and assisting participants in the estimation of the consumed food quantity [42]. The software EvalFINUT® updated with data from USDA (U.S. Department of Agriculture) and BEDCA ("Base de Datos Española de Composición de Alimentos") was used to calculate energy and micronutrient (i.e., vitamin D, calcium and phosphorus) intake derived from the 24-hour recalls.

2.4. *Physical Activity Assessment*

Physical activity levels were objectively assessed with a wrist-worn accelerometer (ActiGraph GT3X+, Pensacola, FL, United States) for 7 consecutive days (24 hours/day) [40]. The sampling frequency was previously set at 100 Hz to store raw accelerations [43]. The ActiLife v.6.13.3 software (ActiGraph, Pensacola, FL, United States) and the GGIR package (v.1.5-12[2]) in R (v.3.1.2[3]) were used to process these files [44,45]. The participants came to the laboratory and specific information about how to wear the accelerometer was given. They were also reminded to remove it only during water-based activities such as swimming or bathing. Only the participants who wore the accelerometer for ≥16 hours/day for 4 days (including 1 weekend day) were included in the analysis.

2.5. *Blood Samples Assessment*

A 10 mL peripheral blood sample was taken from the antecubital vein after overnight fasting. It was collected using the Vacutainer SST system (Becton Dickinson, Plymouth, UK) in ethylenediamine tetra-acetic acid-containing tubes. Blood samples were centrifuged at four thousand revolution per minute for seven minutes at 4 °C and stored at −80 °C. Plasma levels of 1,25$(OH)_2$D were measured using a DiaSorin Liaison®immunochemiluminometric analyzer (DiaSorin Ltd, Wokingham, Berkshire, UK) and expressed in pg/mL.

2.6. *Statistical Analysis*

Data were checked for normality with the use of distribution plots (i.e., visual check of histograms, and Q-Q plots) and the Shapiro-Wilk test. The descriptive parameters were reported as mean and standard deviation.

Differences between sexes were examined using an independent samples T test. Given that no interaction for sex was observed ($p > 0.05$), data are presented for men and women together. Simple linear regression models were built to test the association of 1,25$(OH)_2$D and body composition outcomes (i.e., BMI, LMI, FMI, and BMD). We also performed multiple linear regression models to analyze these associations controlling for age (Model 1), sex (Model 2), and age and sex (Model 3). Additionally, we also adjusted these models for total energy, vitamin D, calcium, phosphorus intake and/or physical activity levels (i.e., light, moderate-vigorous and total physical activity). To test whether 1,25(OH)$_2$D was different across body weight status (i.e., normal-weight, overweight and obese individuals), an analysis of variance (ANOVA) was conducted. Moreover, we performed an analysis of covariance to test the differences of 1,25(OH)$_2$D across weight status adjusting for age and sex.

Data were analyzed with the use of the Statistical Package for Social Sciences (SPSS, v. 22.0, IBM SPSS Statistics, IBM Corporation, Armonk, NY, USA). Graphical plots were built using the GraphPad Prism 5 (GraphPad Software, San Diego, CA, USA). The level of significance was fixed at <0.05.

3. Results

Table 1 shows the descriptive parameters of our study participants by sex. No significant differences in 1,25(OH)$_2$D were observed between men and women (p = 0.576).

Table 1. Descriptive characteristics of participants.

	N	All		*N*	Men		*N*	Women	
Age (years)	73	53.7	(5.1)	34	54.6	(5.2)	39	53	(5.0)
Body composition parameters									
Body mass index (kg/m^2)	73	26.7	(3.8)	34	28.3	(3.6)	39	25.3	(3.3) *
Lean mass (kg)	73	43.2	(11.7)	34	53.9	(6.5)	39	34.1	(5.8) *
Lean mass index (kg/m^2)	73	15.2	(2.9)	34	17.5	(2.0)	39	13.2	(1.8) *
Fat mass (%)	73	40.1	(8.9)	34	34.7	(8.0)	39	44.5	(7.4) *
Fat mass (kg)	73	30.1	(8.5)	34	30.9	(9.8)	39	29.2	(7.1)
Fat mass index (kg/m^2)	73	10.8	(3.1)	34	10.0	(3.2)	39	11.4	(2.9)
Bone mineral density (g/cm^2)	73	1.1	(0.1)	34	1.2	(0.1)	39	1.0	(0.1) *
Dietary intake									
Total Energy intake (kcal/day)	72	2071.7	(455.4)	34	2312.1	(402.9)	38	1854.6	(390.3) *
Vitamin D intake (µg/day)	72	5.0	(6.0)	34	3.8	(3.3)	38	6.1	(7.6)
Calcium intake (mg/day)	72	763.4	(340.5)	34	867.3	(396.9)	38	670.5	(251.4) *
Phosphorus intake (mg/day)	72	1324.7	(558.9)	34	1507.6	(689.6)	38	1161.0	(342.2) *
Physical activity parameters									
LPA (min/day)	70	173.7	(45.4)	33	169.9	(52.7)	37	178.0	(40.7)
MVPA (min/day)	70	95.8	(35.6)	33	96.4	(37.1)	37	96.6	(35.7)
Total PA (min/day)	70	269.5	(75.1)	33	265.2	(79.3)	37	273.3	(72.0)
Blood parameters									
1,25 Dihydroxyvitamin D (pg/ml)	73	40.3	(14.1)	34	38.3	(13.4)	39	42.0	(14.6)

Dara are presented as means (standard deviation). Abbreviations: LPA, light physical activity; MVPA, moderate-vigorous physical activity; PA, physical activity. * Significance differences between sexes (p < 0.05) obtained by the independent sample T test.

Figure 1 shows the associations between 1,25(OH)$_2$D and body composition related parameters. There was a significant negative association of 1,25(OH)$_2$D with BMI ($\beta = -0.274$, $R^2 = 0.075$, $p = 0.019$, Figure 1A), LMI ($\beta = -0.268$, $R^2 = 0.072$, $p = 0.022$, Figure 1B) and BMD ($\beta = -0.325$, $R^2 = 0.105$, $p = 0.005$, Figure 1D), which persisted after including age, sex, and age and sex in the model (all $p \leq 0.042$, Table 2). 1,25(OH)$_2$D was not significantly associated with FMI ($\beta = -0.080$, $R^2 = 0.006$, $p = 0.502$; Figure 1C), which did not change adjusting for age, sex, and age and sex (all $p \geq 0.35$, Table 2). The results remained unchanged after further adjusting for total energy, vitamin D, calcium, phosphorus intake and/or physical activity levels (i.e., light, moderate-vigorous and total physical activity) (data not shown, all $p > 0.1$).

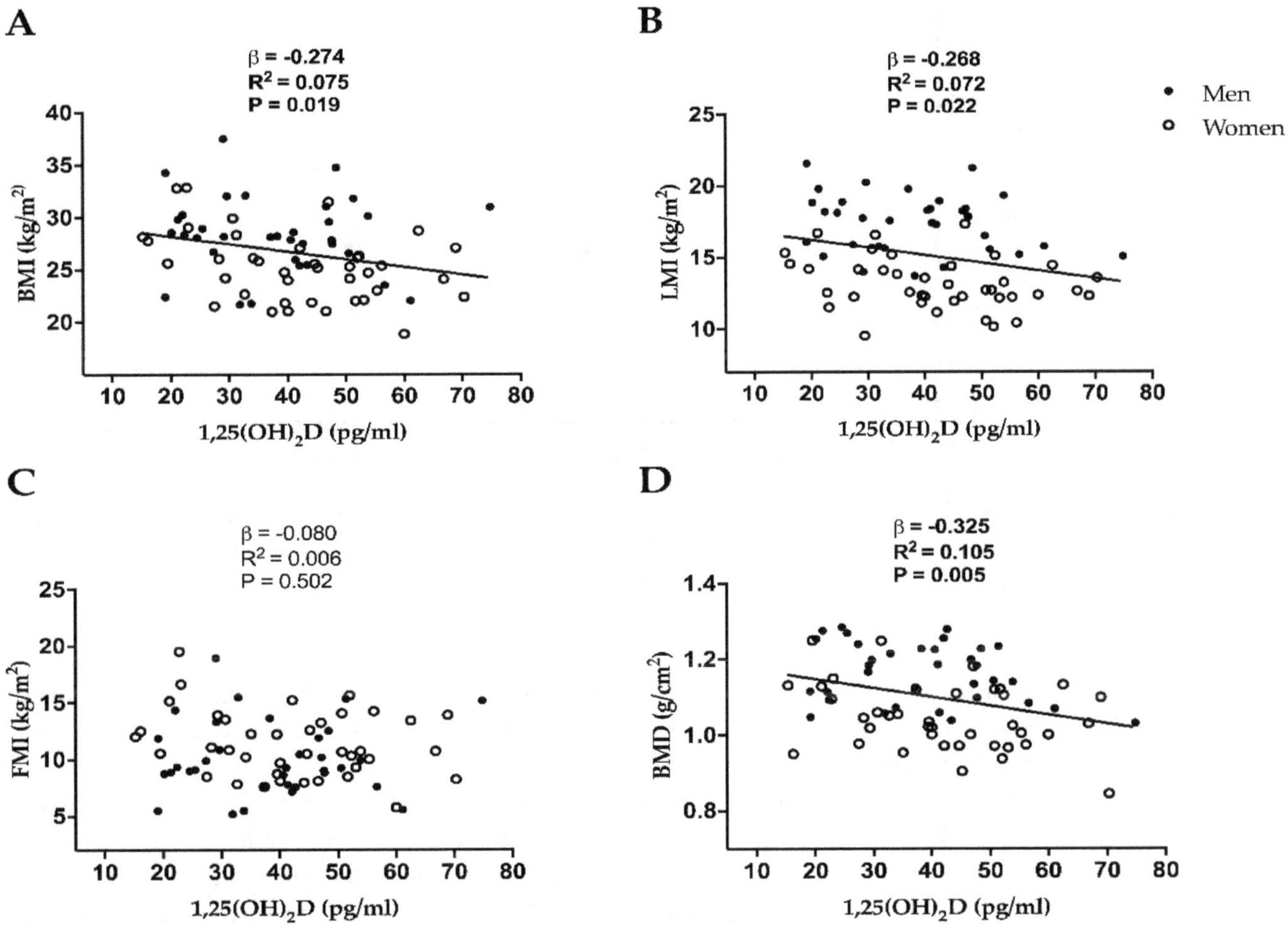

Figure 1. Simple linear regression graphs between 1,25-Dihydroxyvitamin D (1,25(OH)$_2$D) and body mass index (BMI) (**A**), lean mass index (LMI) (**B**), fat mass index (FMI) (**C**), and bone mineral density (BMD) (**D**) in middle-aged sedentary adults. β (standardized regression coefficient), R^2, and P from a simple linear regression analysis.

Table 2. Association of 1,25-Dihydroxyvitamin D with body mass index, lean mass index, fat mass index and bone mineral density.

	1,25-Dihydroxyvitamin D					
	Model 1		Model 2		Model 3	
	p value	β	*p* value	β	*p* value	β
Body mass index (kg/m^2)	**0.020**	−0.274	**0.040**	−0.263	**0.042**	−0.262
Lean mass index (kg/m^2)	**0.023**	−0.269	**0.030**	−0.383	**0.032**	−0.383
Fat mass index (kg/m^2)	0.505	−0.080	0.354	−0.112	0.356	−0.113
Bone mineral density (g/cm^2)	**0.005**	−0.325	**0.009**	−0.370	**0.009**	−0.377

Model 1 was adjusted for age; Model 2 was adjusted for sex; and Model 3 was adjusted for age and sex. *p* value of multiple-regression analysis. β (standardized regression coefficient). Values in bold indicate significance differences ($p < 0.05$).

ANOVA revealed no significant differences in 1,25(OH)$_2$D across body weight status (45.3 ± 13.3 pg/mL in normal-weight, 37.8 ± 13.1 pg/mL in overweight and 38.4 ± 16.7 pg/mL in obese individuals; Figure 2), which persisted after including age and sex as a covariate (44.8 ± 13.1 pg/mL in normal-weight; 37.9 ± 12.3 pg/mL in overweight and 38.9 ± 14.0 in obese individuals; $p = 0.2$).

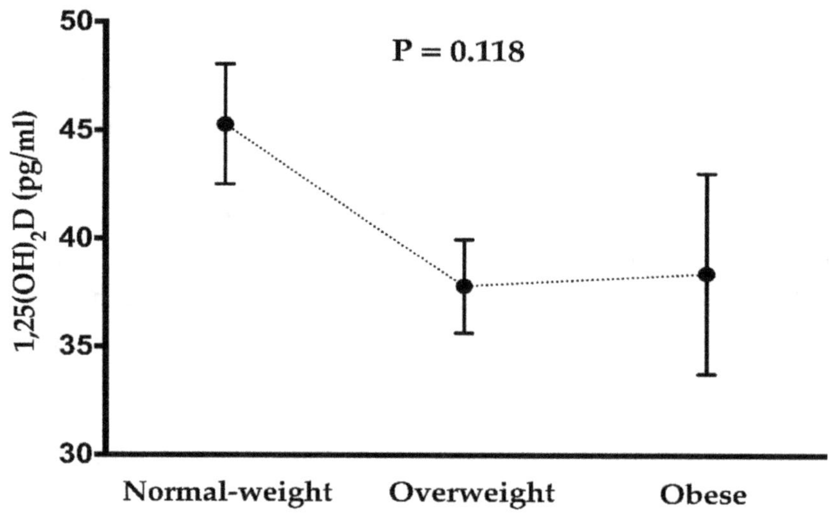

Figure 2. 1,25-Dihydroxyvitamin D (1,25(OH)$_2$D) by body weight status categories in middle-aged adults. Values are presented as means and standard error. p value obtained from the analysis of the variance to compare 1,25(OH)$_2$D across weight status (normal-weight, over-weight, and obese).

4. Discussion

The main results of the present study suggest that 1,25(OH)$_2$D is negatively associated with BMI, LMI and BMD independently of age and sex, whereas no association was found between 1,25(OH)$_2$D and FMI in middle-aged sedentary adults.

There is a controversy in the scientific literature regarding the 1,25(OH)$_2$D status of obese individuals. It has been described in classical studies that there are greater levels of 1,25(OH)$_2$D (~20 to 30%) in both obese men and women [25–28,46]. However, although we did not find any significant differences between BMI groups, we observed that overweight and obese individuals have ~16.6% and ~15.3% lower 1,25(OH)$_2$ than normal-weight individuals, which agrees with a previous large cohort that reported a ~18% lower 1,25(OH)$_2$D in the obese group compared with their lean counterparts [23,24]. These discrepancies between studies cannot be attributed to the individual´s age, sex and/or BMI, since the participants had similar biological characteristics. A seasonal effect might explain these controversial results as the 1,25(OH)$_2$D assessment was conducted in winter months [46] or spring months [27] in some studies, while others did not control the season in which the blood samples were taken [24]. Given that the effects of ultraviolet ray exposure on 25(OH)D could be different for obese and lean individuals, the time of the year when the study was conducted may be of importance. However, previous studies have suggested that the season of the year does not present the same influence on 1,25(OH)$_2$D as it has on 25(OH)D [47]. The different 1,25(OH)$_2$D assay methods used across the studies could be one important factor to consider. While older studies applied radioreceptor assays [25–28,46] in which lipid interferences have been described when samples are not pure enough [48], more recent studies including our own study used modern immuno assays for the assessment of 1,25(OH)$_2$D [30,32]. Taken all together, it is likely that obese subjects present low 1,25(OH)$_2$D. This fact could be explained because obesity is associated with poor levels of 25(OH)D, and it has been demonstrated that 1,25(OH)$_2$D depends on substrate availability [23,49]. A higher fat body mass offers a greater distribution space for both fat-soluble compounds. Additionally, obese individuals are usually exposed to negative lifestyle factors (i.e., unhealthy dietary habits and sedentary behaviour, among others), [50] and to lower sunlight exposure [51]. These lifestyle factors have been shown to have a negative influence on vitamin D status [52,53].

The use of 25(OH)D as a key marker of vitamin D status has logical advantages summarized as greater serum stability and a longer half-life than other markers (e.g., 1,25(OH)$_2$D) [22]. However, it is important to consider that it is biologically inactive and therefore could not be the best vitamin D function indicator [54]. The shorter half-life of 1,25(OH)$_2$D could be one of the reasons why the relationship of 1,25(OH)$_2$D and lean body mass has not been deeply studied. Hassan-Smith et al. reported a positive association between 1,25(OH)$_2$D and lean body mass [29]. These findings differ from those observed in our study in which we obtained higher 1,25(OH)$_2$D in individuals with lower lean body mass. These discrepancies could be explained by the different biological characteristics of the subjects of the study (i.e., our cohort was older than the Hassan-Smith et al. study [29]) and by the different assay methods used to determine 1,25(OH)$_2$D. New studies measuring 1,25(OH)$_2$D are necessary to clarify this issue.

We also found a negative association between 1,25(OH)$_2$D and BMD in our study cohort which concurs with a previous study that reported a positive association of 1,25(OH)$_2$D and the bone resorption marker β-cTX [32]. These results are consistent with the notion that 1,25(OH)$_2$D increases bone resorption via stimulating intestinal calcium absorption after calcium intake [32]. Moreover, recent animal and in vitro studies have proposed that 1,25(OH)$_2$D has a direct effect on osteoclasts inducing bone resorption by its interaction with the receptor activator of nuclear factor-κβ/receptor activator of nuclear factor-κβ ligand signaling pathway [55,56]. Taking this into consideration, an inverse association would be expected between 1,25(OH)$_2$D and bone mineral density. In addition, it seems plausible that 1,25(OH)$_2$D is produced when BMD is low and once BMD is recovered 25 (OH)D is transformed into the inactive 24,25(OH)$_2$D. Although this argument could explain our findings, further intervention studies are needed to understand this issue.

Our study has some limitations. The cross-sectional design does not allow ascribing causality to the observed relationships. Further, our study population was limited to sedentary healthy middle-aged adults (45–65 years old) and hence these results may not be generalizable to younger, older, and/or physically active individuals. This study, like most clinical studies, was based on a single assay of 1,25(OH)$_2$D. We did not assess the 24-hydroxyvitamin D$_2$ plasma levels. In addition, a whole-body DXA scan was conducted, so future studies are necessary to investigate whether spine and hip bone mineral density have the same association pattern. Finally, due to the relatively small sample size of the current study, the data should be interpreted with caution. One of the strengths of this study is that body composition was measured using a gold-standard technology, such as dual-energy X-ray absorptiometry. In addition, the measurement of objective physical activity data and dietary intake to be used as covariates represent further strengths.

5. Conclusions

In conclusion, our results suggest that 1,25(OH)$_2$D could be negatively associated with BMI, LMI and BMD independently of age and sex, while no significant relationship was obtained between 1,25(OH)$_2$D and FMI in middle-aged sedentary adults. Intervention studies are needed to understand whether changes in body composition status are associated with changes in 1,25(OH)$_2$D in this age-population.

Author Contributions: Conceptualization, A.D.-l.-O., L.J.-F., M.J.C., L.G.-M., Á.G. and F.J.A.-G.; methodology, A.D.-l.-O., L.J.-F. and F.J.A.-G.; formal analysis, A.D.-l.-O. and F.J.A.-G.; writing—Original draft, A.D.-l.-O. and F.J.A.-G.; writing—review and editing, A.D.-l.-O., L.J.-F., L.G.-M., Á.G., M.J.C. and F.J.A.-G.

Acknowledgments: The authors would like to thank all the participants that took part in the study for their time and effort. We are grateful to Ana Yara Postigo Fuentes for her assistance with the English language. This study is part of a PhD Thesis conducted in the Official Doctoral Program in Biomedicine of the University of Granada, Spain.

References

1. Jin, K.; Simpkins, J.W.; Ji, X.; Leis, M.; Stambler, I. The Critical Need to Promote Research of Aging and Aging-related Diseases to Improve Health and Longevity of the Elderly Population. *Aging Dis.* **2015**, *6*, 1–5. [CrossRef] [PubMed]
2. Fulop, T.; Larbi, A.; Witkowski, J.M.; McElhaney, J.; Loeb, M.; Mitnitski, A.; Pawelec, G. Aging, frailty and age-related diseases. *Biogerontology* **2010**, *11*, 547–563. [CrossRef] [PubMed]
3. Hamer, M.; O'Donovan, G. Sarcopenic obesity, weight loss, and mortality: The English Longitudinal Study of Ageing. *Am. J. Clin. Nutr.* **2017**, *106*, 125–129. [CrossRef] [PubMed]
4. Kohara, K. Sarcopenic obesity in aging population: Current status and future directions for research. *Endocrine* **2014**, *45*, 15–25. [CrossRef] [PubMed]
5. Hirschfeld, H.P.; Kinsella, R.; Duque, G. Osteosarcopenia: Where bone, muscle, and fat collide. *Osteoporos. Int.* **2017**, *28*, 2781–2790. [CrossRef]
6. Prado, C.M.; Purcell, S.A.; Alish, C.; Pereira, S.L.; Deutz, N.E.; Heyland, D.K.; Goodpaster, B.H.; Tappenden, K.A.; Heymsfield, S.B. Implications of low muscle mass across the continuum of care: A narrative review. *Ann. Med.* **2018**, *50*, 675–693. [CrossRef]
7. Harvey, N.; Dennison, E.; Cooper, C. Osteoporosis: Impact on health and economics. *Nat. Rev. Rheumatol.* **2010**, *6*, 99. [CrossRef]
8. Withrow, D.; Alter, D.A. The economic burden of obesity worldwide: A systematic review of the direct costs of obesity. *Obes. Rev.* **2011**, *12*, 131–141. [CrossRef]
9. Bruyère, O.; Beaudart, C.; Ethgen, O.; Reginster, J.-Y.; Locquet, M. The health economics burden of sarcopenia: A systematic review. *Maturitas* **2018**, *119*, 61–69. [CrossRef]
10. Holick, M.F.; Chen, T.C. Vitamin D deficiency: A worldwide problem with health consequences. *Am. J. Clin. Nutr.* **2008**, *87*, 1080S–1086S. [CrossRef]
11. Bischoff-Ferrari, H.A.; Dawson-Hughes, B.; Staehelin, H.B.; Orav, J.E.; Stuck, A.E.; Theiler, R.; Wong, J.B.; Egli, A.; Kiel, D.P.; Henschkowski, J. Fall prevention with supplemental and active forms of vitamin D: A meta-analysis of randomised controlled trials. *BMJ* **2009**, *339*, b3692. [CrossRef] [PubMed]
12. Looker, A.C. Serum 25-hydroxyvitamin D and risk of major osteoporotic fractures in older U.S. adults. *J. Bone Miner. Res.* **2013**, *28*, 997–1006. [CrossRef] [PubMed]
13. Zittermann, A.; Gummert, J.F. Nonclassical vitamin D action. *Nutrients* **2010**, *2*, 408–425. [CrossRef] [PubMed]
14. Autier, P.; Boniol, M.; Pizot, C.; Mullie, P. Vitamin D status and ill health: A systematic review. *Lancet Diabetes Endocrinol.* **2014**, *2*, 76–89. [CrossRef]
15. Cranney, A.; Horsley, T.; O'Donnell, S.; Weiler, H.; Puil, L.; Ooi, D.; Atkinson, S.; Ward, L.; Moher, D.; Hanley, D.; et al. Effectiveness and safety of vitamin D in relation to bone health. *Evid. Rep. Technol. Assess. (Full. Rep.)* **2007**, 1–235.
16. Visser, M.; Deeg, D.J.H.; Lips, P. Low vitamin D and high parathyroid hormone levels as determinants of loss of muscle strength and muscle mass (sarcopenia): The Longitudinal Aging Study Amsterdam. *J. Clin. Endocrinol. Metab.* **2003**, *88*, 5766–5772. [CrossRef]
17. Afzal, S.; Brondum-Jacobsen, P.; Bojesen, S.E.; Nordestgaard, B.G. Vitamin D concentration, obesity, and risk of diabetes: A mendelian randomisation study. *lancet. Diabetes Endocrinol.* **2014**, *2*, 298–306. [CrossRef]
18. Holick, M.F. Vitamin D deficiency. *N. Engl. J. Med.* **2007**, *357*, 266–281. [CrossRef]
19. Norman, A.W. From vitamin D to hormone D: Fundamentals of the vitamin D endocrine system essential for good health. *Am. J. Clin. Nutr.* **2008**, *88*, 491S–499S. [CrossRef]
20. Jenkinson, C.; Taylor, A.E.; Hassan-Smith, Z.K.; Adams, J.S.; Stewart, P.M.; Hewison, M.; Keevil, B.G. High throughput LC-MS/MS method for the simultaneous analysis of multiple vitamin D analytes in serum. *J. Chromatogr. B Anal. Technol. Biomed. Life Sci.* **2016**, *1014*, 56–63. [CrossRef]
21. Casetta, B.; Jans, I.; Billen, J.; Vanderschueren, D.; Bouillon, R. Development of a method for the quantification of 1alpha,25(OH)2-vitamin D3 in serum by liquid chromatography tandem mass spectrometry without derivatization. *Eur. J. Mass Spectrom. (Chichester Eng.)* **2010**, *16*, 81–89. [CrossRef] [PubMed]
22. Lips, P. Relative value of 25(OH)D and 1,25(OH)2D measurements. *J. Bone Miner. Res.* **2007**, *22*, 1668–1671. [CrossRef] [PubMed]
23. Konradsen, S.; Ag, H.; Lindberg, F.; Hexeberg, S.; Jorde, R. Serum 1,25-dihydroxy vitamin D is inversely associated with body mass index. *Eur. J. Nutr.* **2008**, *47*, 87–91. [CrossRef] [PubMed]

24. Parikh, S.J.; Edelman, M.; Uwaifo, G.I.; Freedman, R.J.; Semega-Janneh, M.; Reynolds, J.; Yanovski, J.A. The relationship between obesity and serum 1,25-dihydroxy vitamin D concentrations in healthy adults. *J. Clin. Endocrinol. Metab.* **2004**, *89*, 1196–1199. [CrossRef]
25. Bell, N.H.; Epstein, S.; Greene, A.; Shary, J.; Oexmann, M.J.; Shaw, S. Evidence for alteration of the vitamin D-endocrine system in obese subjects. *J. Clin. Investig.* **1985**, *76*, 370–373. [CrossRef]
26. Hey, H.; Stokholm, K.H.; Lund, B.; Lund, B.; Sorensen, O.H. Vitamin D deficiency in obese patients and changes in circulating vitamin D metabolites following jejunoileal bypass. *Int. J. Obes.* **1982**, *6*, 473–479.
27. Liel, Y.; Ulmer, E.; Shary, J.; Hollis, B.W.; Bell, N.H. Low circulating vitamin D in obesity. *Calcif. Tissue Int.* **1988**, *43*, 199–201. [CrossRef]
28. Kerstetter, J.; Caballero, B.; O'Brien, K.; Wurtman, R.; Allen, L. Mineral homeostasis in obesity: Effects of euglycemic hyperinsulinemia. *Metabolism* **1991**, *40*, 707–713. [CrossRef]
29. Hassan-Smith, Z.K.; Jenkinson, C.; Smith, D.J.; Hernandez, I.; Morgan, S.A.; Crabtree, N.J.; Gittoes, N.J.; Keevil, B.G.; Stewart, P.M.; Hewison, M. 25-hydroxyvitamin D3 and 1,25-dihydroxyvitamin D3 exert distinct effects on human skeletal muscle function and gene expression. *PLoS ONE* **2017**, *12*, e0170665. [CrossRef]
30. Marantes, I.; Achenbach, S.J.; Atkinson, E.J.; Khosla, S.; Melton III, L.J.; Amin, S. Is vitamin D a determinant of muscle mass and strength? *J. Bone Miner. Res.* **2011**, *26*, 2860–2871. [CrossRef]
31. Fujiyoshi, A.; Polgreen, L.E.; Hurley, D.L.; Gross, M.D.; Sidney, S.; Jacobs, D.R.J. A cross-sectional association between bone mineral density and parathyroid hormone and other biomarkers in community-dwelling young adults: The CARDIA study. *J. Clin. Endocrinol. Metab.* **2013**, *98*, 4038–4046. [CrossRef] [PubMed]
32. Vanderschueren, D.; Pye, S.R.; O'Neill, T.W.; Lee, D.M.; Jans, I.; Billen, J.; Gielen, E.; Laurent, M.; Claessens, F.; Adams, J.E.; et al. Active vitamin D (1,25-dihydroxyvitamin D) and bone health in middle-aged and elderly men: The European Male Aging Study (EMAS). *J. Clin. Endocrinol. Metab.* **2013**, *98*, 995–1005. [CrossRef] [PubMed]
33. Swanson, C.M.; Srikanth, P.; Lee, C.G.; Cummings, S.R.; Jans, I.; Cauley, J.A.; Bouillon, R.; Vanderschueren, D.; Orwoll, E.S.; Nielson, C.M. Associations of 25-Hydroxyvitamin D and 1,25-Dihydroxyvitamin D with Bone Mineral Density, Bone Mineral Density Change, and Incident Nonvertebral Fracture. *J. Bone Miner. Res.* **2015**, *30*, 1403–1413. [CrossRef] [PubMed]
34. Orwoll, E.; Kane-Johnson, N.; Cook, J.; Roberts, L.; Strasik, L.; McClung, M. Acute parathyroid hormone secretory dynamics: Hormone secretion from normal primate and adenomatous human tissue in response to changes in extracellular calcium concentration. *J. Clin. Endocrinol. Metab.* **1986**, *62*, 950–955. [CrossRef] [PubMed]
35. Stone, K.; Bauer, D.C.; Black, D.M.; Sklarin, P.; Ensrud, K.E.; Cummings, S.R. Hormonal predictors of bone loss in elderly women: A prospective study. The Study of Osteoporotic Fractures Research Group. *J. Bone Miner. Res.* **1998**, *13*, 1167–1174. [CrossRef]
36. Cummings, S.R.; Browner, W.S.; Bauer, D.; Stone, K.; Ensrud, K.; Jamal, S.; Ettinger, B. Endogenous hormones and the risk of hip and vertebral fractures among older women. Study of Osteoporotic Fractures Research Group. *N. Engl. J. Med.* **1998**, *339*, 733–738. [CrossRef]
37. Lips, P.; Netelenbos, J.C.; Jongen, M.J.; van Ginkel, F.C.; Althuis, A.L.; van Schaik, C.L.; van der Vijgh, W.J.; Vermeiden, J.P.; van der Meer, C. Histomorphometric profile and vitamin D status in patients with femoral neck fracture. *Metab. Bone Dis. Relat. Res.* **1982**, *4*, 85–93. [CrossRef]
38. Fontana, L.; Kennedy, B.K.; Longo, V.D.; Seals, D.; Melov, S. Medical research: Treat ageing. *Nature* **2014**, *511*, 405–407. [CrossRef]
39. Belsky, D.W.; Caspi, A.; Houts, R.; Cohen, H.J.; Corcoran, D.L.; Danese, A.; Harrington, H.; Israel, S.; Levine, M.E.; Schaefer, J.D.; et al. Quantification of biological aging in young adults. *Proc. Natl. Acad. Sci. USA* **2015**, *112*, E4104–E4110. [CrossRef]
40. Amaro-Gahete, F.J.; De-la-O, A.; Jurado-Fasoli, L.; Espuch-Oliver, A.; Robles-Gonzalez, L.; Navarro-Lomas, G.; de Haro, T.; Femia, P.; Castillo, M.J.; Gutierrez, A. Exercise training as S-Klotho protein stimulator in sedentary healthy adults: Rationale, design, and methodology. *Contemp. Clin. Trials Commun.* **2018**, *11*, 10–19. [CrossRef]
41. Halliday, T.M.; Davy, B.M.; Clark, A.G.; Baugh, M.E.; Hedrick, V.E.; Marinik, E.L.; Flack, K.D.; Savla, J.; Winett, S.; Winett, R.A. Dietary intake modification in response to a participation in a resistance training program for sedentary older adults with prediabetes: Findings from the Resist Diabetes study. *Eat. Behav.* **2014**, *15*, 379–382. [CrossRef] [PubMed]

42. López, M.D.R.; Martín-Lagos, R.A.; Martin-Lagos, R.A. *Guía para Estudios Dietéticos: Álbum Fotográfico de Alimentos*; Editorial Universidad de Granada: Granada, Spain, 2010; ISBN 9788433851673.
43. Migueles, J.H.; Cadenas-Sanchez, C.; Ekelund, U.; Delisle Nystrom, C.; Mora-Gonzalez, J.; Lof, M.; Labayen, I.; Ruiz, J.R.; Ortega, F.B. Accelerometer Data Collection and Processing Criteria to Assess Physical Activity and Other Outcomes: A Systematic Review and Practical Considerations. *Sports Med.* **2017**, *47*, 1821–1845. [CrossRef] [PubMed]
44. Hildebrand, M.; Hansen, B.H.; van Hees, V.T.; Ekelund, U. Evaluation of raw acceleration sedentary thresholds in children and adults. *Scand. J. Med. Sci. Sports* **2017**, *27*, 1814–1823. [CrossRef] [PubMed]
45. Hildebrand, M.; VAN Hees, V.T.; Hansen, B.H.; Ekelund, U. Age group comparability of raw accelerometer output from wrist- and hip-worn monitors. *Med. Sci. Sports Exerc.* **2014**, *46*, 1816–1824. [CrossRef]
46. Zamboni, G.; Soffiati, M.; Giavarina, D.; Tato, L. Mineral metabolism in obese children. *Acta Paediatr. Scand.* **1988**, *77*, 741–746. [CrossRef]
47. Zittermann, A. Vitamin D in preventive medicine: Are we ignoring the evidence? *Br. J. Nutr.* **2003**, *89*, 552–572. [CrossRef]
48. Clarke, A.D.; Rowbury, C.S. Removal of lipids before liquid chromatography of vitamin D in serum. *Clin. Chem.* **1985**, *31*, 657–658.
49. Zittermann, A. Vitamin D and disease prevention with special reference to cardiovascular disease. *Prog. Biophys. Mol. Biol.* **2006**, *92*, 39–48. [CrossRef]
50. Mozaffarian, D. Foods, obesity, and diabetes-are all calories created equal? *Nutr. Rev.* **2017**, *75*, 19–31. [CrossRef]
51. Vimaleswaran, K.S.; Berry, D.J.; Lu, C.; Tikkanen, E.; Pilz, S.; Hiraki, L.T.; Cooper, J.D.; Dastani, Z.; Li, R.; Houston, D.K.; et al. Causal relationship between obesity and vitamin D status: Bi-directional Mendelian randomization analysis of multiple cohorts. *PLoS Med.* **2013**, *10*, e1001383. [CrossRef]
52. Skaaby, T.; Husemoen, L.L.N.; Thuesen, B.H.; Pisinger, C.; Hannemann, A.; Jorgensen, T.; Linneberg, A. Longitudinal associations between lifestyle and vitamin D: A general population study with repeated vitamin D measurements. *Endocrine* **2016**, *51*, 342–350. [CrossRef] [PubMed]
53. Need, A.G.; Morris, H.A.; Horowitz, M.; Nordin, C. Effects of skin thickness, age, body fat, and sunlight on serum 25-hydroxyvitamin D. *Am. J. Clin. Nutr.* **1993**, *58*, 882–885. [CrossRef] [PubMed]
54. Ryan, Z.C.; Craig, T.A.; Folmes, C.D.; Wang, X.; Lanza, I.R.; Schaible, N.S.; Salisbury, J.L.; Nair, K.S.; Terzic, A.; Sieck, G.C. 1α, 25-dihydroxyvitamin D3 regulates mitochondrial oxygen consumption and dynamics in human skeletal muscle cells. *J. Biol. Chem.* **2016**, *291*, 1514–1528. [CrossRef] [PubMed]
55. Lieben, L.; Carmeliet, G.; Masuyama, R. Calcemic actions of vitamin D: Effects on the intestine, kidney and bone. *Best Pract. Res. Clin. Endocrinol. Metab.* **2011**, *25*, 561–572. [CrossRef]
56. Lips, P. Vitamin D physiology. *Prog. Biophys. Mol. Biol.* **2006**, *92*, 4–8. [CrossRef]

11

Barriers towards Sun Exposure and Strategies to Overcome these Barriers in Female Indoor Workers with Insufficient Vitamin D

Nurul Nadiah Shahudin [1,2], Mohd Jamil Sameeha [2], Arimi Fitri Mat Ludin [3], Zahara Abdul Manaf [3], Kok-Yong Chin [4] and Nor Aini Jamil [2,*]

1 Faculty of Sports Sciences & Recreation, Universiti Teknologi MARA (UiTM) Cawangan Pahang (Kampus Jengka), Pahang 26400, Malaysia; p97542@siswa.ukm.edu.my
2 Centre for Community Health Studies (ReaCH), Faculty of Health Sciences, Universiti Kebangsaan Malaysia, Kuala Lumpur 50300, Malaysia; sameeha@ukm.edu.my
3 Centre for Healthy Ageing and Wellness (H-CARE), Faculty of Health Sciences, Universiti Kebangsaan Malaysia, Kuala Lumpur 50300, Malaysia; arimifitri@ukm.edu.my (A.F.M.L.); zaharamanaf@ukm.edu.my (Z.A.M.)
4 Department of Pharmacology, Faculty of Medicine, Universiti Kebangsaan Malaysia, Cheras 56000, Malaysia; gabrielchinky@gmail.com
* Correspondence: ainijamil@ukm.edu.my

Abstract: The prevalence of vitamin D insufficiency is significant even in tropical countries such as Malaysia. Sun exposure is the primary source of vitamin D for most people due to limited intakes of food containing vitamin D and supplements. This study explored the perception of barriers towards sun exposure and strategies to overcome these barriers among vitamin D insufficient women workers in Kuala Lumpur, Malaysia. Twenty-five female indoor workers with serum 25-hydroxyvitamin D < 50 nmol/L participated in seven focus group discussions (FGDs). Barriers towards sun exposure were lack of accurate knowledge of vitamin D, health concern towards sun exposure, time constraints, desire to have fair and beautiful skin, sedentary lifestyle, indoor workplace, weather, lack of social support, living arrangement, safety concerns, and religious or cultural practices. The improvement strategies were classified into lifestyle changes and workplace opportunity for sun exposure. Public education on safe sun exposure to produce an optimal level of vitamin D is necessary. Future studies should evaluate the effectiveness of sunlight exposure program at workplace for the high-risk vitamin D deficiency group.

Keywords: vitamin D; sunlight exposure; barriers; indoor workers; female; focus group discussion

---

1. Introduction

Vitamin D insufficiency remains to be a concerning health issue worldwide due to its high prevalence among populations from various countries, cultural backgrounds and age groups [1], including tropical countries receiving substantial amount of sun exposure throughout the year [2]. However, the significant health impact of low vitamin D status remains unclear. Although incidence of rickets and osteomalacia are increasing in certain places, these conditions remain relatively rare worldwide [3,4]. The clinical evidence of vitamin D deficiency and nonskeletal health is not yet validated [5]. In countries where dietary vitamin D food intake and supplements are limited [6], and fortification of food with vitamin D is not compulsory, sunlight exposure is the primary source of vitamin D among the populations [6,7]. Government bodies often establish sun exposure guidelines to ensure a balance between the beneficial and harmful effects of sunlight [7]. However, it is almost impossible to provide guidance that fulfils all aspects because several factors can influence the cutaneous synthesis of vitamin D such as the zenith angle and latitude, different times of the day, air pollution, skin pigmentation, body surface area exposed when outdoors and age [8,9]. Currently, there are no sun exposure guidelines in Malaysia [10].

Previous studies around the world suggest that vitamin D deficiency is attributed to limited sun exposure, lack of dietary vitamin D food intake [11,12], urbanization [12], air pollution [13], obesity [14] and sedentary lifestyle [15]. It has been speculated that the excess body fat retains vitamin D in the body fat compartments resulting in decreased bioavailability of vitamin D among the obese individuals. This could also explain the lower vitamin D status among females compared to males as a result of higher body fat mass in females [16]. The limited sun exposure, especially in tropical countries, such as Malaysia, Thailand, Saudi Arabia and Iran, is mainly due to sun avoidance practice that is influenced by cultural, racial and religious backgrounds [2,6,8,9]. Malaysia is a unique multi-racial country, which is mainly composed of Malays, Chinese and Indians with various skin types. The high-risk groups of vitamin D insufficiency in Malaysia are children [17], adolescents [18,19], females [19–21], urban population [17,21], indoor workers [6,21], obese [17,18] and Indian and Malay ethnicities due to higher skin pigmentation and clothing styles (especially among Malay women wearing full-body garments) [2,6,17,19].

Cutaneous synthesis of vitamin D through outdoor activities and sun-bathing is widely practice by the westerners [9,11,22]. However, this practice was not popular among the vast majority of the Asian populations [23–25]. Sun-bathing and outdoor activities for sports and recreation are uncommon and not part of Asian culture [26,27]. Incidental sun exposure might occur while commuting to and from destinations, especially amongst those using public transportation. However, due to urbanization, most Asians are passive commuters and indoor workers [23,27].

A recent study on knowledge, attitude and practice conducted among high-risk female office workers in Kuala Lumpur, Malaysia suggested that further investigation into the factors contributing to vitamin D deficiency is essential as they have a moderate attitude and practice towards sunlight exposure and dietary intake of vitamin D [10]. This information that could be garnered from such studies would provide practical recommendations to the public and health agencies to prevent vitamin D deficiency among the Malaysian population. The current study is an extension of the previous study [10], which aimed to explore the perceived barriers towards sun exposure and strategies to overcome these barriers among indoor women workers with insufficient vitamin D status in Kuala Lumpur, Malaysia.

2. Materials and Methods

2.1. Study Participants

The participants from this study were derived from a recent study conducted among women office workers working in a medical university and teaching hospital in Kuala Lumpur, Malaysia [10]. In brief, they were indoor women workers with insufficient vitamin D level (serum 25-hydroxyvitamin D (25OHD) concentration <50 nmol/L) [28] and aged between 18 and 59 years. Indoor workers are defined as those working in an indoor setting for at least four days a week. Purposive sampling technique was used to ensure participants were recruited from four groups: (i) administrative staff (clerical staff, administrative staff assistants and lab technicians); (ii) executive (officers and top management employees); (iii) academicians (lecturers, senior lecturers and professors); and (iv) clinicians (medical assistants, nurses and doctors). Pregnant, lactating, or menopause women were excluded from this study. This study was approved by the Research Ethics Committees of Universiti Kebangsaan Malaysia (approval code: UKM PPI/111/8/JEP-2019-116).

2.2. Focus Group Discussion (FGD)

The FGDs were conducted in Bahasa Malaysia between October and November 2019 in a meeting room. All participants answered basic questionnaires and had given their written informed consent prior to participating in the FGD. Each FGD was led by a trained moderator (NNS), monitored by an experienced qualitative researcher (MJS) and observed by a research assistant. The moderator audiotaped all sessions using a video recorder (Sony, ICD-UX560F, Japan), while the research assistant was tasked with taking notes and recording descriptions of the participants' non-verbal behaviors. These notes offered as a backup to resolve any issues regarding audio clarity and to monitor participants' body language during the session.

The moderator first explained the purpose of the discussion, rules and regulations of FGD, followed by asking a series of specific, predetermined questions (Table 1). Two main topics were discussed, namely (i) barriers to receiving adequate sun exposure to synthesise vitamin D; and (ii) strategies to improve their vitamin D insufficiency. All participants were encouraged to share their ideas and opinions, and suitable probes were used to obtain in-depth findings. Recruitment was stopped when no new relevant information emerged due to data saturation.

Table 1. Focus Group Discussion Questions.

Topic	Questions
Barriers	(1) Internally, what do you think leads to your vitamin D insufficiency? (2) Externally, what do you think contributes to your vitamin D insufficiency? (3) What prevents or restricts you from sun exposure on weekdays? (4) What prevents or constraints you from sun exposure on weekends?
Improvement Strategy	(1) Do you want to improve your vitamin D status? (2) What are you going to do to improve your vitamin D level? (3) What type of activities do you want your employer to do to promote workplace sun exposure? (4) Can you suggest a suitable workplace intervention program? (frequency, intensity, type and time)

2.3. Data Coding and Analysis

The Consolidated Criteria for Reporting Qualitative Research (COREQ) framework [29] was used to guide the reporting of the findings. Audio recordings were transcribed verbatim. The transcripts were thematically analyzed using NVivo version 12 [30]. Each transcript was reviewed line-by-line and codes were categorized concurrently by three coders (NNS, NAJ and MJS). The identified codes were either single words (e.g., hot, beauty) or short phrases (e.g., sunscreen usage) that captured the essence of the excerpts [31]. Subsequently, the codes were grouped under broad domains of the discussion guide and theoretical constructs (e.g., time constraints). The discrepancies in coding were discussed with the research team (NNS, NAJ, MJS, AFML and ZAM) until a mutual agreement was achieved for the final nodes as described by Hadi and Closs [32]. As all researchers had expertise in nutrition and exercise health, they attempted to suspend their perspectives to avoid biases and focused on participants' statements that described their perceptions and experiences during the FGD.

2.4. Trustworthiness

To ensure the quality and trustworthiness of this study, multiple approaches were used. Prolonged engagement with study participants helped to gain their trust and establish rapport [32], as the researcher worked with the same participants during the preliminary study in February to May 2019 [10], until the FGD session conducted in October 2019. An audit trail was used to improve the quality of the instrument [32]. The lead researcher (NNS) met with supervisors (NAJ & MJS) after the first two FGDs to discuss possible questions to be revised and checked on probes improvement. Furthermore, peer debriefing was applied where the weekly meetings were conducted between NAJ, MJS and NNS to discuss on data analysis and interpretations continuously throughout the research process. Lastly, thick description of this study was presented in the methodology section to obtain external validity to ensure that this study could be transferable to other settings, situations and populations [32].

3. Results

Twenty-five female indoor workers took part in seven FGDs. Each group contained three to five participants and ranged from 45 min to 1 h in duration. Table 2 shows the participants' characteristics. Majority of the participants were between 30 and 39 years old (64%), married (64%), had a diploma or a higher education background (80%) and worked as an administrative staff (76%). Most of them had low to middle household-income (92%).

Table 2. Participants' Characteristics.

Variable	*n*	(%)	Mean	SD
Age				
18–29 years	3	12%	35.6	5.8
30–39 years	16	64%		
40–49 years	6	24%		
Marital Status				
Single	6	24%		
Married	16	64%		
Divorced/widowed	3	12%		
Education				
Secondary school	5	20%		
Diploma	10	40%		
Bachelor or higher	10	40%		
Occupation				
Administrative staff	19	76%		
Executive	1	4%		
Academician	3	12%		
Clinician	2	8%		
Household Monthly Income (MYR *)				
Low (<3860)	12	48%		
Middle (3860–8319)	11	44%		
High (>8319)	2	8%		

* MYR: Malaysia Ringgit.

3.1. Barriers towards Sun Exposure

A total of eleven perceived barriers towards sun exposure for adequate vitamin D status were identified and categorized into internal and external factors (Table 3). Five themes were recognized from the internal factor, including lack of knowledge due to misinformation about how vitamin D is synthesized upon exposure to sunlight or ultraviolet B (UVB) irradiation. Health concern was another barrier towards sun exposure, which was further classified into pre-existing medical conditions and risks for skin cancer. Other internal barriers towards sun exposure were time constraints associated with family and work commitments, desires to have fair and beautiful skin and sedentary lifestyles.

Table 3. Themes for barriers towards sunlight exposure.

Factor	Themes	Quotes
Internal factor	Lack of knowledge	"I got my vitamin D synthesized when I was driving. The sun rays were felt through the windscreen of my car," (33 years old, clinician). "Vitamin D sun is the morning sun. The afternoon and evening sun do not help to produce vitamin D, right?" (27 years old, administrative staff).
	Health concern	"If we are exposed under the sun, will it cause skin cancer? That is why I prefer to stay indoors" (49 years old, administrative staff). "I have this stigma that sunlight can make me fall sick, get fever or headache, regardless whether it is in the morning, afternoon or evening's sunlight," (41 years old, administrative staff). "I can't stand with the hot sun these days. It is so much different compared to younger days, and the heat was unbearable. I believe the sun rays these days is harmful and can cause cancer. It is because of the thinning ozone," (32 years old, administrative staff). "I am a patient of cardiovascular disease. I had a minor stroke two years ago. That is why I didn't go out much these days. Whenever I walk, I tend to get tired quickly, thus making me feel lazy (to walk)," (44 years old, administrative staff). "I am very much an indoor person because my health doesn't permit (me to exercise). I must be cautious whenever (I'm) outside because my respiratory system is very sensitive. For example, if I were to go out at the park, it needs to be somewhere dust-free and less polluted because I can get sick quickly and (it) may cause prolonged cough for months," (34 years old, executive).
	Time constraints	"I don't have enough time to go out after work. There are times when I would only reach home at 7.00 p.m. due to heavy traffic," (34 years old, administrative staff). I don't have time to do any activities before or after work because I stay far from the office, approximately 30 km away. I usually reach home in an hour. Sometimes, I have to travel for 2 h," (32 years old, administrative staff). "No time to go out on weekdays. I must fetch the kids after work. Once I reach home, I need to cook and do all the house chores. As for the weekends, I will do major cleaning, cooking and spend some family time at home. Plus, my husband works on the weekends. Most of the time, I just let the kids play at the car porch (covered) instead of going out," (35 years old, administrative staff). "I don't have time to do any outdoor activities on the weekends because I have part-time work commitment as a phlebotomist," (33 years old, administrative staff).
	Desire to have fair and beautiful skin	"I wear long sleeves whenever I'm out because it's hot and I'm afraid of becoming dark," (37 years old, clinician). "I used to have a lot of freckles. My beautician said the UV rays could cause freckles. That is why I avoid sun exposure," (35 years old, administrative staff). "I think because of ageing, I have been consistently using SPF moisturizer for the past three years to keep hydrated. So, I can avoid wrinkles and dry skin," (42 years old, administrative staff).
	Sedentary lifestyle	"I don't do any outdoor activities. The most I would do on the weekends is to hang out at eateries," (33 years old, administrative staff). "I often spend time at home on the weekend watching television," (24 years old, administrative staff). "I don't know why, but even when I had the chance (to go outdoor), I prefer to stay at home or indoor activity," (42 years old, administrative staff).

Table 3. *Cont.*

Factor	Themes	Quotes
External factor	Indoor workplace	"I am confined indoors during work from 8.00 a.m. to 5.00 p.m. So, sun exposure is limited during the weekdays. I normally take my lunch in the office or cafe, which is in the same building. So, there is no reason for me to go out," (41 years old, administrative staff). "I work in a diagnostic lab that is in the basement. I don't see the sun during working hours," (32 years old, clinician).
	Weather	"Malaysia's weather is so hot. So, I prefer to stay indoors," (33 years old, clinician). "Our weather is so unpredictable, especially during the rainy season. I skip being outdoors and choose to spend the time at my favorite eateries instead," (37 years old, administrative staff).
	Lack of social support	"My husband works during the weekends. Normally, I would wait for his off days to go for an outing. Otherwise, I just spend time with my son at home," (35 years old, administrative staff). "I am single and don't have a lot of friends. I will only go out to the park if my nephews or nieces come over to visit me. I wish to go out more often, but I don't have anyone to go with," (37 years old, academician). "My husband is not an outdoor person. He loves to go shopping and eat at the mall. So, I have no choice but to follow him as we normally go there at least twice a week," (32 years old, executive).
	Living arrangement	"I stay in a high-rise apartment, and there is no direct sunlight coming in. I don't get sunlight because my apartment doesn't come with a balcony. I even have to dry my clothes inside," (32 years old, administrative staff). "I stay at an apartment on the fourth floor, and I don't go out often even during the weekends, just too lazy to go down," (31 years old, clinician). "I stayed in a sub-urban landed property. I don't get direct sunlight in my house compound. There are a lot of big trees surrounding my house,"(44 years old, administrative staff).
	Safety concern	"I prefer indoor activities instead of outdoors because of safety reasons. For example, if you were to go out during the early mornings at the park, it tends to be too quiet. I am scared to go there alone," (38 years old, administrative staff).
	Culture and religious practices	"I enjoy outdoor activities, but I don't like it when men are staring at me (in public)," (32 years old, executive). "I am particular in covering my aurah (part of the body that is prohibited from being revealed to other men for Muslim women). I was active before, doing workout and even join an aerobic class. However, I will make sure that I follow the rules (only exposing the face and both hands up to the wrists)," (42 years old, administrative staff).

For the external factor, six themes emerged including indoor workplaces, hot weather and unpredictable climate change. Lack of social support from the spouse, family members or friends to do outdoor activity together reduced the participants' interest to be exposed to the sun. Limited direct access to the sun at home as a result of living arrangement, house design and location of the house situated in the city were also mentioned. Finally, safety concerns and cultural and religious practices among Muslim women were also barriers towards sunlight exposure.

3.2. Strategy to Overcome the Barrier towards Sun Exposure

The discussion on the strategies to overcome the barrier towards sun exposure was classified into two factors (Table 4). The first is focusing on the personal improvement strategies that the participants were willing to perform on their own by changing their sun exposure behaviors to improve their vitamin D status. Suggestions included increasing outdoor activities during the weekends, practicing appropriate sunscreen usage, clothing adjustments that increase body surface area (BSA) exposed to sunlight, and improving their time management. The second part of the discussion is followed by suggestions for a suitable intervention program to be conducted by employers. The recommendations were categorized based on themes which include types, frequency, intensity and time that can be done based on workplace settings. Figure 1 summarizes the factors of barriers towards sun exposure and improvement strategies as identified by the indoor female workers in this study.

Table 4. Themes for strategies to overcome the barrier.

Factor	Themes	Quotes
Personal Improvement	Increase outdoor activity	"I am unsure whether I can do it on weekdays, but I will do more outdoor activities on the weekends. Maybe later in the afternoons after I am done with household chores," (35 years old, executive). "I need to make some changes, for example, do outdoor activities," (42 years old, administrative staff). "Outdoor outing with the family, for example a trip to the National Zoo. Not only we get to expose under the sun, but also (we) can spend quality time with the family,"(31 years old, administrative staff).
	Practice appropriate sunscreen usage	"The least I can do is to reduce my sunscreen usage, not to apply too thick, especially in the mornings," (27 years old, administrative staff).
	Clothing adjustment	"I think I need to wear short-sleeved clothing instead of long-sleeved when I do my exercise so that I absorb more (sunlight)," (37 years old, clinician). "Just open (rolled up her sleeves) and expose it," (49 years old, administrative staff).
	Time management	"I will do house chores at night. So, I can go out during the day," (32 years old, administrative staff).
Intervention Program at Workplace	Type of activity	"Walking around the campus. For example, aim for the daily 10,000 steps," (37 years old, academician). "Maybe just stay out, like sun-bathing with clothes on," (32 years old, administrative staff). "Group activity such as treasure hunt around the campus," (32 years old, administrative staff). "I guess an outdoor aerobic such as Zumba is the most suitable activity and we have done it before," (33 years old, clinician). "I think leisure activities like 'tele-match' and family day is suitable," (42 years old, administrative staff). "Maybe organize a run (paused) like the fun run. If it is conducted on weekends, we can include our family members too," (33 years old, administrative staff). "If we take a look at the current surrounding, I think outdoor cleaning activity is suitable as one of the methods to obtain sunlight," (33 years old, administrative staff). "Maybe the employer can provide an outdoor workstation that allows the staff to bring their laptop and do their work outdoors. Apart from the lab work which needs to be done indoors, I can do report writing and administrative related work outdoors," (41 years old, administrative staff).
	Frequency	"I think once a week is fine. If it's more than that, two or three times a week, that's a bit too frequent. It will disrupt my work, and I believe my employer will not approve it," (37 years old, administrative staff). "Twice a week is sufficient," (24 years old, administrative staff). "I think once a week is not sufficient, maybe around two to three times a week," (32 years old, administrative staff).

Table 4. *Cont.*

Factor	Themes	Quotes
	Intensity	"I prefer to do light exercise. I don't want to be drenched in sweat in the morning and I need to do work after that," (37 years old, academician). "The exercise intensity should be moderate. So, we can maintain our fitness apart from getting sun exposure. I think it can be boring if it's too slow and relaxed," (34 years old, administrative staff). "I prefer low intensity, more relax," (32 years old, administrative staff). "I prefer moderate (intensity) and gradually increase the intensity. Not only we get the benefit of sun exposure, but also at the same time (we) can improve our cardiovascular fitness," (38 years old, administrative staff).
	Duration and time of the day	"I think the best time to do the program is between 8.00 a.m. to 9.00 a.m. before we start work. It is inconvenient to work, stop for exercise, then work again," (42 years old, administrative staff). "Evening session is suitable, about 5.30 p.m. It is more relaxing to do exercise once the work is done," (33 years old, administrative staff). "10.30 a.m. onwards is suitable as normally we are less occupied around that time," (32 years old, administrative staff). "The first two hours between 8.00 a.m.–10.00 a.m. is fine to me," (33 years old, administrative staff). "I think I can spare 15 min for that (intervention)," (24 years old, administrative staff). "Half an hour is workable for me," (34 years old, administrative staff). "30 min is not enough, at least one hour per session," (34 years old, administrative staff).

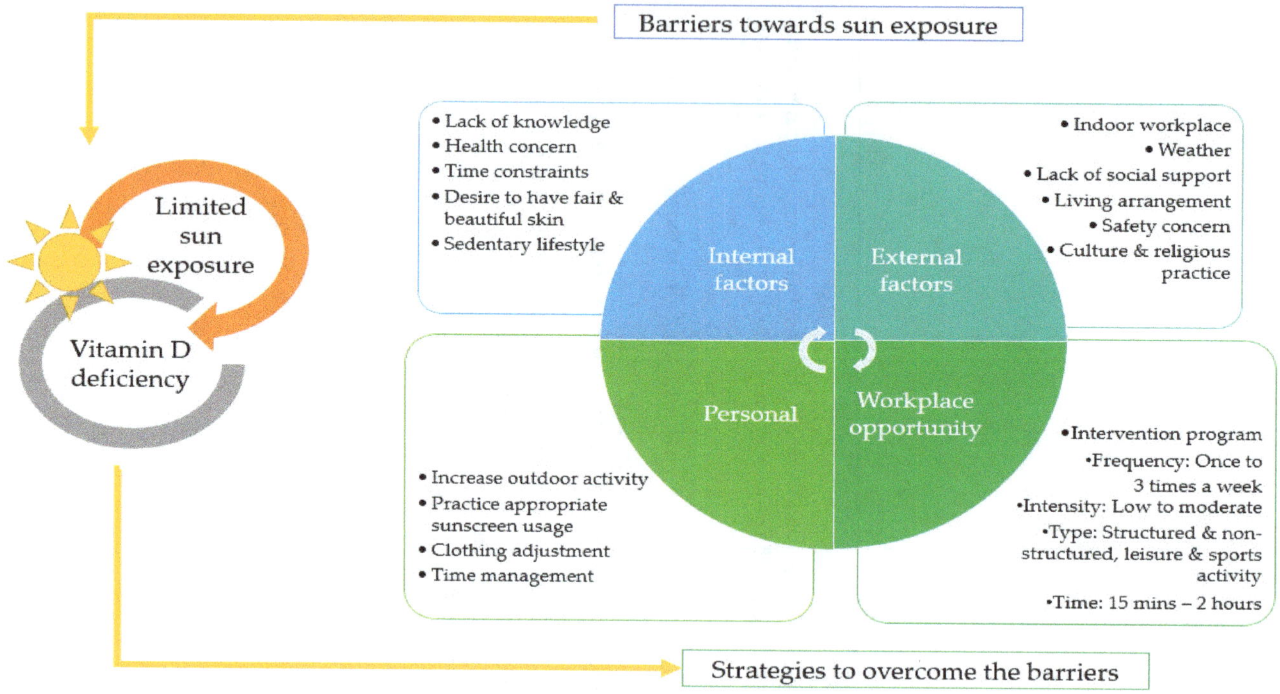

Figure 1. Barriers and improvement strategies to improve sun exposure for vitamin D.

4. Discussion

This study used a qualitative method of FGD to explore the barriers and improvement strategies towards sun exposure among women working indoors in the capital city of Malaysia with insufficient vitamin D status. The study provides new knowledge in this area, with practical messages that can be applied to the population at risk of vitamin D deficiency with a similar demographic background.

Lack of knowledge is on the top of the list for barriers towards sun exposure. We found that most of the participants had a misconception on the metabolism of vitamin D including how vitamin D is synthesized, and the differences between ultraviolet A (UVA) and UVB radiation. UVB is the sources of cutaneous synthesis of vitamin D and it cannot penetrate glass [11]. The participants assumed that the UVA they are exposed to while driving in the car and sitting by office window (with glasses) might provide them with vitamin D. A previous study done in a Malaysian sub-urban setting among post-menopausal Malay women found that poor knowledge on vitamin D influenced their sun exposure behavior [33]. The similarity of the findings could be owing to the lack of knowledge regarding vitamin D health benefits compared to other groups of vitamins among both urban and sub-urban females in Malaysia [1,6,33].

Health concerns to sun exposure, particularly increased risk of skin cancer, were mentioned in the FGD. According to the Global Cancer Observatory 2018 report, skin cancer was the 30th most common cancer in Malaysia and is not as prevalent as other cancers [34]. Most participants believed that they are susceptible to skin cancer due to the thinning of the ozone layer. They were not aware that skin cancer is not prevalent among Malaysians, especially the Malays. Our participants practiced poor sun protection behaviors, such as inappropriate amount and timing of sunblock application. They usually apply sunblock once in the morning together with their makeup before going to work. This finding is consistent with a previous study of skin cancer prevention practice among 400 university students in Kuala Lumpur, with the majority of the subjects being Malay women [35]. The study found that only 43.5% of the participants used sunblock, often applying them inadequately and forgetting to reapply after swimming, sweating, or other activities after the sunblock is degraded or washes-off [35]. A cross-sectional study in Queensland, Australia where the highest rate of skin cancer in the world reported that participants from low-income household tend to have uncertainty and concern about vitamin D and sun exposure [36]. Both studies suggested that sun protection education is needed in these populations to address the misunderstanding about skin cancer risk and improve the skin protection practice [25,35]. Some participants in our study also perceived that dizziness and fever were direct results of sun exposure, despite the lack of scientific evidence. This assumption also led to sunlight avoidance among our study participants.

Time constraint was frequently mentioned by the participants that caused limited sun exposure. All of the subjects in this study were working women in the urban area, who thrive to balance between work and family. This finding is consistent with a recent study among employees in Kuala Lumpur, who associated 'lack of time' with being busy with work, house chores and other family commitments [37]. A recent review highlighted that limited time spent outdoors among the urban population was due to their working nature, increased screen time and less manual work undertaken outdoor compared to rural population [12]. The majority of our participants drove to work. A typical driving scenario in the urban area encompasses a mixture of standstill traffic and slow traffic, depending on the route and time of the day [38]. Our participants spent on average around 1 to 1.5 h to commute daily to work. Once they reached home, they were bound to do house chores, further limiting their sunlight exposure time. Similar experiences were shared by women in eight European countries, whereby gender inequality and expectations of married working women, especially mothers, are higher in balancing work-family commitments compared to their counterparts [39].

The subjects of this study also expressed aesthetic concerns about sunlight exposure. This finding echoed previous reports among Asians, whereby a fair skin tone is often associated with beauty [25,40]. Common remarks such as fear of becoming dark, having freckles, sunburn and makeup usage, influenced sun avoidance behavior, especially among women [25]. Apart from sun protection cream, most moisturizers, foundation cream and compact powder these days, come with an added sun protection factor (SPF). The subjects surveyed also indicated a preference to stay indoors. A sedentary lifestyle has long been associated with vitamin D deficiency, physical inactivity, and health-related problems such as obesity and diabetes [2,19,20]. While the mechanism underlying the association between vitamin D and obesity is still uncertain, the low vitamin D status in obese individuals could be due to their sedentary lifestyle and low outdoor activity, vitamin D sequestration in adipose tissue, or simply a volumetric dilution effect [14]. A population study in Malaysia reported that only 14% of adults in Malaysia ever exercised and the majority spent 74% of the day being sedentary such as watching television, lying down, or hanging out to have drinks [41]. These factors are also correlated with our participants' social support given by their spouse, friends and employers [42]. It was previously reported that single individuals preferred to stay at home when there was no company while married couples with kids mainly adhered to their family commitments [37].

Being bounded indoors at their workplace as well as living arrangements are among the external factors leading to a lack of sunlight exposure. On average, indoor workers spend eight hours a day at the office for five days a week during the day. A similar investigation in Singapore found that indoor workers were among the high-risk group for vitamin D deficiency, probably because UVB is filtered by the glass window of the office [43]. Similar to other densely populated cities like Hong Kong and Singapore, the majority of the populations in Kuala Lumpur live in high-rise buildings [44], due to higher land costs. Low-income groups typically reside in a flat unit or a low-cost apartment with basic facilities, whereas the middle- and high-income groups may opt to live in a condominium with full facilities such as a playground, in-house park for jogging or walking, tennis court and swimming pool. The majority of our participants who lived in high-rise buildings mentioned that they either did not receive direct sunlight from their unit, or did not have sports or recreational facilities from their surrounding vicinity to encourage them to go out. A study among Saudi women attributed the lack of sun exposure to the modern house designs. Currently, the house design in Saudi has changed towards closed and high rise buildings built without a balcony, thus, limiting their sun exposure compared to living in a home with older designs that often incorporate a courtyard that allows sun ray to enter the house [45]. Apart from geographical reasons, the external barrier was influenced by cultural and religious practices similar to those of Muslims in our study. The Malays in Malaysia are generally

Muslims. As a Muslim woman, specific clothing guidelines commonly observed based on Quranic teachings allows only the face and hands to be exposed when in public [45,46]. Our participants further highlighted that religious restrictions that affect their actions and activities in public also limit their sun exposure.

Outdoor safety is an emerging barrier towards sun exposure among our subjects. The rising cost of living in Kuala Lumpur has given rise to an increased crime rate in the vicinity. Based on the criminal index in Malaysia from the year 2009 to 2015, 16,034 street crime investigations were carried on snatch thefts, robberies and similar offences [47]. These crimes were almost exclusively targeted on women walking alone in open areas [47]. Our participants mentioned that they too felt worried and insecure about being outdoors, even in public parks.

Strategies to tackle the barriers to sun exposure were mentioned by the participants through two factors: personal improvement and workplace opportunity. First and foremost, most of the participants agreed that they need to change their lifestyle to improve their vitamin D status. An educational program is essential for the promotion and enhancement of personal improvements to sunlight exposure. Besides, participants also believed that employers could play an essential role in promoting sun exposure at the workplace. Activities such as Zumba, aerobics and light exercise may be suitable to be conducted at workplace to promote both sunlight exposure and physical activity. Various timing and frequency proposed by the participants, ranging from 15 min to 2 h, once to three times a week. Besides, employers could also provide outdoor workstations that allow for sun exposure while being at work whenever necessary. These suggestions, however, would be subject to approval by the employer and improvements in existing organizational policies. A structured program of gradual increment from low to high intensity activities for 30–60 min was suggested in previous study among desk-based employees in Kuala Lumpur, Malaysia [37]. However, dietary vitamin D intake and supplements may be recommended to make up the shortfall from sunlight exposure, especially among those who have limited sunlight exposure, for whatever reasons they may have. A recent data showed a positive association between adherence to the Mediterranean diet and vitamin D status that could be explained by the synergistic anti-inflammatory and antioxidant effects of its high consumption of whole grain and plant-based food and moderate intake of fish, white meat, and eggs [48].

This study provides insight into the barriers towards sun exposure among vitamin D insufficiency women. However, several limitations were noted in this study. Firstly, it was conducted in one institution, with an uneven representatives from four target groups; administrators, executives, academicians and clinicians, due to time and work commitment constraints. Therefore, the findings in this study mainly reflect the perceptions of the administrator group. This study was also conducted among the Malay women population only, thus, it does not reflect the perception of other ethnic groups in Malaysia. Future studies should explore the barriers towards sun exposure among other at-risk groups, such as shift workers in Malaysia to understand their perspective on this matter. Furthermore, an intervention study should be performed to assess the effectiveness of sunlight exposure program in the workplace in improving vitamin D status of female indoor workers in Malaysia.

5. Conclusions

The Malay female indoor workers with insufficient vitamin D level reported that the barriers to sun exposure were influenced by both internal and external factors, such as work commitments, environment, and social factors. An educational program should be mooted in spreading accurate information on the importance of sun exposure and the best practice for optimal level of vitamin D. Working women should also take the initiative to maximize their sun exposure during the weekends. Apart from lifestyle changes, employers also can play an active role in promoting positive sun exposure at the workplace by organizing outdoor activities. Regardless, further evaluation on the effectiveness of sunlight exposure program among female indoor workers remains necessary.

Author Contributions: Conceptualization, N.N.S., M.J.S., A.F.M.L. and N.A.J.; formal analysis, N.N.S. and M.J.S.; funding acquisition, N.A.J.; investigation, N.N.S.; methodology, N.N.S., M.J.S. and N.A.J.; software, N.N.S., M.J.S. and N.A.J.; supervision, M.J.S. and N.A.J.; validation, M.J.S., A.F.M.L., Z.A.M. and N.A.J.; writing—original draft, N.N.S.; writing—review and editing, M.J.S., A.F.M.L., Z.A.M., K.-Y.C. and N.A.J. All authors have read and agreed to the published version of the manuscript.

Acknowledgments: We would like to thank all the study participants for their contributions in this study. Thanks are also extended to Nur Syazwani binti Mastor and Nurul Nabila binti Md Yusuf who assisted with the logistics and preparation.

References

1. Scott, D.; Ebeling, P.R. Vitamin D and public health. *Int. J. Environ. Res. Public Health* **2019**, *16*, 848. [CrossRef]
2. Shafinaz, I.S.; Moy, F.M. Vitamin D level and its association with adiposity among multi-ethnic adults in Kuala Lumpur, Malaysia: A cross sectional study. *BMC Public Health* **2016**, *16*, 232. [CrossRef] [PubMed]
3. Creo, A.L.; Thacher, T.D.; Pettifor, J.M.; Strand, M.A.; Fischer, P.R. Nutritional rickets around the world: An update. *Paediatr. Int. Child Health* **2016**, *37*, 84–98. [CrossRef] [PubMed]
4. Bouillon, R.; Antonio, L. Nutritional rickets: Historic overview and plan for worldwide eradication. *J. Steroid Biochem. Mol. Biol.* **2020**, *198*, 105563. [CrossRef] [PubMed]
5. Rosen, C.J.; Adams, J.S.; Bikle, D.D.; Black, D.M.; Demay, M.B.; Manson, J.E.; Murad, M.H.; Kovacs, C.S. The nonskeletal effects of vitamin D: An Endocrine Society scientific statement. *Endocr. Rev.* **2012**, *33*, 456–492. [CrossRef] [PubMed]
6. Abd Aziz, N.H.; Yazid, N.A.; Abd Rahman, R.; Abd Rashid, N.; Wong, S.K.; Mohamad, N.V.; Lim, P.S.; Chin, K.-Y. Is first trimester maternal 25-hydroxyvitamin D level related to adverse maternal and neonatal pregnancy outcomes? A prospective cohort study among Malaysian Women. *Int. J. Environ. Res. Public Health* **2020**, *17*, 3291. [CrossRef]
7. Bonevski, B.; Bryant, J.; Lambert, S.; Brozek, I.; Rock, V. The ABC of vitamin D: A qualitative study of the knowledge and attitudes regarding vitamin D deficiency amongst selected population groups. *Nutrients* **2013**, *5*, 915–927. [CrossRef]
8. Farrar, M.D.; Webb, A.R.; Kift, R.; Durkin, M.T.; Allan, D.; Herbert, A.; Berry, J.L.; Rhodes, L.E. Efficacy of a dose range of simulated sunlight exposures in raising vitamin D status in South Asian adults: Implications for targeted guidance on sun exposure. *Am. J. Clin. Nutr.* **2013**, *97*, 1210–1216. [CrossRef]
9. Wacker, M.; Holick, M.F. Sunlight and vitamin D: A global perspective for health. *Derm. Endocrinol.* **2013**, *5*, 51–108. [CrossRef]
10. Jamil, N.A.; Shahudin, N.N.; Abdul Aziz, N.S.; Chew, J.Q.; Wan Aminuddin, W.A.A.; Mat Ludin, A.F.; Chin, K.Y.; Abdul Manaf, Z.; Mat Daud, N. Knowledge, attitude and practice related to vitamin D and its relationship with vitamin D status among Malay female office workers. *Int. J. Environ. Res. Public Health* **2019**, *16*, 4735. [CrossRef]
11. Holick, M.F. Vitamin D deficiency. *N. Engl. J. Med.* **2007**, *357*, 266–281. [CrossRef] [PubMed]
12. Mendes, M.M.; Darling, A.L.; Hart, K.H.; Morse, S.; Murphy, R.J.; Lanham-New, S.A. Impact of high latitude, urban living and ethnicity on 25-hydroxyvitamin D status: A need for multidisciplinary action? *J. Steroid Biochem. Mol. Biol.* **2019**, *188*, 95–102. [CrossRef] [PubMed]
13. Barrea, L.; Savastano, S.; Di Somma, C.; Savanelli, M.C.; Nappi, F.; Albanese, L.; Colao, A. Low serum vitamin D-status, air pollution and obesity: A dangerous liaison. *Rev. Endocr. Metab. Disord.* **2017**, *18*, 207–214. [CrossRef] [PubMed]
14. Savastano, S.; Barrea, L.; Savanelli, M.C.; Nappi, F.; Somma, C.D.; Orio, F.; Colao, A. Low vitamin D status and obesity: Role of nutritionist. *Rev. Endocr. Metab. Disord.* **2017**, *18*, 215–225. [CrossRef]
15. Awad, A.B.; Alappat, L.; Valerio, M. Vitamin D and metabolic syndrome risk factors: Evidence and mechanisms. *Crit. Rev. Food Sci. Nutr.* **2012**, *52*, 103–112. [CrossRef]
16. Muscogiuri, G.; Barrea, L.; Somma, C.D.; Laudisio, D.; Salzano, C.; Pugliese, G.; Alteriis, G.D.; Colao, A.; Savastan, S. Sex differences of vitamin D status across BMI classes: An observational prospective cohort study. *Nutrients* **2019**, *11*, 3034. [CrossRef]

17. Poh, B.K.; Rojroongwasinkul, N.; Nguyen, B.K.L.; Sandjaja; Ruzita, A.T.; Yamborisut, U.; Hong, T.N.; Ernawati, F.; Deurenberg, P.; Parikh, P. 25-hydroxy-vitamin D demography and the risk of vitamin D insufficiency in the South East Asian Nutrition Surveys (SEANUTS). *Asia Pac. J. Clin. Nutr.* **2016**, *25*, 538–548. [PubMed]
18. Khor, G.L.; Chee, W.S.S.; Shariff, Z.M.; Poh, B.K.; Arumugam, M.; Rahman, J.A.; Theobald, H.E. High prevalence of vitamin D insufficiency and its association with BMI-for-age among primary school children in Kuala Lumpur, Malaysia. *BMC Public Health* **2011**, *11*, 95. [CrossRef] [PubMed]
19. Quah, S.W.; Abdul Majid, H.; Al-Saddat, N.; Yahya, A.; Su, T.T.; Jalaludin, M.Y. Risk factors of vitamin D deficiency among 15-year-old adolescents participating in the Malaysian Health and Adolescents Longitudinal Research Team Study (MyHeARTs). *PLoS ONE* **2018**, *13*, e0200736. [CrossRef]
20. Moy, F.M. Vitamin D status and its associated factors of free-living Malay adults in a tropical country, Malaysia. *J. Photochem. Photobiol.* **2011**, *104*, 444–448. [CrossRef]
21. Nurbazlin, M.; Chee, W.S.S.; Rokiah, P.; Tan, A.T.B.; Chew, Y.Y.; Siti Nusaibah, A.R.; Chan, S.P. Effects of sun exposure on 25(OH) vitamin D concentration in urban and rural women in Malaysia. *Asia Pac. J. Clin. Nutr.* **2013**, *22*, 391–399. [PubMed]
22. Gilchrest, B.A. Sun exposure and vitamin D sufficiency. *Am. J. Clin. Nutr.* **2008**, *88*, 570S–577S. [CrossRef] [PubMed]
23. Nimitphong, H.; Holick, M.F. Vitamin D status and sun exposure in southeast Asia. *Derm. Endocrinol.* **2013**, *5*, 34–37. [CrossRef]
24. Man, R.E.K.; Li, L.J.; Cheng, C.Y.; Wong, T.Y.; Lamoureux, E.; Sabanayagam, C. Prevalence and determinants of suboptimal vitamin D levels in a multiethnic Asian population. *Nutrients* **2017**, *9*, 313. [CrossRef] [PubMed]
25. Jang, H.; Koo, F.K.; Ke, L.; Clemson, L.; Cant, R.; Fraser, D.R.; Seibel, M.J.; Tseng, M.; Mpofu, E.; Mason, R.S.; et al. Culture and sun exposure in immigrant East Asian women living in Australia. *Women Health* **2013**, *53*, 504–518. [CrossRef] [PubMed]
26. Aman, M.S.; Fauzee, M.S.O.; Mohamed, M. The understanding of meaning and cultural significance of leisure, recreation and sport in Malaysia towards capitalizing human resources. *J. Glob. Bus.* **2007**, *3*, 129–135.
27. Nguyen, H.T.T.; von Schoultz, B.; Nguyen, T.V.; Dzung, D.N.; Duc, P.T.M.; Thuy, V.T.; Hirschberg, A.L. Vitamin D deficiency in northern Vietnam: Prevalence, risk factors and associations with bone mineral density. *Bone* **2012**, *51*, 1029–1034. [CrossRef]
28. Ross, A.C.; Manson, J.E.; Abrams, S.A.; Aloia, J.F.; Brannon, P.M.; Clinton, S.K.; Durazo-Arvizu, R.A.; Gallagher, J.C.; Gallo, R.L.; Jones, G.; et al. The 2011 report on dietary reference intakes for calcium and vitamin D from the Institute of Medicine: What clinicians need to know. *J. Clin. Endocrinol. Metab.* **2011**, *96*, 53–58. [CrossRef]
29. Tong, A.; Sainsbury, P.; Craig, J. Consolidated criteria for reporting qualitative research (COREQ): A 32-item checklist for interviews and focus groups. *Int. J. Qual. Health Care* **2007**, *19*, 349–357. [CrossRef]
30. *NVivo Qualitative Data Analysis Software*, version 12; QSR International (UK) Limited: Cheshire, UK, 2019.
31. Fereday, J.; Muir-Cochrane, E. Demonstrating rigor using thematic analysis: A hybrid approach of inductive and deductive coding and theme development. *Int. J. Qual. Methods* **2006**, *5*, 80–92. [CrossRef]
32. Hadi, M.A.; Closs, S.J. Ensuring rigour and trustworthiness of qualitative research in clinical pharmacy. *Int. J. Clin. Pharm.* **2016**, *38*, 641–646. [CrossRef]
33. Istiany, A.; Rahman, S.A.; Kasim, Z.K.; Swee, W.C.S.; Yassin, Z.; Parid, A.M. Effect of nutrition education and sun exposure on vitamin D Status among post-menopausal Malay women. *Int. J. Sci. Eng. Investig.* **2012**, *1*, 91–97.
34. World Health Organization. Cancer Today Population Fact Sheet (Malaysia). 2019. Available online: https://gco.iarc.fr/today/data/factsheets/populations/458-malaysia-fact-sheets.pdf (accessed on 10 April 2020).
35. Al-Naggar, R.A.; Bobryshev, Y.V. Practice of skin cancer prevention among young Malaysian. *Community Med. Health Educ.* **2012**, *2*, 2. [CrossRef]
36. Youl, P.H.; Janda, M.; Kimlin, M. Vitamin D and sun protection: The impact of mixed public health messages in Australia. *Int. J. Cancer* **2008**, *124*, 1963–1970. [CrossRef]
37. Zahara, A.M.; Abdul Hadi, R.; Arimi Fitri, M.L.; Siti Munirah, A.B. Motivations, barriers and preferences to exercise among overweight and obese desk-based employees. *Int. J. Sport Exerc. Psychol.* **2020**, 1–15. [CrossRef]

38. Abas, M.A.; Rajoo, S.; Zainal Abidin, S.F. Development of Malaysian urban drive cycle using vehicle and engine parameters. *Transp. Res. Part D Transp. Environ.* **2018**, *63*, 388–403. [CrossRef]
39. Beham, B.; Drobnič, S.; Präg, P.; Baierl, A.; Lewis, S. Work-to-family enrichment and gender inequalities in eight European countries. *Int. J. Hum. Resour. Manag.* **2020**, *31*, 589–610. [CrossRef]
40. Blebil, A.Q.; Dujaili, J.A.; Teoh, E.; Wong, P.S.; Bhuvan, K.C. Assessment of awareness, knowledge, attitude, and the practice of vitamin D among the general public in Malaysia. *J. Karnali Acad. Health Sci.* **2019**, *2*, 171–180. [CrossRef]
41. Poh, B.K.; Safiah, M.Y.; Tahir, A.; Siti Haslinda, M.D.; Siti Norazlin, N.; Norimah, A.K.; Wan Manan, W.M.; Mirnalini, K.; Zalilah, M.S.; Azmi, M.Y.; et al. Physical activity pattern and energy expenditure of Malaysian adults: Findings from the Malaysian Adult Nutrition Survey (MANS). *Mal. J. Nutr.* **2010**, *16*, 13–37.
42. Waters, C.N.; Ling, E.P.; Chu, A.H.Y.; Ng, S.H.X.; Chia, A.; Lim, Y.W.; Müller-Riemenschneider, F. Assessing and understanding sedentary behaviour in office-based working adults: A mixed-method approach. *BMC Public Health* **2016**, *16*, 360. [CrossRef]
43. Divakar, U.; Sathish, T.; Soljak, M.; Bajpai, R.; Dunleavy, G.; Visvalingam, N.; Nazeha, N.; Soh, C.K.; Christopoulos, G.; Car, J. Prevalence of vitamin D deficiency and its associated work-related factors among indoor workers in a multi-ethnic southeast Asian country. *Int. J. Environ. Res. Public Health* **2020**, *17*, 164. [CrossRef] [PubMed]
44. Wahab, S.R.H.A.; Ani, A.I.C.; Sairi, A.; Tawil, N.M.; Razak, M.Z.A. Classification of high-rise residential building facilities: A descriptive survey on 170 housing scheme in Klang Valley. *MATEC Web Conf.* **2016**, *66*, 00103. [CrossRef]
45. Aljefree, N.; Lee, P.; Ahmed, F. Exploring knowledge and attitudes about vitamin D among adults in Saudi Arabia: A qualitative study. *Healthcare* **2017**, *5*, 76. [CrossRef] [PubMed]
46. Jamil, N.A.; Yew, M.H.; Noor Hafizah, Y.; Gray, S.R.; Poh, B.K.; Macdonald, H.M. Estimated vitamin D synthesis and dietary vitamin D intake among Asians in two distinct geographical locations (Kuala Lumpur, 3°N v. Aberdeen, 57°N) and climates. *Public Health Nutr.* **2018**, *21*, 3118–3124. [CrossRef] [PubMed]
47. Latimaha, R.; Bahari, Z.; Ismail, N.A. Examining the linkages between street crime and selected state economic variables in Malaysia: A panel data analysis. *J. Ekon. Malays.* **2019**, *53*, 59–72.
48. Barrea, L.; Muscogiuri, G.; Laudisio, D.; Pugliese, G.; de Alteriis, G.; Colao, A.; Savastano, S. Influence of the Mediterranean Diet on 25-hydroxyvitamin D levels in adults. *Nutrients* **2020**, *12*, 1439. [CrossRef]

12

Calcitriol and Calcidiol Can Sensitize Melanoma Cells to Low–LET Proton Beam Irradiation

Ewa Podgorska [1,†], Agnieszka Drzal [1,†], Zenon Matuszak [2], Jan Swakon [3], Andrzej Slominski [4], Martyna Elas [1] and Krystyna Urbanska [1,*]

1 Faculty of Biochemistry, Biophysics and Biotechnology, Jagiellonian University, Gronostajowa 7 Street, Krakow 30-387, Poland; ewa.podgorska@doctoral.uj.edu.pl (E.P.); agnieszka.drzal@doctoral.uj.edu.pl (A.D.); martyna.elas@uj.edu.pl (M.E.)
2 Department of Medical Physics and Biophysics, Faculty of Physics and Applied Computer Science, AGH University of Science and Technology, al. A. Mickiewicza 30, Krakow 30-059, Poland; zenon.matuszak@fis.agh.edu.pl
3 Polish Academy of Sciences, Institute of Nuclear Physics, Krakow 31-342, Poland; jan.swakon@ifj.edu.pl
4 Department of Dermatology, Comprehensive Cancer Center Cancer Chemoprevention Program, University of Alabama at Birmingham, Birmingham, AL 35294, USA; aslominski@uabmc.edu
* Correspondence: krystyna.urbanska@uj.edu.pl
† These authors contributed equally to this work.

Abstract: Proton beam irradiation promises therapeutic utility in the management of uveal melanoma. Calcitriol (1,25(OH)$_2$D$_3$)—the biologically active metabolite of vitamin D$_3$—and its precursor, calcidiol (25(OH)D$_3$), exert pleiotropic effects on melanoma cells. The aim of the study was to evaluate the effect of both calcitriol and calcidiol on melanoma cell proliferation and their response to proton beam irradiation. Three melanoma cell lines (human SKMEL-188 and hamster BHM Ma and BHM Ab), pre-treated with 1,25(OH)$_2$D$_3$ or 25(OH)D$_3$ at graded concentrations (0, 10, 100 nM), were irradiated with 0–5 Gy and then cultured in vitro. Growth curves were determined by counting the cell number every 24 h up to 120 h, which was used to calculate surviving fractions. The obtained survival curves were analysed using two standard models: linear-quadratic and multi-target single hit. Calcitriol inhibited human melanoma proliferation at 10 nM, while only calcidiol inhibited proliferation of hamster lines at 10 and 100 nM doses. Treatment with either 1,25(OH)$_2$D$_3$ or 25(OH)D$_3$ radio sensitized melanoma cells to low doses of proton beam radiation. The strength of the effect increased with the concentration of vitamin D$_3$. Our data suggest that vitamin D$_3$ may be an adjuvant that modifies proton beam efficiency during melanoma therapy.

Keywords: vitamin D$_3$; proton beam radiotherapy; melanoma; in vitro

---

1. Introduction

Because of their high incidence, mortality rates and resistance to the therapy, melanomas are still one the most challenging cancer types for researchers and clinicians [1,2]. Over the last decade, our understanding of the molecular principles regulating melanoma behaviour has improved significantly, leading to new therapies [3,4]. However, even with the new therapeutic approaches the problem of limited efficacy and selective responsiveness of patients still remains [5]. Therefore, new creative approaches and their combinations are required.

Accumulating evidence from a variety of epidemiological and experimental studies confirms in vitro and in vivo anticancer activity of vitamin D$_3$ [6–9]. Those studies indicate that biologically active vitamin D$_3$ derivatives may lower the incidence, and inhibit the progression, of various tumours, including melanoma [10–12] and sensitize them to radiotherapy [13–18]. Moreover, there are reports of an inverse relationship between patient survival and melanoma thickness and 25(OH)D_3 serum levels, polymorphisms in the genes encoding the vitamin D receptor (VDR), the vitamin D binding protein, expression of the VDR and CYP27B1 expression [19–25] and complex relations with CYP24A1 [26]. Additionally, it was proposed that VDR plays a role in the development and progression of melanocytic tumours [27].

So far, no studies have been published on a combination of vitamin D_3 and proton beam irradiation, a therapy with superior dose distribution compared to photon radiation, which is commonly used in the treatment of uveal melanoma. However, reports on the differences in the level of production of free radicals, cell cycle, cell migration inhibition and apoptotic signalling between photon and proton beam radiotherapy [28–32] suggest possible differences in the effect of their combination with vitamin D_3.

This work aims to examine the influence of calcitriol (1,25$(OH)_2D_3$) and calcidiol (25(OH)D_3) on the proliferation and response to proton beam radiotherapy of three melanoma cell lines: human SKMEL-188 and hamster BMH Ma and BHM Ab. In the light of existing evidence, we hypothesize that vitamin D_3 can sensitize melanoma cells to radiation, thus enhancing its effectiveness. Two different models, linear-quadratic and single hit multi-target, were fitted to analyse the surviving curves of the tested melanoma cell lines exposed to combined treatment and to get the most comprehensive picture of proton radiation dose response.

2. Results

2.1. Impact of Two Metabolites of Vitamin D_3 on Melanoma Cell Proliferation

1,25$(OH)_2D_3$ and 25(OH)D_3 affected the growth rate of melanoma cells in culture (Figure 1). In the case of calcitriol, only human SKMEL-188 melanoma cells showed a significant decrease in growth rate, after treatment with the concentration of 10 nM, with BHM Ma and BHM Ab hamster lines showing no major changes in the rate of proliferation. Calcidiol, on the other hand, slightly but significantly stimulated proliferation of SKMEL-188 cells at the concentration of 100 nM, with both BHM Ma and BHM Ab hamster cells showing an inhibition of proliferation at 10 and 100 nM concentrations.

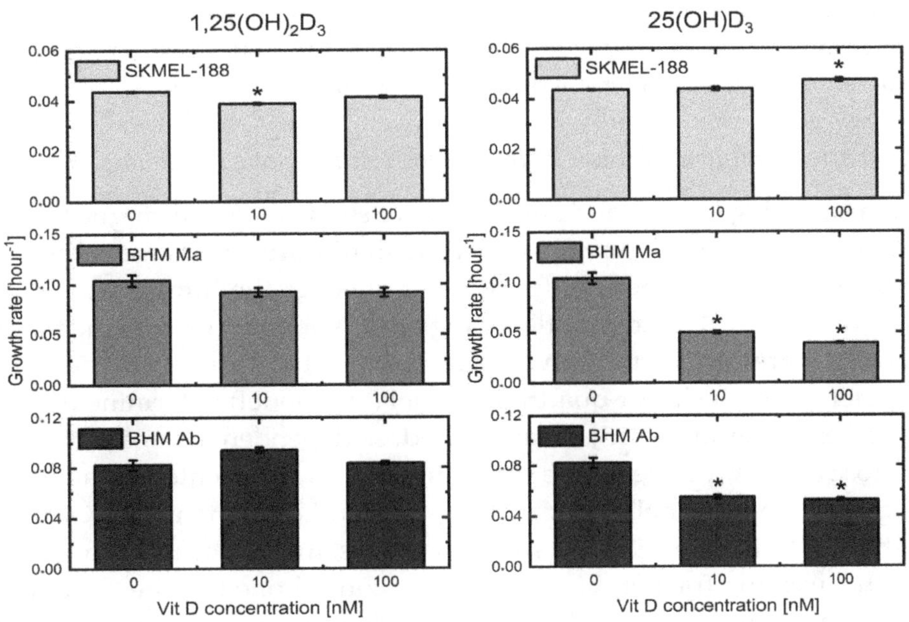

Figure 1. The impact of calcitriol (1,25$(OH)_2D_3$) and calcidiol (25(OH)D_3) on the proliferation of human SKMel-188 and hamster BHM Ma and BHM Ab melanoma cells. Growth rate was calculated from exponential fitting to cell number, counted every 24 h for 4 days in culture. * denotes statistical significance $p < 0.05$ against control (0 nM of vitamin D_3 derivative).

There were also significant differences in basal growth rates between the tested melanoma cell lines. Both hamster lines showed similar proliferation rates (approximately 0.09 h^{-1}), while the human SKMEL-188 cells divided almost two times slower. Such differences may be one of the factors influencing response to the vitamin D_3 metabolites.

2.2. *Proton Beam Radiosensitivity of Melanoma Cells*

Melanoma cell lines are characterized by different radiosensitivity to proton beam therapy (Figure 2), with the highest level of cell killing seen in BHM amelanotic Ab cells. BHM melanotic Ma and SKMEL-188 cells show similar survival curves. Similar differences in response to radiation between BHM Ma and BHM Ab cells were reported for X ray irradiation, where pigmented cells (BHM Ma) were 2.4 times more radio resistant than the unpigmented (BHM Ab) ones [33]. In the case of proton radiation this characteristic is less pronounced but still marked with the ratio of mean lethal dose of 1.56.

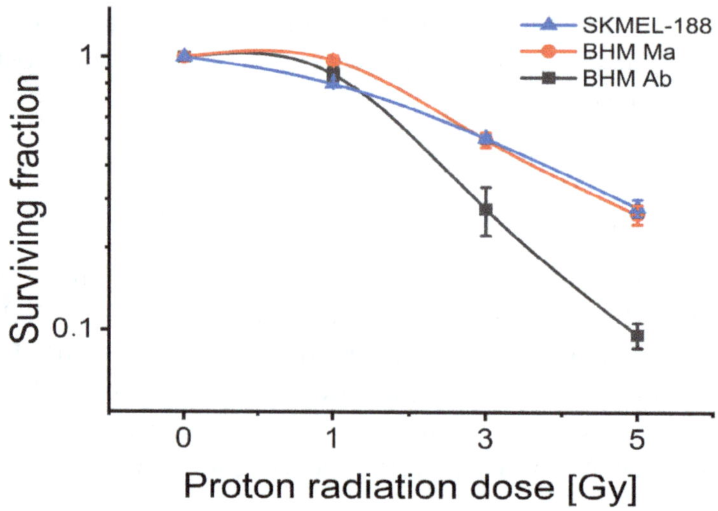

Figure 2. Proton beam radiosensitivity of SKMel-188, BHM Ma and BHM Ab melanoma cells. Surviving fraction was determined from the model described by Buch et al. [34], based on the experimental data from cell number, counted every 24 h for 4 days in culture after irradiation.

2.3. *Vitamin D_3 Derivatives Influence Proton Beam Radiosensitivity of Melanoma Cells*

Changes in both surviving fraction and survival curve shape can be distinguished after pre-treatment with both vitamin D_3 metabolites (Figure 3). The most significant effects are seen for both vitamin D_3 derivatives in hamster melanoma lines, with a weaker effect in the human line. Furthermore, higher doses of 25(OH)D_3 cause in BHM Ma cells a flattening of the survival curve in the region of higher doses (3–5 Gy). Those changes are consistent with the data from fitted survival models. It has been shown that α and β parameters from the linear-quadratic model (LQ model) determine the effectiveness at low and high radiation doses, respectively [35]. Vitamin D_3 dose dependent decrease in surviving fraction for proton irradiation dose of 1 Gy, visible on the survival curve, is represented by an increase in the values of parameter α (Figure 4, upper panel). For calcitriol, no significant change in α was detected at 10 nM dose for SKMEL-188 and BHM Ma cells. On survival curves, that concentration was slightly protective for cancer cells, with surviving fraction higher than the control one but the effect was not statistically significant. The most effective dose was 100 nM. Calcidiol has a clear dose dependent effect on the radiosensitivity of the studied melanoma cell lines, with the highest concentration being the most effective one. An increase in parameter β, indicating higher effectiveness of high doses of radiation, occurs only for calcitriol pre-treatment: 10 nM dose in BHM Ma and BHM Ab cells (Figure 4, lower panel). The same dose leads to a noticeable decrease in surviving fraction on survival curves. The tested doses were within the range of the normal serum level of calcitriol, which is between 50–120 nM.

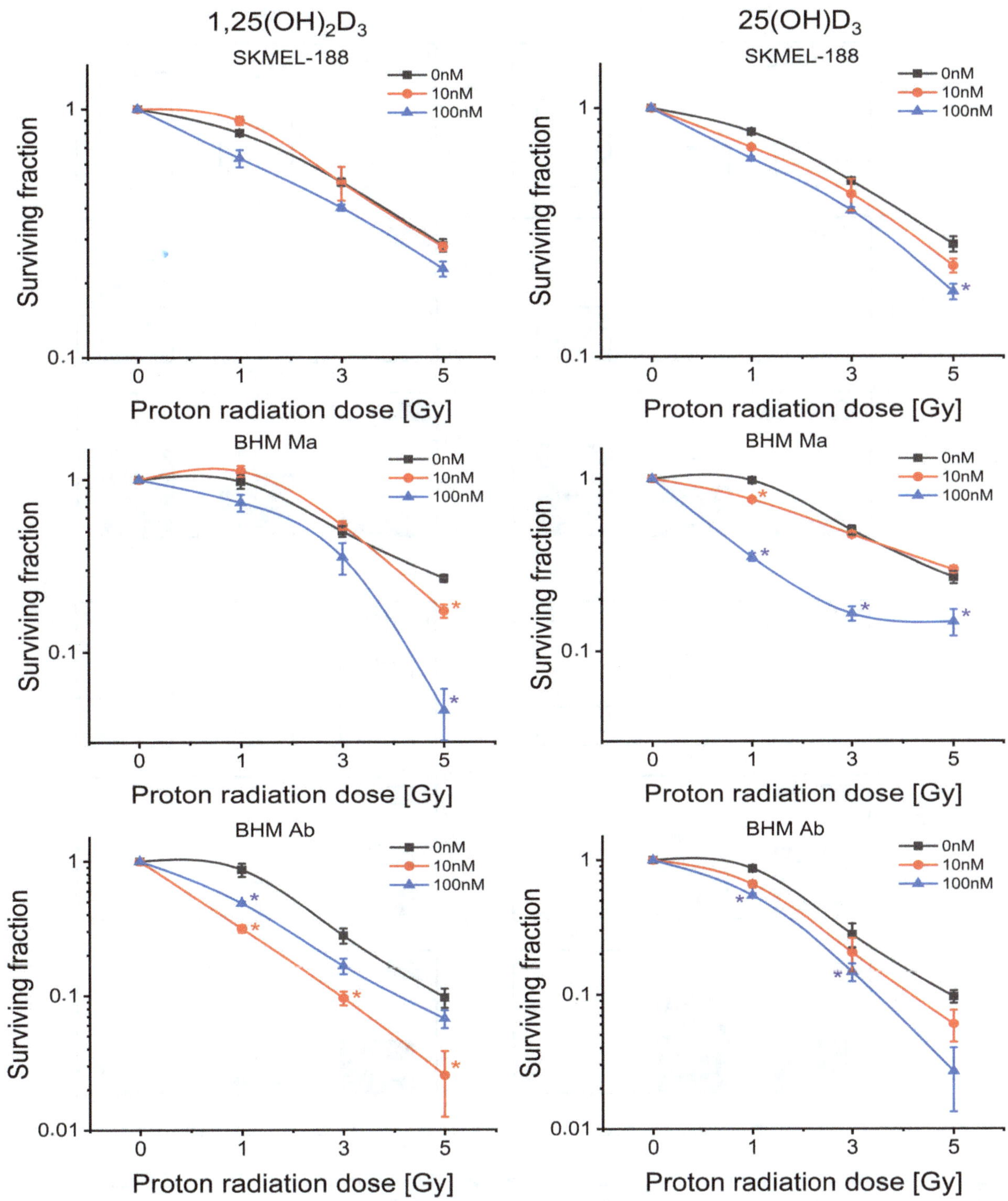

Figure 3. The effect of calcitriol ($1,25(OH)_2D_3$) and calcidiol ($25(OH)D_3$) on the cellular response to proton beam irradiation of human SKMel-188 and hamster BHM Ma and BHM Ab melanoma cells. Surviving fraction was determined from the model described by Buch et al. [34], based on the experimental data from cell number, counted every 24 h for 4 days in culture after irradiation. * denotes statistical significance $p < 0.05$ against irradiated control.

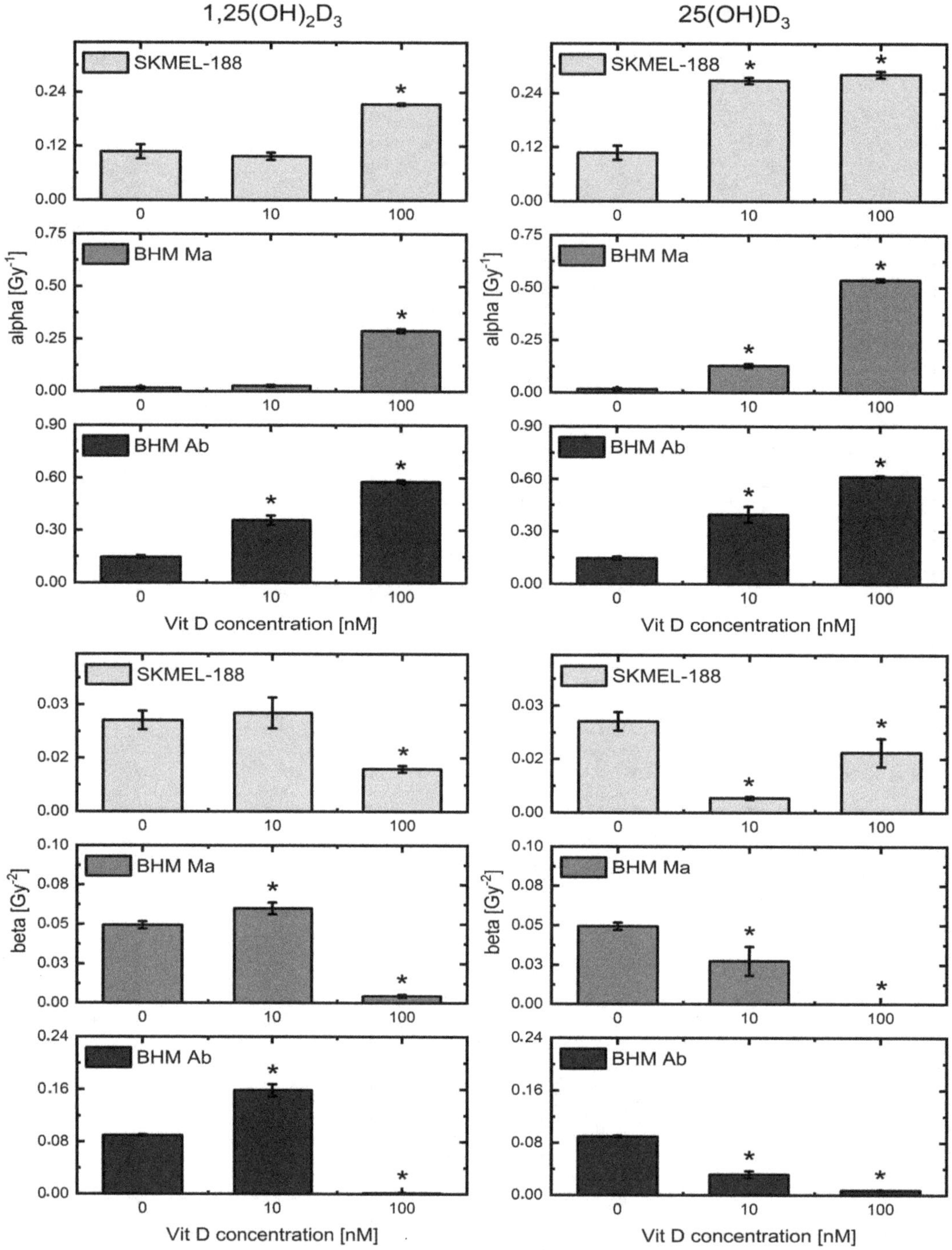

Figure 4. Coefficients α (**upper** panel) and β (**lower** panel) from linear-quadratic model calculated for cells pre-treated with calcitriol ($1{,}25(OH)_2D_3$) and calcidiol ($25(OH)D_3$) and irradiated with proton beam. Surviving fraction was determined from the model described by Buch et al. [34], based on the experimental data from SKMel-188, BHM Ma and BHM Ab cell number, counted every 24 h for 4 days in culture after irradiation. * denotes statistical significance $p < 0.05$ against control (0 nM of vitamin D_3 derivative).

Results from the second model applied to survival data, single hit multi-target, are in agreement with data from the LQ model. Changes in the calculated parameters n and D_0 are shown in Figure 5. Parameter n, indicating the required number of hits for cell death and being sensitive to the effectiveness of low radiation doses, shows an opposite trend to parameter α from the LQ model. An increase in α goes together with a decrease in n, which is consistent with vitamin D_3 metabolites radiosensitizing cells to low doses of proton beam irradiation. The second parameter, mean lethal dose D_0, describes the average effect of radiation, without distinction between low and high doses [36]. Only several groups were characterized by a decrease in that parameter in comparison to the control, representing the process of radiosensitization by the tested vitamin D_3 analogues. Among them, there were groups treated with 100 nM of calcitriol, the most effective treatment in enhancing the efficiency of low radiation doses. This indicates that the highest influence of vitamin D_3 analogues on the averaged effects relates to the response to low doses of proton radiation.

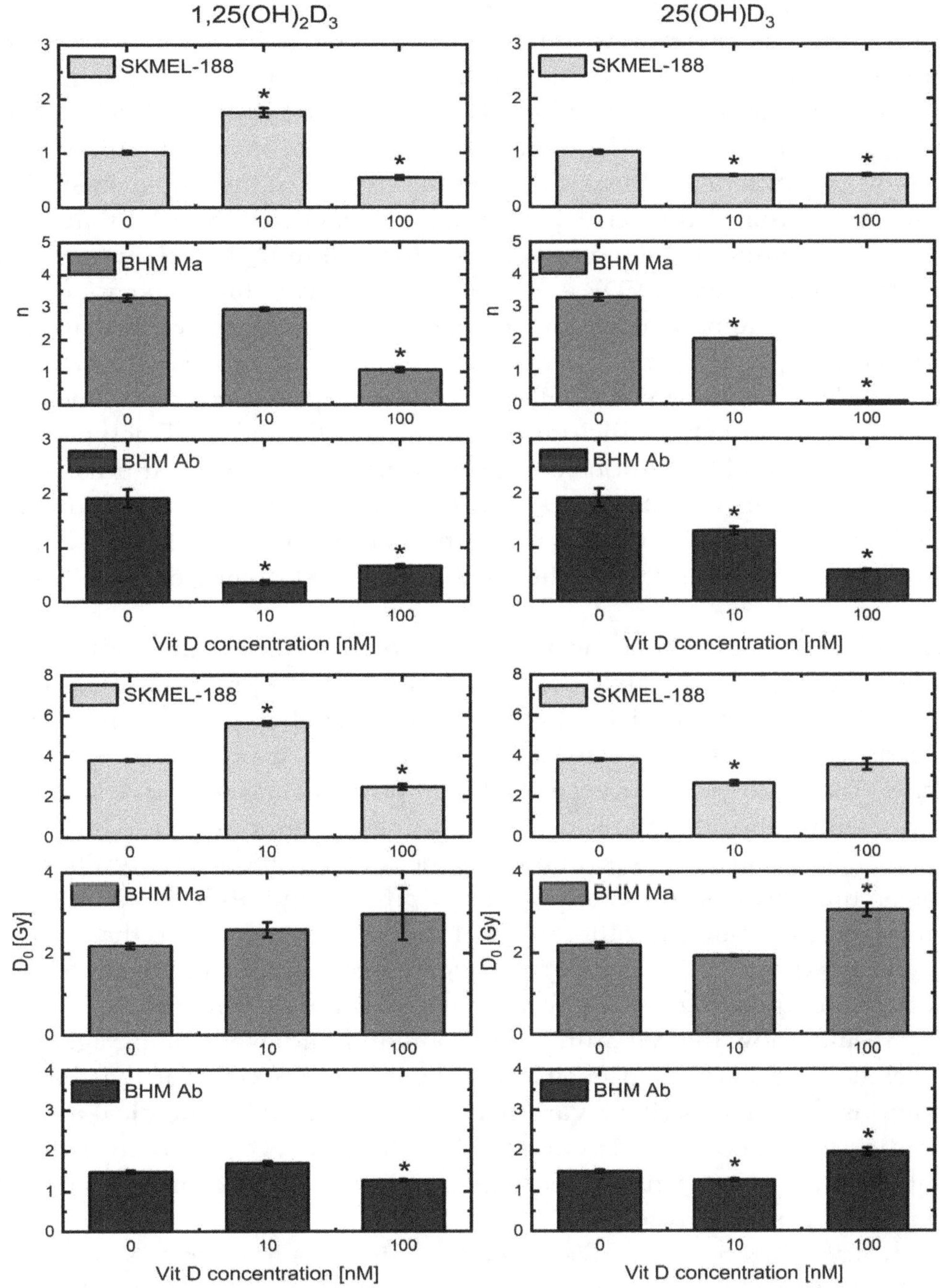

Figure 5. Coefficients n (**upper** panel) and D_0 (**lower** panel) from multi-target single hit model calculated for cells pre-treated with calcitriol ($1,25(OH)_2D_3$) and calcidiol ($25(OH)D_3$) and irradiated with proton beam. Surviving fraction was determined from the model described by Buch et al. [34], based on the experimental data from SKMel-188, BHM Ma and BHM Ab cell number, counted every 24 h for 4 days in culture after irradiation. * denotes statistical significance $p < 0.05$ against control (0 nM of vitamin D_3 derivative).

3. Discussion

Current pre-clinical and clinical reports show that vitamin D_3 has overall anticancer properties [6–8]. The finding is also supported by a strong correlation between higher serum 25(OH)D_3 level and lower incidence of breast [37,38], colon [39], lung [40], prostate [41] and melanoma [10] and by the antiproliferative and pro-differentiative action of vitamin D_3 and its analogues towards multiple cancer cell lines [42–47]. Interestingly, not all cancer cell lines do respond to vitamin D_3 [20,48–51], which also included melanoma lines [41,50] and such responsiveness can depend on the culture conditions [11].

In the present study, we demonstrate differential effects of the biologically active form of vitamin D_3, calcitriol and its precursor calcidiol, on the proliferation rate of three melanoma cell lines: human SKMEL-188 and hamster BHM Ma and BHM Ab (Figure 1). Only SKMEL-188 cells responded to lower doses of 1,25(OH)$_2$$D_3$ with inhibition of growth rate, which was consistent with other reports [22,52]. However, inhibition of proliferation by calcidiol, with no effect in the case of calcitriol in both BHM Ma and BHM Ab cells requires further explanation. It has been proposed that one of the factors influencing the responsiveness of melanoma cell lines to vitamin D_3 is melanin pigmentation [53,54], which would explain the decrease in VDR expression with concomitant decrease in anti-proliferative response to 1,25(OH)$_2$$D_3$ in human melanoma. It is possible that a similar mechanism could underlie the resistance of BHM Ma, which produces melanin pigment also when cultured in a medium with low tyrosine content [55]. However, since BHM Ab cells were pre-selected for amelanotic phenotype by culturing in DMEM, other factors, including a defect in VDR or a high activity of CYP24A1 that inactivates 1,25(OH)$_2$$D_3$ could be responsible for the differential effects. It must also be noted that there are alternative receptors for vitamin D_3 derivatives that could affect responsiveness to active forms of vitamin D_3 (reviewed in [9,10]). Therefore, proper understanding of these differential effects would require additional studies, involving the identification and cloning of hamster nuclear receptors for vitamin D_3.

Vitamin D_3 enhances the of anticancer drugs such as doxorubicin, cisplatin, gemcitabine or cyclophosphamide [56–58] and sensitizes cancer cells to ionizing radiation [12–18]. In this paper, we focus on combining calcitriol or calcidiol with proton beam therapy. That mode of cancer therapy is commonly used for the treatment of tumours located near or on critical organs, because of its dosimetric benefits. Thanks to the occurrence of a Bragg peak, there is no exit dose normally deposited by photon therapy within the healthy tissue surrounding the tumour [59]. Accumulating evidence suggests that even with relative biological effectiveness of 1.1, there are significant differences in biological effects on tumour cells between low-energy protons and photon radiation [60]. As regards the combination of proton beam radiotherapy and vitamin D_3 treatment, the most crucial aspects appear to be the increased production of reactive oxygen species (ROS) and the differences in cell cycle inhibition and apoptotic signalling, all implicated in the response to vitamin D_3.

Overall, our results show that vitamin D_3 is a potential radiosensitizing agent in proton beam irradiation of melanoma cells. Radiosensitization is a complex concept that has many different interpretations and is used to describe a variety of interactions at biochemical and biological level. Alterations in radiosensitization are demonstrated in the SF curve; a downward or leftward shift of the curve implies a radiosensitizing interaction, while an upward or rightward shift implies a radioprotective influence on the treated cells.

Generally, radiosensitization is conventionally defined as an increased amount of radiation-induced cell death resulting from exposure to a second agent, after correction for the cytotoxicity of the agent (in our case vitamin D_3, nontoxic in the tested concentrations). Considering the changes in shape and the above-mentioned shift in SF suggests that both calcitriol and calcidiol are radiosensitizing agents, within the range of the concentrations used. Radiosensitization by vitamin D_3 is particularly visible for low radiation doses, for which we a decrease or elimination of the shoulder on the SF curve is observed (Figure 3). The effect of radiosensitization is also visible at high radiation doses of about 5 Gy. The surviving fraction values of the cells are lower than the analogous values for SF curve obtained for the exposure without vitamin D_3. Some of the observed survival-dose dependencies, in particular for

BHM Ma cells pre-treated with 100 nM of calcidiol, do not resemble the commonly found SF curves with the shoulder in the low dose area and with a linear course for zero for high doses. In this case, we observe a gradual disappearance of the effect the radiation dose has on the number of killed cells. The SF curve gradually flattens (upward-bending) and the number of surviving cells does not decrease with increasing dose. The effect is the reason for the unusual values of some coefficients characterizing survival curves of such non-classical forms of SF, for example, close to zero β values (see Figure 4). The phenomenon (upward-bending of SF) has already been observed during the He-3 irradiation of the V79 cells but the authors interpreted it as an artefact [61]. More recent theoretical studies linked that effect mainly with the repair processes in irradiated cells [62,63]. Nevertheless, the theory is formal and does not explain the upward-bending effect of SF curves with the help of probable molecular mechanisms involved in the repair of irradiated cells. In our work, the upward-bending effect was only observed in the presence of vitamin D_3 derivatives. Therefore, it might be due to the radioprotective properties of vitamin D_3. Probable targets of such interaction include ATM and mTor, which are directly related to the process of DNA repair and cell proliferation [64–66]. Thus, the radiosensitization effect of high vitamin D_3 doses would be classified as radiosensitization by targeting the response to DNA damage.

In conclusion, our data suggest that active forms of vitamin D may improve the effectiveness of proton therapy. They also support further in vivo studies on use of vitamin D as adjuvant during radiotherapy of melanoma.

4. Materials and Methods

4.1. Cell Lines

Human SKMEL-188 melanoma cell line, a gift from Dr Chakraborty, Yale University, was established from a human metastatic melanoma and then maintained in our laboratories as a continuous cell line [67,68].

BHM Ma, Bomirski Hamster Melanoma—pigmented subline, is a stable transplantable tumour cell line that was derived by Dr Andrzej Bomirski in Gdansk, Poland, from a spontaneous hamster melanoma in 1959 [69].

BHM Ab, Bomirski Hamster Melanoma—non-pigmented subline, arose in 1963 by spontaneous alteration of a black tumour (BHM Ma). The amelanotic subline of Bomirski Hamster Melanoma results in non-pigmented tumours in hamsters. The tumours are malignant, dedifferentiated, fast-growing and metastasizing [69]. The cells isolated from those tumours by means of a non-enzymatic method undergo rapid pigmentation in primary cultures in media containing high concentrations of L-tyrosine [70,71]. The level of pigmentation depends on the culture medium; in DMEM with 10% of foetal bovine serum (FBS) the cells are pigmented, while in media low in L-tyrosine, such as Ham's F10, they are amelanotic [72]. However, culturing for prolonged period in DMEM leads to the selection for an amelanotic phenotype that is stable in cell culture [73]. This type of preselected cells was used in the experiments.

4.2. Cell Culture

For each cell line, a different culture medium was used: for BHM Ma—RPMI, for BHM Ab—DMEM and for SKMEL-188 Ham's F10 medium supplemented with glucose, L-glutamine and pyridoxine hydrochloride. The cells were cultured in 75 cm^2 flasks in culture medium supplemented with 10% of FBS (Gibco—Thermofisher Scientific, Waltham, MA, USA) and antibiotics (Sigma, St. Luis, MO, USA) and grown until 70% confluent. The calcitriol or calcidiol (Sigma, St. Louis, MO, USA) was dissolved in 100% ethanol to obtain 100 μM stocks. After that stocks were diluted in media to obtain 10 and 100 nM. Concentration of ethanol in media never exceeded 1%. The cells were incubated with vitamin D compounds for 24 h before irradiation. To study the influence of calcitriol or calcidiol on cell proliferation, cell growth curves were determined by manual counting the cells growing with vitamin D_3 metabolites at different concentrations every 24 h up to 120 h. Counts were performed with the use of haemocytometer, by triplicate by one analyst under a 40× objective according to the standard methodology. Influence on cell response to proton radiation was tested by cultivating cells for 24 h prior to irradiation in a culture medium with 10% FBS, antibiotics and vitamin D_3 metabolites as indicated.

4.3. Irradiation Procedure

The irradiation was performed at the Institute of Nuclear Physics of the Polish Academy of Sciences (IFJ PAN) in Krakow uses he Proteus C-235 cyclotron produced proton beam. The 230 MeV proton beam, after degradation to 70 MeV, was delivered to the treatment room with a small field horizontal beam line. The passive scattering technique and rotating energy modulator were used to forming the irradiation field. A 40 mm diameter, fully modulated proton beam with energy of 61 MeV, spread-out Bragg Peak (SOBP) with 31.5 mm range and 31.5 mm modulation (measured in water), was used for cell irradiation. Dose of 1, 3, or 5 Gy at dose rates of 1 Gy/min, 2 Gy/min and 6.6 Gy/min respectively, were delivered to the samples. The dose averaged LET_d calculated at the depth of 15.8 mm in the SOBP that is, at the centre of the cell container position, was 2.8 keV/µm. The dosimetry was performed according to the recommendations of IAEA TRS-398 protocol [74]. A semiflex ionisation chamber with 0.125 cm^3 active volume and a PTW reference class UNIDOS Webline electrometer calibrated at the IFJ PAN with ^{60}Co radiation source were used. A dedicated PMMA phantom with a holder for the Eppendorf container was used during irradiation. Cells were irradiated in Eppendorf tubes positioned in the phantom, orthogonally to the direction of the proton beam. Cell suspension in phosphate buffer saline (PBS) at 1 × 106 cells/mL was transported on ice between the facilities, including the untreated (non-irradiated) control. Cells were transferred to the culture medium and placed at 1 × 105 cell/mL in 24-well plates. Every 24 h, for 5 days, cells from 6 wells were removed and counted. The experiment was repeated 3 times for each cell line tested.

4.4. Data Analysis

Data from cell counting was used to determine cell growth rates, doubling times and surviving fractions. Since the cells in most of the experimental groups exhibited logistic growth, the first step was to establish the duration of exponential growth phase (96 h). Then, growth rates (gr):

$$N_t = N_0 e^{gr \cdot t} \tag{1}$$

and doubling times ($t_{doubling\ time}$):

$$t_{doubling\ time} = \frac{\ln(2)}{gr} \tag{2}$$

where calculated by exponential function fitting, using the nonlinear least squares method. Additionally, time delay for irradiated groups was calculated as previously described [34]. Those values were used to calculate surviving fractions:

$$SF = 2^{-\frac{t_{delay}}{t_{doubling\ time}}} \tag{3}$$

Establishing the relationship between the physical conditions of irradiation and its biological effects is a starting point for any radiobiological experiment. Such relations are known as survival curves and presented as the dependence of cell survival probability (Surviving Fractions—SF) on the absorbed radiation dose (in Gy). Many theoretical models of ionizing radiation–induced cell killing have been proposed and described in literature but because the fundamental mechanisms leading to lethal cell damage are not well understood, the models have semi-empirical character and many limitations [36]. Our experimental survival curves were analysed within framework of two classical models describing the response of cells populations to ionizing radiation (IR). The models have a few basic assumptions in common: cell inactivation is treated as a multistep process, cells are killed by energy absorption deposited in a sensitive volume of the cell and radiation-induced lethal events have Poisson distribution. The first one is a "molecular model," widely known as the linear-quadratic model (LQ):

$$SF(D) = e^{-(\alpha D+\beta D^2)} \tag{4}$$

describing the logarithmic plot of SF in linear and quadratic dose–dependent terms, where D is the absorbed dose. The experimentally determined parameters α and β are interpreted as rates of cell annihilation by a single-hit and double-hit mechanism, respectively. Molecular interpretation of LQ model is based on the following assumptions: DNA is a critical target, radiation produces the breakage in DNA strands, the broken bonds in DNA strand can be repaired and the critical damage leading to cell death is a double strand break (DSB), resulting in non-repairable lesions. The linear part (α) represents a lethal lesion produced by a direct induction of DSB (one track hit) and the quadratic term (β) is a result of two single strand breaks (SSB) which could be repaired (a sub-lethal lesion).

The second model used for analysis of our survival curves is a multitarget–single hit (MTSH) model:

$$SF(D) = 1 - (1 - e^{-\frac{D}{D_0}})^n \tag{5}$$

$D_0 = 1/k$ is the dose for $1/e$ survival in the linear portion of the plot, where k—inactivation constant for each target (or mean lethal dose), n—target multiplicity, number of targets per cell that must be inactivated for cell death.

Radiation survival curves are presented as log-linear plots of surviving fraction and dose, respectively; surviving fraction is plotted along the vertical axis (normalized to unity when $D = 0$), radiation dose is plotted along the horizontal axis.

Both models were fitted to the dose dependence of survival fraction, using the nonlinear least squares method. All analyses were carried out with in-house written Matlab (2014b, MathWorks, Natick, MA, USA) scripts. Optimization of the fitting procedures (both for growth and survival curves) was conducted until mean R-squared from all curves was higher than 0.9. Besides parameters values, their standard errors were calculated and used for the calculation of weighted mean and its error within experimental groups.

4.5. Statistical Analysis

Results were presented as weighted mean and weighted mean error. All analyses were performed with STATISTICA 13 software (Stat-Soft Inc., Tulsa, OK, USA), with the use of weights computed during the fitting procedure. For each parameter, Shapiro-Wilk normality test and Levene's test were used to determine a normal distribution and equality of variances, respectively. Depending on the data, a one-way ANOVA, followed by post-hoc Tukey's HSD test or Kruskal–Wallis H test, followed by Dunn's test was performed. p values smaller than 0.05 were considered statistically significant.

5. Conclusions

We conclude that the effect of vitamin D_3 metabolites on the proliferation and response to proton radiation in the studied melanoma cell lines is not straightforward. As regards cell proliferation, the impact of melanin content and other factors such as VDR, CYP27A1, CYP27B1 and CYP24A1 gene expressions as well as VDR localization and interaction with other receptors should be considered in the differential responses of cells to calcitriol and calcidiol. The studied vitamin D_3 derivatives have proven to be potent radiosensitizers in proton therapy. Radiosensitization by vitamin D_3 was particularly visible for low radiation doses. Interestingly, for higher doses the observed upward-bending of SF curves in the presence of vitamin D_3 implies involvement of repair mechanisms and interaction between VDR and radiation-induced signalling pathways. Our results indicate the need for a further investigation of the underlying molecular mechanisms and suggest that vitamin D_3 can be a promising agent, capable of modifying proton beam therapy efficacy and thus offering a new option in cancer therapy.

Author Contributions: E.P. and A.D. performed the experiments and analysed the results, Z.M. tested different models for data fitting, J.S. performed proton beam dosimetry and cell irradiation, A.S. contributed towards discussion of the results and revised the manuscript, M.E. edited and revised the text, K.U. was responsible for the concept of the paper.

Abbreviations

ATM	Ataxia-telangiectasia mutated kinase
BHM	Bomirski hamster melanoma
CSDA	Continues slowing down approximation
DSB	Double strand break
IR	Ionizing radiation
LQ	Linear-quadratic
mTor	Mammalian target of rapamycin
MTSH	Multitarget—single hit
SF	Surviving fraction
SOBP	Spread-out bragg peak
SSB	Single strand break
VDR	Vitamin D receptor

References

1. Matthews, N.H.; Li, W.-Q.; Qureshi, A.A.; Weinstock, M.A.; Cho, E. Epidemiology of Melanoma. In *Cutaneous Melanoma: Etiology and Therapy*; Codon Publications: Brisbane, Australia, 2017.
2. Slominski, A.T.; Carlson, J.A. Melanoma resistance: A bright future for academicians and a challenge for patient advocates. *Mayo Clin. Proc.* **2014**, *89*, 429–433. [CrossRef] [PubMed]
3. Rajkumar, S.; Watson, I.R. Molecular characterisation of cutaneous melanoma: Creating a framework for targeted and immune therapies. *Br. J. Cancer* **2016**, *115*, 145–155. [CrossRef] [PubMed]
4. Su, M.Y.; Fisher, D.E. Immunotherapy in the Precision Medicine Era: Melanoma and Beyond. *PLoS Med.* **2016**, *13*, e1002196. [CrossRef] [PubMed]
5. Levesque, M.P.; Cheng, P.F.; Raaijmakers, M.I.G.; Saltari, A.; Dummer, R. Metastatic melanoma moves on: Translational science in the era of personalized medicine. *Cancer Metastasis Rev.* **2017**, *36*, 7–21. [CrossRef] [PubMed]
6. Ordonez-Moran, P.; Larriba, M.J.; Pendas-Franco, N.; Aguilera, O.; Gonzalez-Sancho, J.M.; Munoz, A. Vitamin D and cancer: An update of in vitro and in vivo data. *Front. Biosci.* **2005**, *10*, 2723–2749. [CrossRef] [PubMed]
7. Feldman, D.; Krishnan, A.V.; Swami, S.; Giovannucci, E.; Feldman, B.J. The role of vitamin D in reducing cancer risk and progression. *Nat. Rev. Cancer* **2014**, *14*, 342–357. [CrossRef] [PubMed]
8. Grant, W.B. Roles of Solar UVB and Vitamin D in Reducing Cancer Risk and Increasing Survival. *Anticancer Res.* **2016**, *36*, 1357–1370. [PubMed]
9. Slominski, A.T.; Brozyna, A.A.; Zmijewski, M.A.; Józwicki, W.; Jetten, A.M.; Mason, R.S.; Tuckey, R.C.; Elmets, C.A. Vitamin D signalling and melanoma: Role of Vitamin D and its receptors in melanoma progression and management. *Lab. Investig.* **2017**, *97*, 706–724. [CrossRef] [PubMed]
10. Slominski, A.T.; Brożyna, A.A.; Skobowiat, C.; Zmijewski, M.A.; Kim, T.K.; Janjetovic, Z.; Oak, A.S.; Jozwicki, W.; Jetten, A.M.; Mason, R.S.; et al. On the role of classical and novel forms of vitamin D in melanoma progression and management. *J. Steroid Biochem. Mol. Biol.* **2018**, *177*, 159–170. [CrossRef] [PubMed]

11. Wasiewicz, T.; Szyszka, P.; Cichorek, M.; Janjetovic, Z.; Tuckey, R.C.; Slominski, A.T.; Zmijewski, M.A. Antitumor effects of vitamin D analogues on hamster and mouse melanoma cell lines in relation to melanin pigmentation. *Int. J. Mol. Sci.* **2015**, *16*, 6645–6667. [CrossRef] [PubMed]
12. Polar, M.K.; Gennings, C.; Park, M.; Gupta, M.S.; Gewirtz, D.A. Effect of the vitamin D_3 analog ILX 23-7553 on apoptosis and sensitivity to fractionated radiation in breast tumour cells and normal human fibroblasts. *Cancer Chemother. Pharmacol.* **2003**, *51*, 415–421. [CrossRef] [PubMed]
13. Sundaram, S.; Sea, A.; Feldman, S.; Strawbridge, R.; Hoopes, P.J.; Demidenko, E.; Binderup, L.; Gewirtz, D.A. The combination of a potent vitamin D_3 analog, EB 1089, with ionizing radiation reduces tumour growth and induces apoptosis of MCF-7 breast tumour xenografts in nude mice. *Clin. Cancer Res.* **2003**, *9*, 2350–2356. [PubMed]
14. Wang, Z.; Liu, J.; Si, S.; Xu, B.; Wang, Y.; Ren, Y.; Dai, Z.; Cui, D.; Su, X.; Song, S. Vitamin D improves the sensitization of lung cancer to radiotherapy. *Int. J. Clin. Exp. Med.* **2017**, *10*, 4921–4928.
15. Sundaram, S.; Gewirtz, D.A. The vitamin D_3 analog EB 1089 enhances the response of human breast tumor cells to radiation. *Radiat. Res.* **1999**, *152*, 479–486. [CrossRef] [PubMed]
16. Chaudhary, M.; Sundaram, S.; Gennings, C.; Carter, H.; Gewirtz, D.A. The vitamin D_3 analog, ILX-23-7553, enhances the response to Adriamycin and irradiation in MCF-7 breast tumor cells. *Cancer Chemother. Pharmacol.* **2001**, *47*, 429–436. [CrossRef]
17. Weitsman, G.E.; Koren, R.; Zuck, E.; Rotem, C.; Liberman, U.A.; Ravid, A. Vitamin D sensitizes breast cancer cells to the action of H_2O_2: Mitochondria as a convergence point in the death pathway. *Free Radic. Biol. Med.* **2005**, *39*, 266–278. [CrossRef] [PubMed]
18. Dunlap, N.; Schwartz, G.G.; Eads, D.; Cramer, S.D.; Sherk, A.B.; John, V.; Koumenis, C. 1α,25-Dihydroxyvitamin D_3 (calcitriol) and its analogue, 19-nor-1α,25$(OH)_2D_2$, potentiate the effects of ionising radiation on human prostate cancer cells. *Br. J. Cancer* **2003**, *89*, 746–753. [CrossRef] [PubMed]
19. Slominski, A.T.; Brozyna, A.; Jozwicki, W.; Tuckey, R.C. Vitamin D as an adjuvant in melanoma therapy. *Melanoma Manag.* **2015**, *2*, 1–4. [CrossRef] [PubMed]
20. Wu, W.; Beilhartz, G.; Roy, Y.; Richard, C.L.; Curtin, M.; Brown, L.; Cadieux, D.; Coppolino, M.; Farach-Carson, M.C.; Nemere, I.; et al. Nuclear translocation of the 1,25D_3-MARRS (membrane associated rapid response to steroids) receptor protein and NFκB in differentiating NB4 leukemia cells. *Exp. Cell Res.* **2010**, *316*, 1101–1108. [CrossRef] [PubMed]
21. Tan, C.; De Noronha, R.G.; Roecker, A.J.; Pyrzynska, B.; Khwaja, F.; Zhang, Z.; Zhang, H.; Teng, Q.; Nicholson, A.C.; Giannakakou, P.; et al. Identification of a novel small-molecule inhibitor of the hypoxia-inducible factor 1 pathway. *Cancer Res.* **2005**, *65*, 605–612. [CrossRef] [PubMed]
22. Skobowiat, C.; Oak, A.S.W.; Kim, T.-K.; Yang, C.H.; Pfeffer, L.M.; Tuckey, R.C.; Slominski, A.T. Noncalcemic 20-hydroxyvitamin D_3 inhibits human melanoma growth in in vitro and in vivo models. *Oncotarget* **2016**, *8*, 9823–9834. [CrossRef] [PubMed]
23. Brozyna, A.A.; Jozwicki, W.; Janjetovic, Z.; Slominski, A.T. Expression of vitamin D receptor decreases during progression of pigmented skin lesions. *Hum. Pathol.* **2011**, *42*, 618–631. [CrossRef] [PubMed]
24. Brozyna, A.A.; Jóźwicki, W.; Janjetovic, Z.; Slominski, A.T. Expression of the vitamin D-activating enzyme 1α-hydroxylase (CYP27B1) decreases during melanoma progression. *Hum. Pathol.* **2013**, *44*, 374–387. [CrossRef] [PubMed]
25. Brozyna, A.A.; Jóźwicki, W.; Slominski, A.T. Decreased VDR expression in cutaneous melanomas as marker of tumor progression: New data and analyses. *Anticancer Res.* **2014**, *34*, 2735–2744. [PubMed]
26. Brożyna, A.A.; Jochymski, C.; Janjetovic, Z.; Jóźwicki, W.; Tuckey, R.C.; Slominski, A.T. CYP24A1 expression inversely correlates with melanoma progression: Clinic-pathological studies. *Int. J. Mol. Sci.* **2014**, *15*, 19000–19017. [CrossRef] [PubMed]
27. Chagani, S.; Kyryachenko, S.; Yamamoto, Y.; Kato, S.; Ganguli-Indra, G.; Indra, A.K. In vivo Role of Vitamin D Receptor Signaling in UVB-Induced DNA Damage and Melanocyte Homeostasis. *J. Investig. Dermatol.* **2016**, *136*, 2108–2111. [CrossRef] [PubMed]
28. Girdhani, S.; Sachs, R.; Hlatky, L. Biological Effects of Proton Radiation: What We Know and Don't Know. *Radiat. Res.* **2013**, *179*, 257–272. [CrossRef] [PubMed]
29. Gerelchuluun, A.; Hong, Z.; Sun, L.; Suzuki, K.; Terunuma, T.; Yasuoka, K.; Sakae, T.; Moritake, T.; Tsuboi, K. Induction of in situ DNA double-strand breaks and apoptosis by 200 MeV protons and 10 MV X-rays in human tumour cell lines. *Int. J. Radiat. Biol.* **2011**, *87*, 57–70. [CrossRef] [PubMed]

30. Jasińska-Konior, K.; Pochylczuk, K.; Czajka, E.; Michalik, M.; Romanowska-Dixon, B.B.; Swakoń, J.; Urbańska, K.; Elas, M.; Jasinska-Konior, K.; Pochylczuk, K.; et al. Proton beam irradiation inhibits the migration of melanoma cells. *PLoS ONE* **2017**, *12*, e0186002. [CrossRef] [PubMed]
31. Grosse, N.; Fontana, A.O.; Hug, E.B.; Lomax, A.; Coray, A.; Augsburger, M.; Paganetti, H.; Sartori, A.A.; Pruschy, M. Deficiency in homologous recombination renders mammalian cells more sensitive to proton versus photon irradiation. *Int. J. Radiat. Oncol. Biol. Phys.* **2014**, *88*, 175–181. [CrossRef] [PubMed]
32. Antoccia, A.; Sgura, A.; Berardinelli, F.; Cavinato, M.; Cherubini, R.; Gerardi, S.; Tanzarella, C. Cell Cycle Perturbations and Genotoxic Effects in Human Primary Fibroblasts Induced by Low-energy Protons and X/γ-rays. *J. Radiat. Res.* **2009**, *50*, 457–468. [CrossRef] [PubMed]
33. Śniegocka, M.; Podgórska, E.; Plonka, P.M.; Elas, M.; Romanowska-Dixon, B.; Szczygiel, M.; Żmijewski, M.A.; Cichorek, M.; Markiewicz, A.; Brożyna, A.A.; et al. Transplantable melanomas in hamsters and gerbils as models for human melanoma. Sensitization in melanoma radiotherapy—From animal models to clinical trials. *Int. J. Mol. Sci.* **2018**, *19*, 1048. [CrossRef] [PubMed]
34. Buch, K.; Peters, T.; Nawroth, T.; Sänger, M.; Schmidberger, H.; Langguth, P. Determination of cell survival after irradiation via clonogenic assay versus multiple MTT Assay—A comparative study. *Radiat. Oncol.* **2012**, *7*, 1. [CrossRef] [PubMed]
35. Franken, N.A.P.; Oei, A.L.; Kok, H.P.; Rodermond, H.M.; Sminia, P.; Crezee, J.; Stalpers, L.J.A.; Barendsen, G.W. Cell survival and radiosensitisation: Modulation of the linear and quadratic parameters of the LQ model (Review). *Int. J. Oncol.* **2013**, *42*, 1501–1515. [CrossRef] [PubMed]
36. Bodgi, L.; Canet, A.; Pujo-Menjouet, L.; Lesne, A.; Victor, J.-M.; Foray, N. Mathematical models of radiation action on living cells: From the target theory to the modern approaches. A historical and critical review. *J. Theor. Biol.* **2016**, *394*, 93–101. [CrossRef] [PubMed]
37. Mehta, R.G.; Hussain, E.A.; Mehta, R.R.; Das Gupta, T.K. Chemoprevention of mammary carcinogenesis by 1α-hydroxyvitamin D5, a synthetic analog of Vitamin D. *Mutat. Res.* **2003**, *523–524*, 253–264. [CrossRef]
38. Welsh, J.; Wietzke, J.A.; Zinser, G.M.; Byrne, B.; Smith, K.; Narvaez, C.J. Vitamin D-3 Receptor as a Target for Breast Cancer Prevention. *J. Nutr.* **2003**, *133*, 2425S–2433S. [CrossRef] [PubMed]
39. Lamprecht, S.A.; Lipkin, M. Chemoprevention of colon cancer by calcium, vitamin D and folate: Molecular mechanisms. *Nat. Rev. Cancer* **2003**, *3*, 601–614. [CrossRef] [PubMed]
40. Nakagawa, K. 1,25-Dihydroxyvitamin D_3 is a preventive factor in the metastasis of lung cancer. *Carcinogenesis* **2004**, *26*, 429–440. [CrossRef] [PubMed]
41. Krishnan, A.V.; Medicine, S.; Feldman, D. Vitamin D Analogs in Cancer Prevention and Therapy. **2003**, *164*. [CrossRef]
42. Szyszka, P.; Zmijewski, M.A.; Slominski, A.T. New vitamin D analogs as potential therapeutics in melanoma. *Expert Rev. Anticancer Ther.* **2012**, *12*, 585–599. [CrossRef] [PubMed]
43. Moreno, J.; Krishnan, A.V.; Feldman, D. Molecular mechanisms mediating the anti-proliferative effects of Vitamin D in prostate cancer. *J. Steroid Biochem. Mol. Biol.* **2005**, *97*, 31–36. [CrossRef] [PubMed]
44. Banerjee, P.; Chatterjee, M. Antiproliferative role of vitamin D and its analogs—A brief overview. *Mol. Cell. Biochem.* **2003**, *253*, 247–254. [CrossRef] [PubMed]
45. Thill, M.; Woeste, A.; Reichert, K.; Fischer, D.; Rody, A.; Friedrich, M.; Köster, F. Vitamin D inhibits ovarian cancer cell line proliferation in combination with celecoxib and suppresses cyclooxygenase-2 expression. *Anticancer Res.* **2015**, *35*, 1197–1203. [PubMed]
46. Chen, J.; Wang, J.; Kim, T.K.; Tieu, E.W.; Tang, E.K.Y.; Lin, Z.; Kovacic, D.; Miller, D.D.; Postlethwaite, A.; Tuckey, R.C.; et al. Novel vitamin D analogs as potential therapeutics: Metabolism, toxicity profiling and antiproliferative activity. *Anticancer Res.* **2014**, *34*, 2153–2164. [PubMed]
47. Kozielewicz, P.; Grafton, G.; Kutner, A.; Curnow, S.J.; Gordon, J.; Barnes, N.M. Novel vitamin D analogues; cytotoxic and anti-proliferative activity against a diffuse large B-cell lymphoma cell line and B-cells from healthy donors. *J. Steroid Biochem. Mol. Biol.* **2016**, *164*, 98–105. [CrossRef] [PubMed]
48. Humeniuk-Polaczek, R.; Marcinkowska, E. Impaired nuclear localization of vitamin D receptor in leukemia cells resistant to calcitriol-induced differentiation. *J. Steroid Biochem. Mol. Biol.* **2004**, *88*, 361–366. [CrossRef] [PubMed]
49. Agadir, A.; Lazzaro, G.; Zheng, Y.; Zhang, X.-K.; Mehta, R. Resistance of HBL100 human breast epithelial cells to vitamin D action. *Carcinogenesis* **1999**, *20*, 577–582. [CrossRef] [PubMed]

50. Seifert, M.; Rech, M.; Meineke, V.; Tilgen, W.; Reichrath, J. Differential biological effects of 1,25-dihydroxyVitamin D_3 on melanoma cell lines in vitro. *J. Steroid Biochem. Mol. Biol.* **2004**, *89–90*, 375–379. [CrossRef] [PubMed]
51. Reichrath, J.; Rech, M.; Moeini, M.; Meese, E.; Tilgen, W.; Seifert, M. In vitro comparison of the vitamin D endocrine system in $1,25(OH)_2D_3$-responsive and -resistant melanoma cells. *Cancer Biol. Ther.* **2007**, *6*, 48–55. [CrossRef] [PubMed]
52. Slominski, A.T.; Janjetovic, Z.; Kim, T.K.; Wright, A.C.; Grese, L.N.; Riney, S.J.; Nguyen, M.N.; Tuckey, R.C. Novel vitamin D hydroxyderivatives inhibit melanoma growth and show differential effects on normal melanocytes. *Anticancer Res.* **2012**, *32*, 3733–3742. [PubMed]
53. Sun, J.; Yin, M.; Zhu, S.; Liu, L.; Zhu, Y.; Wang, Z.; Xu, R.X.; Chang, S. Ultrasound-mediated destruction of oxygen and paclitaxel loaded lipid microbubbles for combination therapy in hypoxic ovarian cancer cells. *Ultrason. Sonochem.* **2016**, *28*, 319–326. [CrossRef] [PubMed]
54. Janjetovic, Z.; Brozyna, A.A.; Tuckey, R.C.; Kim, T.K.; Nguyen, M.N.; Jozwicki, W.; Pfeffer, S.R.; Pfeffer, L.M.; Slominski, A.T. High basal NF-κB activity in nonpigmented melanoma cells is associated with an enhanced sensitivity to vitamin D_3 derivatives. *Br. J. Cancer* **2011**, *105*, 1874–1884. [CrossRef] [PubMed]
55. Sarna, M.; Zadlo, A.; Czuba-Pelech, B.; Urbanska, K. Nanomechanical phenotype of melanoma cells depends solely on the amount of endogenous pigment in the cells. *Int. J. Mol. Sci.* **2018**, *19*, 607. [CrossRef] [PubMed]
56. Wietrzyk, J.; Nevozhay, D.; Filip, B.; Milczarek, M.; Kutner, A. The antitumor effect of lowered doses of cytostatics combined with new analogs of vitamin D in mice. *Anticancer Res.* **2007**, *27*, 3387–3398. [PubMed]
57. Pelczynska, M.; Switalska, M.; Maciejewska, M.; Jaroszewicz, I.; Kutner, A.; Opolski, A. Antiproliferative activity of vitamin D compounds in combination with cytostatics. *Anticancer Res.* **2006**, *26*, 2701–2705. [PubMed]
58. Ma, Y.; Yu, W.D.; Trump, D.L.; Johnson, C.S. $1,25D_3$ enhances antitumor activity of gemcitabine and cisplatin in human bladder cancer models. *Cancer* **2010**, *116*, 3294–3303. [CrossRef] [PubMed]
59. Newhauser, W.D.; Zhang, R. The physics of proton therapy. *Phys. Med. Biol.* **2015**, *60*, R155–R209. [CrossRef] [PubMed]
60. Fokas, E.; Kraft, G.; An, H.; Engenhart-Cabillic, R. Ion beam radiobiology and cancer: Time to update ourselves. *Biochim. Biophys. Acta Rev. Cancer* **2009**, *1796*, 216–229. [CrossRef] [PubMed]
61. Folkard, M.; Prise, K.M.; Vojnovic, B.; Newman, H.C.; Roper, M.J.; Michael, B.D. Inactivation of V79 cells by low-energy protons, deuterons and helium-3 ions. *Int. J. Radiat. Biol.* **1996**, *69*, 729–738. [CrossRef] [PubMed]
62. Kundrät, P. Detailed analysis of the cell-inactivation mechanism by accelerated protons and light ions. *Phys. Med. Biol.* **2006**, *51*, 1185–1199. [CrossRef] [PubMed]
63. Kundrát, P.; Lokajíček, M.; Hromčíková, H. Probabilistic two-stage model of cell inactivation by ionizing particles. *Phys. Med. Biol.* **2005**, *50*, 1433–1447. [CrossRef] [PubMed]
64. Trémezaygues, L.; Seifert, M.; Vogt, T.; Tilgen, W.; Reichrath, J. 1,25-Dihydroxyvitamin D_3 modulates effects of ionizing radiation (IR) on human keratinocytes: In vitro analysis of cell viability/proliferation, DNA-damage and -repair. *J. Steroid Biochem. Mol. Biol.* **2010**, *121*, 324–327. [CrossRef] [PubMed]
65. Murray, P.J.; Cornelissen, B.; Vallis, K.A.; Chapman, S.J. DNA double-strand break repair: A theoretical framework and its application. *J. R. Soc. Interface* **2016**, *13*, 20150679. [CrossRef] [PubMed]
66. Murray, D.; Mirzayans, R.; Parliament, M. New insights into patient radiosensitivity in relation to the biology of the ATM protein. *Transl. Cancer Res.* **2016**, *5*, S809–S814. [CrossRef]
67. Janczyk, A.; Wolnicka-Glubisz, A.; Chmura, A.; Elas, M.; Matuszak, Z.; Stochel, G.; Urbanska, K. NO-dependent phototoxicity of Roussin's black salt against cancer cells. *Nitric Oxide Biol. Chem.* **2004**, *10*, 42–50. [CrossRef] [PubMed]
68. Brindell, M.; Kuliś, E.; Elmroth, S.K.C.; Urbańska, K.; Stochel, G. Light-induced anticancer activity of $[RuCl_2(DMSO)_4]$ complexes. *J. Med. Chem.* **2005**, *48*, 7298–7304. [CrossRef] [PubMed]
69. Bomirski, A.; Słominski, A.; Bigda, J. The natural history of a family of transplantable melanomas in hamsters. *Cancer Metastasis Rev.* **1988**, *7*, 95–118. [CrossRef] [PubMed]
70. Słominski, A. Rapid melanization of Bomirski amelanotic melanoma cells in cell culture. *Biosci. Rep.* **1983**, *3*, 189–194. [CrossRef] [PubMed]
71. Słomiński, A. Some properties of Bomirski Ab amelanotic melanoma cells, which underwent spontaneous melanization in primary cell culture—Growth kinetics, cell morphology, melanin content and tumorigenicity. *J. Cancer Res. Clin. Oncol.* **1985**, *109*, 29–37. [CrossRef] [PubMed]

72. Słominski, A.; Moellmann, G.; Kuklinska, E.; Bomirski, A.; Pawelek, J. Positive regulation of melanin pigmentation by two key substrates of the melanogenic pathway, L-tyrosine and L-dopa. *J. Cell Sci.* **1988**, *89*, 287–296. [PubMed]

73. Słomiński, A.; Bomirski, A. Phenotypic changes of Ab hamster melanoma during long-term culture. *Anticancer Res.* **1985**, *5*, 403–409. [PubMed]

74. Boberek, M.; Swakoń, J.; Stolarczyk, L.; Olko Pawełand Waligórski, M. A monitoring system for the 60 MeV radiotherapy proton beam at IFJ PAN using a scintillating screen and a CCD camera. *Rom. Rep. Phys.* **2014**, *66*, 5–15.

13

Vitamin-D Receptor-Gene Polymorphisms Affect Quality of Life in Patients with Autoimmune Liver Diseases

Agnieszka Kempinska-Podhorodecka [1,*], Monika Adamowicz [1], Mateusz Chmielarz [1], Maciej K. Janik [2], Piotr Milkiewicz [2,3] and Malgorzata Milkiewicz [1]

[1] Department of Medical Biology, Pomeranian Medical University, 70-111 Szczecin, Poland; monikadamowicz@gmail.com (M.A.); ch.mateusz94@gmail.com (M.C.); milkiewm@pum.edu.pl (M.M.)

[2] Liver and Internal Medicine Unit, Medical University of Warsaw, 02-097 Warsaw, Poland; mjanik24@gmail.com (M.K.J.); p.milkiewicz@wp.pl (P.M.)

[3] Translational Medicine Group, Pomeranian Medical University, 70-111 Szczecin, Poland

* Correspondence: agnieszkakempinska@interia.eu

Abstract: Vitamin D deficiency has been associated with depressive symptoms and reduced physical functioning. The aim of the study was to characterize the relationship between polymorphisms of the vitamin D receptor (VDR) gene and the quality of life in patients with autoimmune hepatitis (AIH) and primary biliary cholangitis (PBC). Three polymorphisms of the *VDR* gene (*TaqI-rs731236*, *BsmI-rs1544410*, and *ApaI-rs7975232*) were analyzed in patients with AIH (n = 142) and PBC (n = 230) and in healthy individuals (n = 376). Patient quality of life was assessed by validated questionnaires such as Medical Outcomes Study Short-Form 36 (SF-36), State Trait Anxiety Inventory (STAI), Modified Fatigue-Impact Scale (MFIS), Patient-Health Questionnaire 9 (PHQ-9), and PBC-40. The *TaqI* C and *ApaI* A alleles are risk alleles in both AIH and PBC, and a significant dominance of the A allele in *BsmI* was observed in AIH patients. In terms of quality of life, the presence of the CC or CT *TaqI* genotype was associated with emotional reactions, including the fatigue and the cognitive skills of patients with PBC, whereas in the group of AIH patients, homozygotes CC of *TaqI*, AA of *BsmI*, and AA of *ApaI* had worse physical, social, emotional, and mental function. The genetic variations of *VDR* gene can influence individual susceptibility to develop chronic autoimmune liver diseases such as AIH and PBC and affect quality of life.

Keywords: autoimmune hepatitis; primary biliary cholangitis; vitamin D; health-related quality of life; mental well-being

---

1. Introduction

Autoimmune liver diseases, such as primary biliary cholangitis (PBC) and autoimmune hepatitis (AIH), have complex etiologies and are characterized by the progressive destruction of liver structures through autoimmunity mechanisms [1,2]. The vast majority of patients with PBC (80%–90%) are women [3]. The reaction between antimitochondrial antibodies (AMA) and pyruvate dehydrogenase complex-E2 (PDC-E2), located in the inner mitochondrial membrane, underlies the pathogenesis of PBC [4]. The most common clinical symptoms are persistent pruritus and chronic fatigue; however, a substantial percentage of patients may experience no symptoms of liver disease [1]. In biochemistry, elevated alkaline phosphatase and gamma-glutamyltranspeptidase activity, hypercholesterolemia, and often an increase in IgM level are observed. Histologically, the disease is characterized by bile-duct damage leading to chronic cholestasis, progressive fibrosis, and liver cirrhosis [3].

AIH is a disease that affects women more often than men regardless of age or ethnicity [5]. Biochemically, it is characterized by elevated transaminases and hypergammaglobulinemia. It can be divided into two types depending on autoantibodies; Type 1 is the most common and confirmed by the presence of an antinuclear antibody (ANA) or anti-smooth muscle antibody (ASMA). Histologically, AIH is marked by interface hepatitis, emperipolesis, and hepatocyte rosettes [6].

A substantial impairment of health-related quality of life (HRQoL) was reported in both PBC and AIH, with chronic fatigue and depression occurring in a significant proportion of patients with both diseases and pruritus affecting patients with PBC [7,8].

Vitamin D3 inhibits parathyroid-hormone secretion, cell proliferation, and adaptive immunity [9]. The activity of autoimmune diseases is influenced by vitamin-D3 deficiency [10], and this nonclassical effect of vitamin D is associated with the presence of the vitamin-D receptor (VDR) on numerous cells in the immune system. It was demonstrated that vitamin D has an impact on the Th1 lymphocytes responsible for the production of interleukin 2, tumor necrosis factor-alpha (TNA-α), and interferon gamma (IFNγ) [11]. The secretion of these cytokines can inhibit calcitriol (1.25$(OH)_2D_3$—the active metabolite of vitamin D), which translates into the alleviation of the inflammatory reaction. This substance also has a promoting effect on T regulatory cells that are also responsible for turning off the immune-system response, which may be crucial in the treatment of autoimmune diseases associated with excessive responses by the immune system [12]. Furthermore, the presence of VDR was observed on Th2 cells that, after activation, produce interleukins 4 and 10 [13]. Vitamin D enhances the diversification of macrophages and their bactericidal effect; it also inhibits the maturation of dendritic cells, which is essential in autoimmune diseases [14]. Consequently, attempts were made to use vitamin D_3 as a biopreparate capable of treating humans through the immunomodulation of the immune system [15].

Recent studies showed that vitamin D is also involved in neurotransmission and neuroprotection, and its receptor (VDR) is present in brain tissue, like glial cells, hippocampus, thalamus, or neurons [16]. In turn, the polymorphism of the *VDR* gene modulates *VDR* expression that can affect the vitamin D_3 signaling cascade [17,18]. A combination of these factors may suggest the impact of polymorphisms of the *VDR* gene on cognitive dysfunction, thus reducing the quality of life of patients with PBC and AIH.

Therefore, bearing in mind the results of our own study regarding the reduced expression of *VDR* in patients with PBC [19], the clinical symptoms of patients with PBC and AIH (including chronic fatigue and insomnia) [20,21], and reports on the protective effect of vitamin D on vessels and nerves, the aims of this study were characterizing the relationship between *VDR* gene polymorphisms (*BsmI and ApaI*, located in an intron between exons 8 and 9, and *TaqI* C > T located in exon 9) and the HRQoL in patients with a clinical diagnosis of PBC and AIH using validated scale tools and clinical-data forms.

2. Materials and Methods

2.1. Patients

Two-hundred-and-thirty patients with PBC (213 females and 17 males; median age at diagnosis 55; range 28–90 years) and 142 patients with AIH (111 females and 31 males; median age at diagnosis 32; range 24–64 years) were include into this study. Vitamin D supplementation was recommended in all patients with PBC. Main laboratory and demographic data of the included patients are presented at Table 1.

All patients with PBC met The European Association for the Study of the Liver (EASL) criteria for the diagnosis of PBC [22]. One-hundred-and-fifty-eight (68.7%) patients who had histological/clinical/imaging features consistent with liver cirrhosis AIH were diagnosed according EASL's Clinical Practice Guideline [2] for this condition and sixty-five (45.8%) of them had features of liver cirrhosis in histology.

Table 1. Demographic data of analyzed subjects.

Feature	PBC (n = 230)	AIH (n = 142)	Controls (n = 376)
Age (years)	55 (28–90)	32 (24–64)	28 (18–66)
Gender (F/M)	213/17	111/31	344/32
ALT (IU/L) (normal: 5–35)	47.0 (10.0–987.0)	113.8 (1.0–1542.0)	W.N.R.
ALP (IU/L) (normal: 40–120)	286.0 (37.0–1344.0)	100.1 (23.0–344.0)	W.N.R.
GGT, IU/L (normal: 5–35)	177.0 (11.0–1932.0)	102.9 (8.0–766.0)	W.N.R.
Bilirubin (mg/dL) (normal: 0.2–1.0)	0.9 (0.2–45.0)	1.6 (0.2–34.1)	N.D.
Albumin (g/dL) (normal: 3.5–4.5)	4.0 (2.1–5.8)	4.0 (2.0–5.0)	N.D.
Cholesterol (mg/dL) (normal: <190)	217.0 (50.0–1096.0)	182.0 (53.0–319.0)	N.D.
TG (mg/dL) (normal: <150)	105.0 (47.0–681.0)	91.0 (27.0–252.0)	N.D.

PBC: primary biliary cholangitis; AIH: autoimmune; ALT: alanine aminotransferase; ALP: alkaline phosphatase; GGT: gamma-glutamyl transferase; TG: triglycerides; W.N.R.: within normal range; N.D. not done.

A control group of 376 blood donors from the Regional Blood Donor Center in Szczecin (Poland), (344 females and 32 males; median age at enrollment 28; range 18–66 years) was investigated. All participants had a medical check-up. A good state of health was a prerequisite to qualify for blood donation. Each participant provided their written informed consent. All materials were deposited in the Department of Medical Biology, Pomeranian Medical University in Szczecin.

The study was approved by the Bioethical Committee of the Pomeranian Medical University in Szczecin, 2011, no. KB-0012/57/11.

2.2. VDR Genotyping

DNA was extracted from peripheral blood mononuclear cells using the DNeasy Blood and Tissue Kit (Qiagen, Hilden, Germany). Genotyping of three variants of *VDR* gene polymorphism (*TaqI-rs731236, BsmI-rs1544410, ApaI-rs7975232*) was carried out using real-time polymerase chain reaction using TaqMan probes (Applied Biosystems, Foster City, CA, Country; assay ID: C_2404008_10, C_8716062_10, C_28977635_10, respectively). Fluorescence analysis was conducted with Allelic Discrimination 7500 software v.2.0.2.

2.3. Health-Related Quality-of-Life Tools

Medical Outcomes Study Short Form 36 version 1.0 (*SF-36v1*, license no. QM011392-QualityMetric CT133208/OP018661) is a standardized questionnaire that contains 36 questions in 8 domains related to physical health (Physical Functioning, Role-Physical, Bodily Pain, General Health) and psychological well-being (Vitality, Social Functioning, Role-Emotional, Mental Health), which can be calculated in addition to two summary parameters: Physical-Component Summary and Mental-Component Summary [23].

PBC-40 was developed in 2005 and focuses on PBC [24]. The questionnaire consists of 40 questions related to the various aspects of chronic cholestatic liver disease: the worsening of chronic fatigue syndrome; feeling of health; skin pruritus; and cognitive, emotional, and social functions.

The Polish version of the Modified Fatigue-Impact Scale (MFIS) was used to assess the impact of fatigue on AIH patients' life [25]. It is a modified form of the original Fatigue-Impact Scale. The questionnaire that included 21 items and a total MFIS score (range 0–84) is based on three subscales: physical (9 items, score range 0–36), cognitive (10 items, score range 0–40), and psychical (2 items, score range 0–8).

State Trait Anxiety Inventory (STAI) is a tool designed to measure the levels of state and trait anxiety [25]. The Polish version of this questionnaire was used in this study. This 40-item scale includes two subscales, state anxiety (1–20 items) and trait anxiety (20–40 items). Each item is given a weighted score of 1 to 4. Higher score suggests elevated levels of anxiety. Therefore, 0–20 results from both subscales represent no anxiety, a 41–60 score indicates midlevel anxiety, and results from 61 to 80 indicate severe anxiety.

Patient-Health Questionnaire 9 (PHQ-9) is a self-administered screening tool that is used to monitor the severity of depressive symptoms [26]. A questionnaire was validated for Polish population. PHQ-9 scores of 5–9, 10–14, 15–19, and 20–27 are the ranges for mild, moderate, moderately severe, and severe depression, respectively.

In patients with PBC, two questionnaires were used, SF-36 and PBC-40. In patients with AIH, SF-36, MFIS, PHQ-9, and STAI were applied.

2.4. Statistical Analysis

All statistical analyses were carried out using StatView version 5 software (SAS Institute Inc., Carry, NC, USA). The genotype and allelic frequencies were compared using a chi-squared test of association (Pearson). The odds ratio (OR) and 95% confidence interval (CI) for each variable were also estimated. Analysis of genotype frequency in regard to the clinical characteristics and HRQoL assessment of PBC and AIH patients was performed using ANOVA with Fisher's protected least significant difference (PLSD). Data are shown as medians (and ranges) for demographic data, and as means and standard deviations (SD) for continuous variables of assessing HRQoL. *p*-values of less than 0.05 were considered to be statistically significant.

3. Results

The frequencies of all three *VDR* polymorphisms investigated in patients with PBC or AIH showed significant differences in comparison to the control group. The odds ratios (ORs) observed for the presence of these polymorphisms in the diseases and control groups are summarized in Table 2.

Table 2. Genotype counts for vitamin-D receptor (*VDR*) polymorphisms (rs731236, rs1544410, rs7975232) in PBC, AIH, and control subjects.

Frequencies	Controls (%) $n = 376$	PBC (%) $n = 230$	p * PBC vs. Control	χ^2	OR (95% CI)	AIH (%) $n = 142$	p * AIH vs. Control	χ^2	OR (95% CI)
				Taql (rs731236)					
TT (TT)	172 (45.7%)	28 (12.2%)	**<0.001**	72.7	0.2 (0.1–0.3)	48 (33.8%)	**0.01**	6.0	0.6 (0.4–0.9)
CT (tT)	160 (42.6%)	118 (51.3%)	**0.04**	4.4	1.4 (1.0–2.0)	62 (43.7%)	0.8	0.05	1.0 (0.7–1.5)
CC (tt)	44 (11.7%)	84 (36.5%)	**<0.001**	52.8	4.3 (2.9–6.6)	32 (22.5%)	**0.002**	9.7	2.2 (1.3–3.6)
				Bsml (rs1544410)					
AA (BB)	52 (13.8%)	25 (10.9%)	0.3	1.1	0.8 (0.5–1.3)	34 (23.9%)	**0.006**	7.6	2.0 (1.2–3.2)
GA (bB)	173 (46%)	109 (47.4%)	0.7	0.1	1.1 (0.8–1.5)	60 (42.3%)	0.4	0.6	0.9 (0.6–1.3)
GG (bb)	151 (40.2%)	96 (41.7%)	0.7	0.1	1.1 (0.8–1.5)	48 (33.8%)	0.2	1.76	0.8 (0.5–1.1)
				Apal (rs7975232)					
AA (AA)	74 (19.7%)	63 (27.4%)	**0.03**	4.8	1.5 (1.0–2.3)	46 (32.4%)	**0.002**	9.4	2.0 (1.3–3.0)
CA (aA)	196 (52.1%)	111 (48.2%)	0.3	0.8	0.9 (0.6–1.2)	61 (43.0%)	0.06	3.5	0.7 (0.5–1.0)
CC (aa)	106 (28.2%)	56 (24.4%)	0.3	1.0	0.8 (0.6–1.2)	35 (24.6%)	0.4	0.6	0.8 (0.5–1.3)

* Chi-squared test of association (Pearson); PBC: primary biliary cholangitis; AIH: autoimmune hepatitis; OR: odds ratio; CI: confidence interval. Bold font indicates statistical significance.

In PBC patients, the *TaqI* CC and CT genotypes were more prevalent in comparison to controls (36.5% vs. 11.7%, $p < 0.001$, and 51.3% vs. 42.6%, $p = 0.04$, respectively), whereas the TT genotype of *TaqI* was considerably less frequent than in the controls (12.2% vs. 45.7%, $p < 0.001$; Table 2). Similarly, in AIH patients, the *TaqI* CC genotype appeared more often than in the control group (22.5% vs. 11.7%, $p = 0.002$), while the TT was less frequent than in the controls (33.8% vs. 45.7%, $p = 0.01$; Table 2).

Regarding *BsmI* polymorphism, the frequency of the AA genotype was substantially higher in patients with AIH compared to controls (23.9% vs. 13.8%, $p = 0.006$; Table 2). The results of *ApaI* genotyping showed that the AA genotype occurred more frequently in both patients with PBC and AIH (27.4% vs. 19.7% in controls, $p = 0.03$, and 32.4% vs. 19.7% in controls; $p = 0.002$, respectively; Table 2).

Furthermore, analyses of frequencies of each allele in the three polymorphic sites clearly demonstrated that the *TaqI* C and *ApaI* A alleles were more prevalent in both PBC and AIH compared to in healthy individuals. Thus, the distribution of the *TaqI* C allele was 62.0% in PBC and 44.4% in AIH vs. 33.0% in controls (both $p < 0.001$); for the *ApaI* A allele, 51.4% in PBC and 54% in AIH vs. 45.7% in controls, $p = 0.05$ and $p = 0.02$, respectively. Additionally, 45.0% of AIH patients were carriers of the *BsmI* A allele in comparison to 36.8% controls, $p = 0.02$ (Table 3).

Table 3. Allele association for VDR in PBC, AIH, and control subjects.

SNP	Allele	Controls $n = 376$ (%)	PBC $n = 230$ (%)	P * PBC vs. Control	χ^2	OR (95%CI)	AIH $n = 142$ (%)	P * AIH vs. Control	χ^2	OR (95%CI)
TaqI rs731236	T/C (T/t)	504/248 (67.0/33.0)	174/286 (38.0/62.0)	**<0.001**	98.7	3.3 (2.6–4.3)	158/126 (55.6/44.4)	**<0.001**	11.6	1.6 (1.3–2.1)
BsmI rs1544410	A/G (B/b)	277/475 (36.8/63.2)	159/301 (34.6/65.4)	0.4	0.6	1.1 (0.9–1.4)	128/156 (45.0/55.0)	**0.02**	5.9	1.4 (1.1–1.9)
ApaI rs7975232	A/C (A/a)	344/408 (45.7/54.3)	237/223 (51.4/48.6)	**0.05**	3.8	0.8 (0.6–1.0)	153/131 (54.0/46.0)	**0.02**	5.4	1.4 (1.1–1.8)

* Chi-squared test of association (Pearson); PSC: primary biliary cholangitis; AIH: Autoimmune hepatitis; OR: odds ratio; CI: confidence interval. Bold font indicates statistical significance.

In addition, the clinical status and biochemical findings of the patients were examined in relation to *VDR* polymorphism. In PBC patients, *TaqI* and *BsmI* variants were associated with the histological features of cirrhosis regardless of cholestasis and autoimmune parameters in PBC. Thus, in patients with PBC who were cirrhotic at the diagnosis, 52.8% were *TaqI* CC, 39% were CT and 7.5% were TT genotype carriers ($p < 0.0001$ vs. CC). Similarly, in *BmsI* variant, 56.6% of cirrhotics were GG homozygous, 33.9% were GA heterozygous ($p = 0.03$ vs. *GG*), and 9.4% were *AA* homozygotes genotype ($p < 0.0001$ vs. *GG*). Other laboratory markers of the disease severity and enhanced level of AMAs, Gp210, and Sp100 antibodies failed to have any association to the analyzed polymorphisms. In contrast, in the group of AIH patients, the presence of the *VDR* polymorphisms did not correlate with the examined clinical and biochemical features (data not shown).

Regarding the quality of life of PBC patients, several domains of SF-36 and PBC-40 questionnaires were correlated only with the *TaqI* variant of *VDR* polymorphisms. The SF-36 general questionnaire demonstrated that PBC patients with CC and CT genotypes of *TaqI* variants had lower scores for Vitality ($p = 0.01$, and $p = 0.04$, respectively) and Role-Emotional ($p = 0.03$ and $p = 0.04$, respectively) than TT homozygotes did. The results of the PBC-40 questionnaires showed that carriers of CC and CT genotypes had significant cognitive impairment versus the TT genotype ($p = 0.04$ and $p = 0.04$, respectively). Furthermore, PBC patients with the *TaqI* CT genotype suffer from greater fatigue than patients with TT do ($p = 0.04$; Table 4).

In view of the fact that the *TaqI* C allele was associated with the increased risk of cirrhosis as well as reduced quality of life, we did an additional sub-group analysis corresponding to the presence of cirrhosis. We looked at features which came out significant, i.e., vitality and role emotional from SF-36 and cognitive function from PBC40. No significant differences between cirrhotic and non-cirrhotic patients were found, which may suggest that the allele itself, but not the presence of cirrhosis, exerts its negative effect on patients QoL.

Among patients with AIH, health-related quality of life was evaluated by the SF-36, STAI, MFIS, and PHQ-9 questionnaires. Differences between patients in relation to variants of *VDR* polymorphisms were observed only in SF-36 domains. The *TaqI* CC homozygotes scored fewer points for Role-Physical ($p = 0.04$) than the CT heterozygotes did, which, in turn, scored higher than TT homozygotes on Social-Functioning ($p = 0.03$; Table 5).

Table 4. Relationship between *TaqI* polymorphism and features of quality-of-life scales in PBC group.

Domain	*TaqI (rs731236 T/C)*					
	CC (tt)	CT (tT)	TT (TT)	P * CC vs CT	P * CC vs TT	P * TT vs CT
SF-36						
Physical Functioning	57.0 ± 3.2	59.5 ± 2.3	67.0 ± 5.3	0.5	0.09	0.2
Role-Physical	36.5 ± 4.3	34.0 ± 3.7	50.0 ± 8.3	0.6	0.1	0.05
Bodily Pain	54.4 ± 3.2	55.4 ± 2.4	61.0 ± 5.8	0.8	0.3	0.3
General Health	43.4 ± 1.9	43.6 ± 1.7	45.1 ± 3.4	0.9	0.7	0.7
Vitality	44.5 ± 2.4	47.5 ± 1.9	57.0 ± 4.8	0.3	**0.01**	**0.04**
Social Functioning	59.2 ± 3.0	61.2 ± 2.3	69.0 ± 5.3	0.6	0.08	0.1
Role-Emotional	47.4 ± 5.0	49.7 ± 4.2	69.0 ± 7.8	0.7	**0.03**	**0.04**
Mental Health	59.0 ± 2.0	59.9 ± 1.9	67.2 ± 4.3	0.7	0.06	0.09
Physical Component Summary	47.8 ± 2.6	47.8 ± 2.0	55.0 ± 4.7	0.8	0.1	0.1
Mental Component Summary	52.2 ± 2.5	54.4 ± 2.1	65.0 ± 5.0	0.5	0.2	0.4
PBC-40						
Other Symptom	17.0 ± 0.6	17.3 ± 0.5	16.1 ± 1.0	0.6	0.4	0.2
Itch	6.0 ± 0.5	5.4 ± 0.4	5.0 ± 0.9	0.4	0.3	0.6
Fatigue	29.6 ± 1.2	30.4 ± 1.0	26.1 ± 1.8	0.6	0.1	**0.04**
Cognitive function	14.2 ± 0.7	14.1 ± 0.5	11.7 ± 1.0	0.8	**0.04**	**0.04**
Social and Emotional function	31.5 ± 10.7	31.6 ±11.5	28.0 ±11.0	0.9	0.1	0.08

* ANOVA with Fisher's protected least significant difference (PLSD). Letters enclosed in brackets represent previously described nomenclature derived from restriction-fragment length polymorphism (RFLP) analysis. Bold font indicates statistical significance.

Table 5. Relationship between *TaqI* polymorphism and features of quality-of-life scales in AIH group.

Domain	*TaqI (rs731236 T/C)*					
	CC (tt)	CT (tT)	TT (TT)	P * *CC* vs *CT*	P * *CC* vs *TT*	P * *TT* vs *CT*
SF-36						
Physical Functioning	73.0 ± 4.6	79.0 ± 2.8	73.6 ± 3.4	0.2	0.9	0.2
Role-Physical	47.7 ± 7.6	66.1 ± 5.5	55.7 ± 5.8	**0.04**	0.4	0.2
Bodily Pain	67.4 ± 5.2	74.2 ± 3.1	69.4 ± 4.1	0.3	0.7	0.3
General Health	47.5 ± 3.5	49.9 ± 2.5	47.5 ± 3.5	0.6	0.9	0.6
Vitality	53.3 ± 3.5	54.3 ± 2.5	51.6 ± 2.8	0.8	0.7	0.5
Social Functioning	67.2 ± 4.1	75.4 ± 3.2	65.1 ± 3.7	0.1	0.7	**0.03**
Role-Emotional	59.4 ± 7.3	74.7 ± 4.8	68.1 ± 5.8	0.08	0.3	0.4
Mental Health	63.5 ± 2.9	66.3 ± 2.6	61.3 ± 2.5	0.5	0.6	0.2
Physical Component Summary	58.9 ± 4.2	67.3 ± 2.7	61.6 ± 3.5	0.09	0.6	0.2
Mental Component Summary	60.8 ± 3.8	67.7 ± 2.8	61.5 ± 3.0	0.1	0.9	0.1
STAI						
STAI1	47.4 ± 0.8	45.9 ± 0.8	46.2 ± 0.8	0.2	0.4	0.8
STAI2	45.1 ± 0.9	45.3 ± 0.7	46.0 ± 0.8	0.9	0.5	0.5
MFIS						
Physical	13.7 ± 1.6	14.1 ± 1.0	14.1 ± 1.1	0.8	0.9	0.9
Cognitive	13.2 ± 1.6	11.7 ± 0.9	12.2 ± 1.0	0.4	0.6	0.7
Psychosocial	2.8 ± 0.4	2.5 ± 0.2	3.0 ± 0.3	0.4	0.7	0.2
MFIS Score	13.7 ± 1.6	14.1 ± 1.0	14.1 ± 1.1	0.8	0.9	0.9
PHQ-9						
PHQ-9	7.2 ± 0.8	6.0 ± 0.6	7.7 ± 0.8	0.3	0.6	0.08

* ANOVA with Fisher's protected least significant difference (PLSD); The letters enclosed in square brackets represent previously described nomenclature derived from a restriction-fragment length polymorphism (RFLP) analysis. Bold font indicates statistical significance.

The *BsmI* AA homozygotes had lower scores for Physical-Component Summary than the GA heterozygotes did ($p = 0.04$; Table 6).

Table 6. Relationship between *BsmI* polymorphism and features of quality-of-life scales in AIH group.

Domain	*BsmI (rs1544410 A/G)*					
	GG (bb)	GA (bB)	AA (BB)	P * GG vs GA	P * GG vs AA	P * AA vs GA
SF-36						
Physical Functioning	73.9 ± 3.4	80.5 ± 2.5	72.3 ± 4.9	0.1	0.8	0.1
Role-Physical	56.2 ± 5.7	66.7 ± 5.4	49.3 ± 7.6	0.2	0.5	0.05
Bodily Pain	70.3 ± 4.1	73.5 ± 2.9	65.1 ± 5.2	0.5	0.4	0.1
General Health	48.9 ± 3.4	51.0 ± 2.5	46.2 ± 3.7	0.6	0.6	0.3
Vitality	53.3 ± 2.6	54.5 ± 2.4	52.0 ± 3.7	0.7	0.8	0.5
Social Functioning	65.8 ± 3.7	75.2 ± 3.0	67.0 ± 4.2	0.05	0.8	0.1
Role-Emotional	68.7 ± 5.9	75.5 ± 4.7	60.8 ± 7.2	0.4	0.4	0.08
Mental Health	63.5 ± 2.4	67.1 ± 2.4	61.9 ± 3.2	0.3	0.7	0.2
Physical Component Summary	62.3 ± 3.3	67.9 ± 2.5	58.2 ± 4.4	0.2	0.4	**0.04**
Mental Component Summary	62.9 ± 3.0	68.1 ± 2.6	60.4 ± 4.0	0.2	0.6	0.09
STAI						
STAI1	47.1 ± 0.8	45.6 ± 0.8	46.9 ± 0.8	0.1	0.8	0.3
STAI2	46.2 ± 0.8	45.3 ± 0.8	44.7 ± 0.8	0.4	0.2	0.6
MFIS						
Physical	14.0 ± 1.0	14.1 ± 1.0	14.2 ± 1.6	0.9	0.9	0.9
Cognitive	12.4 ± 1.0	11.4 ± 0.8	13.0 ± 1.5	0.5	0.7	0.3
Psychosocial	3.0 ± 0.3	2.6 ± 0.2	2.9 ± 0.4	0.4	0.8	0.6
MFIS Score	29.4 ± 2.0	28.2 ± 1.9	30.1 ± 3.3	0.7	0.9	0.6
PHQ-9						
PHQ-9	7.0 ± 0.8	6.2 ± 0.6	7.4 ± 0.8	0.4	0.7	0.2

* ANOVA with Fisher's protected least-significant difference (PLSD). Letters enclosed in brackets represent previously described nomenclature derived from restriction-fragment length polymorphism (RFLP) analysis. Bold font indicates statistical significance.

The most noticeable differences in quality of life measured by the generic SF-36 were observed in *ApaI* variants of *VDR* polymorphism. *ApaI* AA homozygotes had lower scores for 6 out of 10 factors, namely, Role-Physical ($p = 0.02$), Social Functioning ($p = 0.04$), Role-Emotional ($p = 0.003$), Mental Health ($p = 0.04$), Physical-Component Summary ($p = 0.04$), and Mental-Component Summary ($p = 0.04$) compared to CA heterozygotes (Table 7). Additionally, CA heterozygotes scored more points for Social Functioning ($p = 0.01$) than CC individuals did (Table 7).

Table 7. Relationship between *ApaI* polymorphism and features of quality-of-life scales in AIH group.

Domain	*ApaI (rs7975232 C/A)*					
	CC (aa)	CA (aA)	AA (AA)	P * CC vs CA	P * CC vs AA	P * AA vs CA
SF-36						
Physical Functioning	73.6 ± 4.0	80.5 ± 2.3	74.0 ± 3.9	*0.1*	*0.9*	*0.1*
Role-Physical	56.1 ± 6.9	68.1 ± 5.0	49.5 ± 6.3	*0.2*	*0.5*	***0.02***
Bodily Pain	71.7 ± 4.9	72.7 ± 3.1	67.8 ± 4.1	*0.8*	*0.5*	*0.3*
General Health	47.3 ± 3.8	51.5 ± 2.5	47.5 ± 3.1	*0.3*	*0.9*	*0.3*
Vitality	52.2 ± 3.1	56.5 ± 2.3	50.4 ± 2.8	*0.3*	*0.7*	*0.09*
Social Functioning	63.8 ± 3.9	76.4 ± 2.8	66.6 ± 3.9	***0.01***	*0.6*	***0.04***
Role-Emotional	64.7 ± 6.9	80.6 ± 4.2	58.5 ± 6.1	*0.05*	*0.4*	***0.003***
Mental Health	62.5 ± 2.7	67.8 ± 2.2	60.9 ± 2.9	*0.2*	*0.7*	***0.04***
Physical Component Summary	62.5 ± 2.7	67.9 ± 2.2	60.9 ± 2.9	*0.2*	*0.7*	***0.04***
Mental Component Summary	62.2 ± 3.9	68.2 ± 2.5	58.7 ± 3.5	*0.2*	*0.6*	***0.04***
STAI						
STAI1	46.5 ± 1.0	45.7 ± 0.7	46.9 ± 0.8	*0.5*	*0.7*	*0.2*
STAI2	46.3 ± 0.9	45.2 ± 0.6	45.0 ± 0.8	*0.4*	*0.3*	*0.8*

Table 7. *Cont.*

Domain	*ApaI (rs7975232 C/A)*					
	CC (aa)	CA (aA)	AA (AA)	*p* * CC vs CA	*p* * CC vs AA	*p* * AA vs CA
			MFIS			
Physical	13.2 ± 1.2	14.8 ± 1.0	13.9 ± 1.2	0.3	0.7	0.6
Cognitive	11.5 ± 1.1	12.6 ± 0.9	12.3 ± 1.2	0.5	0.3	0.8
Psychosocial	2.8 ± 0.3	3.0 ± 0.2	2.6 ± 0.3	0.6	0.7	0.3
MFIS Score	27.4 ± 2.4	30.4 ± 1.9	28.8 ± 2.6	0.4	0.8	0.6
			PHQ-9			
PHQ-9	7.1 ± 0.9	6.6 ± 0.6	6.9 ± 0.7	0.7	0.8	0.8

* ANOVA with Fisher's protected least-significant difference (PLSD). Letters enclosed in brackets represent previously described nomenclature derived from restriction-fragment length polymorphism (RFLP) analysis. Bold font indicates statistical significance.

4. Discussion

In this study, we analyzed the prevalence of three common *VDR* polymorphisms (*TaqI-rs731236*, *BsmI-rs1544410*, and *ApaI-rs7975232*) and investigated their potential relationships with the quality of life in a well-characterized cohort of Polish patients with PBC and AIH.

Calcium and vitamin-D supplementation (400–800 IU/day) is recommended to both patients with AIH, who are frequently on long-term steroids, and with PBC, who in their majority are postmenopausal females prone to osteoporosis and impaired vitamin-D absorption secondary to cholestasis. Vitamin D, operating through a nuclear receptor (VDR), is an important modulator of immune processes that adjust both types of immune response [27] by strengthening innate immunity and suppressing acquired immunity reactions [9].

Interestingly, in our study, in the two examined autoimmune liver diseases, both the CC *TaqI* and the AA *ApaI* genotype occurred more frequently than in the controls, and both the C allele of *TaqI* and the A allele of *ApaI* were risk alleles for PBC and AIH. Our results are in contrast to a study in which a significant association of the *TaqI* but not the *ApaI* polymorphism within German AIH patients was reported [28]. However, results from the study that included both patients with AIH and patients with PBC in one merged group showed an increased incidence of the A allele of *ApaI* [29]. These findings may be explained by the genetic heterogeneity that exists in different populations. For instance, the distribution of *BsmI*, *ApaI*, and *TaqI* gene variants was reported to be dissimilar in healthy Chinese controls as compared to healthy Caucasian controls [30]. In our patients with AIH, the A allele and AA genotype of the *BsmI* variant were more prevalent compared to the controls. These results are in a line with reports showing the link between *VDR* polymorphisms and autoimmunity. Thus, the *TaqI, BsmI, and ApaI* polymorphisms of *VDR* gene are the most widely reported as being closely linked with a high risk of autoimmune diseases including PBC [31], multiple sclerosis (*BsmI* AA) [32], Type 1 diabetes (*TaqI* T [33] or *BsmI* AA [34]), and systemic lupus erythematosus (*BsmI* AA) [35,36]. The functional consequence of these *VDR* polymorphisms is important in determining the potential effect on inflammatory mediators in autoimmune diseases. Vitamin D stimulates the development of Th2 cells and the production of anti-inflammatory interleukins. Therefore, reduced signal transduction due to polymorphic variants of the *VDR* gene might skew the immune response to the Th1 pathway that was implicated in the progress of organ-specific autoimmune diseases. *ApaI* and the *BsmI* polymorphisms do not change the amino acid sequence of the VDR protein but may affect gene expression through the alteration of mRNA stability (the disruption of splice sites for mRNA transcription or a change in intronic regulatory elements) [28], and it was demonstrated that the ApaI variant was positively associated with the serum concentration of 25 $(OH)_2D_3$ [37]. Moreover, IFN gamma production upon anti-CD3 stimulation in the AA [BB] genotype of *BsmI* was significantly higher than that in the AG (Bb) and GG (bb) genotype groups, which showed that the polyclonal T-cell response in BB genotype patients was Th1-dominant [34]. In turn, the *TaqI* polymorphism is involved in the regulation of the stability of VDR mRNA, and the TT genotype modulates VDR expression and confers protection against multiple sclerosis [17,28,38].

Our previous report, on a smaller group of PBC patients (n = 143), showed that there is an association between the *TaqI* and *BsmI*, a predisposition to earlier onset of liver damage and a more severe manifestation of disease [39]. In this study on a larger group of PBC patients (n = 230), it was confirmed that the *TaqI CC* and *BsmI GG* genotypes are related to the degree of liver morphologic damage, as assessed by severity of liver fibrosis (Stage IV on histology). On the basis of the results of this study, we validated our previous conclusion that these variants of the *VDR* gene may prompt more severe liver injury and a worse course of primary biliary cholangitis. However, the interpretation of the role of *TaqI and BsmI* variants in the development of liver fibrosis is hindered because only limited information is available on the functional changes induced by these variants of the *VDR* gene.

In general, little is known about the impact of *VDR* polymorphisms on the quality of patients' life since previous studies mostly focused on the prevalence of each polymorphism in autoimmune diseases but not on their relation with the clinical course of the disease [29]. Most studies on the quality of life in patients with PBC or AIH addressed relations between specific aspects of disease, such as fatigue, pruritus, depression, and quality of life after liver transplantation [7,40–49] but not the impact of *VDR* gene polymorphisms.

In this present study, we showed that there is an association between the *TaqI* variant of the *VDR* gene and impaired well-being of patients with PBC, as measured with general and disease-specific questionnaires. The CC of *TaqI* was associated with worse health-related quality of life, as measured by the generic SF-36. This was mainly due to the decrease in subscores of energy and emotional reactions, both associated with fatigue and significant cognitive impairment. Moreover, our analysis of the PBC-40 domains showed that PBC patients' quality of life was significantly impaired in the carriers of CC and CT genotype of *TaqI*, and fatigue and cognitive function were the most affected domains. In contrast to patients with PBC, among AIH patients, all three variants of *VDR* polymorphism, i.e., *TaqI*, *BsmI*, and *ApaI*, affected health-related quality of life. We observed that the CC and CT of *TaqI* were associated with worse physical and social functioning, while the AA genotype of *BsmI* had physical problems and worse overall health. Interestingly, *ApaI* was the polymorphic variant that mostly affected the quality of life of AIH patients. Our study clearly indicated that the AA homozygotes of *ApaI* variant had disturbed or maladaptive emotional responses and mental disorders, while the CC homozygotes scored fewer points for social functioning. We observed a similar phenomenon in patients with another liver disease of presumed autoimmune background, namely, primary sclerosing cholangitis (PSC) [19]. In that group of patients, the SF-36 questionnaire showed that the C allele of *ApaI* was associated with a reduction of physical, emotional, and mental function and worse overall health. Furthermore, the PBC-40 and PBC-27 questionnaires confirmed that the C allele was associated with itching, fatigue, and the impairment of cognitive functions. Correspondingly, individuals who were AA homozygotes (noncarriers of the C allele of *ApaI*) had higher summary scores for the physical and mental disorders measured with SF-36; they suffered less from itching or fatigue and did not have significant cognitive impairment [19]. The observed association between *VDR* polymorphisms and quality of life is of importance to daily clinical practice because patients with AIH struggle with serious symptoms that significantly affect their well-being, including mood disturbance, cognitive dysfunction, chronic fatigue, decreased physical activity, and a high rate of previously unrecognized severe symptoms of depression and anxiety [7,50]; thus, the presence of the CC *ApaI* variant may result in those symptoms worsening.

Perhaps the major limitation of this study, related to its retrospective nature, is the lack of data on Vitamin D serum levels in analyzed patients and thus the inability to correlate these levels with analyzed polymorphisms. This problem has also been noted in other, similar studies. Serum levels of Vitamin D depend not only on whether patient supplements it but also on patient's diet and several other factors. Therefore, normal serum levels of Vitamin D could be related to its regular intake, and this would certainly be independent of the presence of VDR polymorphisms. Judgement based on information provided by the patient regarding Vitamin D/calcium supplementation can also be inaccurate in view of widely reported non-adherence to drugs, which do not directly relieve symptoms such as Vitamin D deficiency or hypertension. Thus, in a real-world situation, it is very difficult to reliably assess relationship between real serum Vitamin D levels and VDR polymorphisms. For the same reason, we were not able to study a direct effect of serum Vitamin D levels on patients QoL.

5. Conclusions

We observed a significant dominance of the CC *TaqI* and AA *ApaI* genotypes in patients with PBC and AIH. Moreover, the impaired quality of life in patients with AIH was significantly associated with the presence of the AA *ApaI* variant of the *VDR* gene. Awareness of this association can contribute to a deeper understanding of the mechanisms responsible for the occurrence of symptoms associated with poorer quality of life, thereby offering the chance to improve the care of AIH patients.

Author Contributions: Conceptualization, A.K.-P. and M.M.; methodology, A.K.-P., M.A., M.C., and M.K.J.; validation, A.K.-P., M.M., and M.K.J.; formal analysis, A.K.-P., M.A., M.C., and M.M.; investigation, P.M.; resources, A.K.-P., M.M., and P.M.; data curation, A.K.-P., M.A., M.K.J., and M.C.; writing—original-draft preparation, A.K.-P. and M.M.; writing—review and editing, all authors; visualization, A.K.-P. and M.A.; supervision, M.M. and P.M.; project administration, A.K.-P., M.M., M.K.J., and P.M.; funding acquisition, A.K.-P., M.M., and P.M. All authors have read and agreed to the published version of the manuscript.

References

1. Hirschfield, G.M.; Dyson, J.K.; Alexander, G.J.M.; Chapman, M.H.; Collier, J.; Hübscher, S.; Pereira, S.P.; Thain, C.; Thorburn, D.; Tiniakos, D.; et al. Primary biliary cholangitis treatment and management guidelines. *Gut* **2018**, *67*, 1568–1594. [CrossRef]
2. Lohse, A.W.; Chazouillères, O.; Dalekos, G.; Drenth, J.; Heneghan, M.; Hofer, H.; Lammert, F.; Lenzi, M. EASL clinical practice guidelines: Autoimmune hepatitis. *J. Hepatol.* **2015**, *63*, 971–1004. [CrossRef]
3. Onofrio, F.Q.; Hirschfield, G.M.; Gulamhusein, A.F. A practical review of primary biliary cholangitis for the gastroenterologist. *Gastroenterol. Hepatol. (NY)* **2019**, *15*, 145–154.
4. Hisamoto, S.; Shimoda, S.; Harada, K.; Iwasaka, S.; Onohara, S.; Chong, Y.; Nakamura, M.; Bekki, Y.; Yoshizumi, T.; Ikegami, T.; et al. Hydrophobic bile acids suppress expression of AE2 in biliary epithelial cells and induce bile duct inflammation in primary biliary cholangitis. *J. Autoimmun.* **2016**, *75*, 150–160. [CrossRef] [PubMed]
5. Puustinen, L.; Barner-Rasmussen, N.; Pukkala, E.; Färkkilä, M. Incidence, prevalence, and causes of death of patients with autoimmune hepatitis: A nationwide register-based cohort study in Finland. *Dig. Liver Dis.* **2019**, *51*, 1294–1299. [CrossRef]
6. Linzay, C.D.; Sharma, B.; Pandit, S. Autoimmune Hepatitis. Available online: https://www.ncbi.nlm.nih.gov/books/NBK459186/ (accessed on 25 July 2020).
7. Janik, M.K.; Wunsch, E.; Raszeja-Wyszomirska, J.; Moskwa, M.; Kruk, B.; Krawczyk, M.; Milkiewicz, P. Autoimmune hepatitis exerts a profound, negative effect on health-related quality of life: A prospective, single-centre study. *Liver Int.* **2019**, *39*, 215–221. [CrossRef]
8. Raszeja-Wyszomirska, J.; Wunsch, E.; Krawczyk, M.; Rigopoulou, E.I.; Kostrzewa, K.; Norman, G.L.; Bogdanos, D.P.; Milkiewicz, P. Assessment of health related quality of life in Polish patients with primary biliary cirrhosis. *Clin. Res. Hepatol. Gastroenterol.* **2016**, *40*, 471–479. [CrossRef]
9. Di Rosa, M.; Malaguarnera, M.; Nicoletti, F.; Malaguarnera, L. Vitamin D3: A helpful immuno-modulator. *Immunology* **2011**, *134*, 123–139. [CrossRef] [PubMed]
10. Gil, Á.; Plaza-Diaz, J.; Mesa, M.D. Vitamin D: Classic and novel actions: Vdre deviation repression. *Ann. Nutr. Metab.* **2018**, *72*, 87–95. [CrossRef] [PubMed]
11. Lemire, J.M.; Archer, D.C.; Beck, L.; Spiegelberg, H.L. Immunosuppressive actions of 1,25-dihydroxyvitamin D3: Preferential inhibition of Th1 functions. *J. Nutr.* **1995**, *125*, 1704S–1708S. [CrossRef] [PubMed]

12. Cantorna, M.T.; Snyder, L.; Lin, Y.D.; Yang, L. Vitamin D and 1,25(OH)2D regulation of t cells. *Nutrients* **2015**, *7*, 3011–3021. [CrossRef] [PubMed]
13. Lemire, J.M.; Adams, J.S.; Kermani-Arab, V.; Bakke, A.C.; Sakai, R.; Jordan, S.C. 1,25-dihydroxyvitamin D3 suppresses human T helper/inducer lymphocyte activity in vitro. *J. Immunol.* **1985**, *134*, 3032–3035. [PubMed]
14. Abbas, A.K.; Murphy, K.M.; Sher, A. Functional diversity of helper T lymphocytes. *Nature* **1996**, *383*, 787–793. [CrossRef] [PubMed]
15. Barchetta, I. Could vitamin D supplementation benefit patients with chronic liver disease? *Gastroenterol. Hepatol. (NY)* **2012**, *8*, 755–757.
16. Cui, X.; Gooch, H.; Petty, A.; McGrath, J.J.; Eyles, D. Vitamin D and the brain: Genomic and non-genomic actions. *Mol. Cell. Endocrinol.* **2017**, *453*, 131–143. [CrossRef]
17. Agliardi, C.; Guerini, F.R.; Saresella, M.; Caputo, D.; Leone, M.A.; Zanzottera, M.; Bolognesi, E.; Marventano, I.; Barizzone, N.; Fasano, M.E.; et al. Vitamin D receptor (VDR) gene SNPs influence VDR expression and modulate protection from multiple sclerosis in HLA-DRB1 * 15-positive individuals. *Brain. Behav. Immun.* **2011**, *25*, 1460–1467. [CrossRef] [PubMed]
18. Mahajan, M.; Sharma, R. Current understanding of role of vitamin D in Type 2 diabetes mellitus. *Int. J. Recent Sci. Res.* **2015**, *6*, 2602–2604.
19. Kempinska-Podhorodecka, A.; Milkiewicz, M.; Jabłonski, D.; Milkiewicz, P.; Wunsch, E. ApaI polymorphism of vitamin D receptor affects health-related quality of life in patients with primary sclerosing cholangitis. *PLoS ONE* **2017**, *12*, e0176264. [CrossRef]
20. Zhao, X.; Wong, P. Managing sleep disturbances in cirrhosis. *Scientifica (Cairo)* **2016**, *2016*, 5. [CrossRef]
21. Purohit, T.; Cappell, M.S. Primary biliary cirrhosis: Pathophysiology, clinical presentation and therapy. *World J. Hepatol.* **2015**, *7*, 926–941. [CrossRef]
22. Hirschfield, G.M.; Beuers, U.; Corpechot, C.; Invernizzi, P.; Jones, D.; Marzioni, M.; Schramm, C. EASL clinical practice guidelines: The diagnosis and management of patients with primary biliary cholangitis. *J. Hepatol.* **2017**, *67*, 145–172. [CrossRef]
23. Ware, J.E.; Sherbourne, C.D. The MOS 36-item short form health status survey (SF-36). *Med. Care* **1992**, *30*, 473–483. [CrossRef] [PubMed]
24. Jacoby, A.; Rannard, A.; Buck, D.; Bhala, N.; Newton, J.L.; James, O.F.W.; Jones, D.E.J. Development, validation, and evaluation of the PBC-40, a disease specific health related quality of life measure for primary biliary cirrhosis. *Gut* **2005**, *54*, 1622–1629. [CrossRef] [PubMed]
25. Fisk, J.D.; Ritvo, P.G.; Ross, L.; Haase, D.A.; Marrie, T.J.; Schlech, W.F. Measuring the functional impact of fatigue: Initial validation of the fatigue impact scale. *Clin. Infect. Dis.* **1994**, *18*, 79–83. [CrossRef]
26. Kroenke, K.; Spitzer, R.L.; Williams, J.B.W. The PHQ-9: Validity of a brief depression severity measure. *J. Gen. Intern. Med.* **2001**, *16*, 606–613. [CrossRef] [PubMed]
27. Yang, C.Y.; Leung, P.S.C.; Adamopoulos, I.E.; Gershwin, M.E. The implication of vitamin D and autoimmunity: A comprehensive review. *Clin. Rev. Allergy Immunol.* **2013**, *45*, 217–226. [CrossRef]
28. Vogel, A.; Strassburg, C.P.; Manns, M.P. Genetic association of vitamin D receptor polymorphisms with primary biliary cirrhosis and autoimmune hepatitis. *Hepatology* **2002**, *35*, 126–131. [CrossRef]
29. Zhong, Z.-X. Polymorphisms in the vitamin D receptor gene and risk of autoimmune liver Diseases: A meta-analysis. *Biomed. J. Sci. Tech. Res.* **2018**, *9*, 1–8. [CrossRef]
30. Fan, L.; Tu, X.; Zhu, Y.; Zhou, L.; Pfeiffer, T.; Feltens, R.; Stoecker, W.; Zhong, R. Genetic association of vitamin D receptor polymorphisms with autoimmune hepatitis and primary biliary cirrhosis in the Chinese. *J. Gastroenterol. Hepatol.* **2005**, *20*, 249–255. [CrossRef]
31. Tanaka, A.; Nezu, S.; Uegaki, S.; Kikuchi, K.; Shibuya, A.; Miyakawa, H.; Takahashi, S.-I.; Bianchi, I.; Zermiani, P.; Podda, M.; et al. Vitamin D receptor polymorphisms are associated with increased susceptibility to primary biliary cirrhosis in Japanese and Italian populations. *J. Hepatol.* **2009**, *50*, 1202–1209. [CrossRef]
32. Niino, M.; Fukazawa, T.; Yabe, I.; Kikuchi, S.; Sasaki, H.; Tashiro, K. Vitamin D receptor gene polymorphism in multiple sclerosis and the association with HLA class II alleles. *J. Neurol. Sci.* **2000**, *177*, 65–71. [CrossRef]
33. Mohammadnejad, Z.; Ghanbari, M.; Ganjali, R.; Afshari, J.T.; Heydarpour, M.; Taghavi, S.M.; Fatemi, S.; Rafatpanah, H. Association between vitamin D receptor gene polymorphisms and type 1 diabetes mellitus in Iranian population. *Mol. Biol. Rep.* **2012**, *39*, 831–837. [CrossRef] [PubMed]

34. Shimada, A.; Kanazawa, Y.; Motohashi, Y.; Yamada, S.; Maruyama, T.; Ikegami, H.; Awata, T.; Kawasaki, E.; Kobayashi, T.; Nakanishi, K.; et al. Evidence for association between vitamin D receptor bsmi polymorphism and type 1 diabetes in Japanese. *J. Autoimmun.* **2008**, *30*, 207–211. [CrossRef] [PubMed]
35. Ozaki, Y.; Nomura, S.; Nagahama, M.; Yoshimura, C.; Kagawa, H.; Fukuhara, S. Vitamin-D receptor genotype and renal disorder in Japanese patients with systemic lupus erythematosus. *Nephron* **2000**, *85*, 86–91. [CrossRef] [PubMed]
36. Huang, C.M.; Wu, M.C.; Wu, J.Y.; Tsai, F.J. Association of vitamin D receptor gene bsmi polymorphisms in Chinese patients with systemic lupus erythematosus. *Lupus* **2002**, *11*, 31–34. [CrossRef]
37. Zhang, J.Z.; Wang, M.; Ding, Y.; Gao, F.; Feng, Y.Y.; Yakeya, B.; Wang, P.; Wu, X.J.; Hu, F.X.; Xian, J.; et al. Vitamin D receptor gene polymorphism, serum 25-hydroxyvitamin D levels, and risk of vitiligo: A meta-analysis. *Medicine* **2018**, *97*, e11506. [CrossRef]
38. Wang, X.; Cheng, W.; Ma, Y.; Zhu, J. Vitamin D receptor gene FokI but not TaqI, ApaI, BsmI polymorphism is associated with hashimoto's thyroiditis: A meta-analysis. *Sci. Rep.* **2017**, *7*, 1–11. [CrossRef]
39. Kempińska-Podhorecka, A.; Wunsch, E.; Jarowicz, T.; Raszeja-Wyszomirska, J.; Loniewska, B.; Kaczmarczyk, M.; Milkiewicz, M.; Milkiewicz, P. Vitamin D receptor polymorphisms predispose to primary biliary cirrhosis and severity of the disease in Polish population. *Gastroenterol. Res. Pract.* **2012**, *2012*, 8. [CrossRef]
40. Huet, P.M.; Deslauriers, J.; Tran, A.; Faucher, C.; Charbonneau, J. Impact of fatigue on the quality of life of patients with primary biliary cirrhosis. *Am. J. Gastroenterol.* **2000**, *95*, 760–767. [CrossRef]
41. Goldblatt, J.; Taylor, P.J.S.; Lipman, T.; Prince, M.I.; Baragiotta, A.; Bassendine, M.F.; James, O.F.W.; Jones, D.E.J. The true impact of fatigue in primary biliary cirrhosis: A population study. *Gastroenterology* **2002**, *122*, 1235–1241. [CrossRef]
42. Navasa, M.; Forns, X.; Sánchez, V.; Andreu, H.; Marcos, V.; Borràs, J.M.; Rimola, A.; Grande, L.; García-Valdecasas, J.C.; Granados, A.; et al. Quality of life, major medical complications and hospital service utilization in patients with primary biliary cirrhosis after liver transplantation. *J. Hepatol.* **1996**, *25*, 129–134. [CrossRef]
43. Younossi, Z.M.; Kiwi, M.L.; Boparai, N.; Price, L.L.; Guyatt, G. Cholestatic liver diseases and health-related quality of life. *Am. J. Gastroenterol.* **2000**, *95*, 497–502. [CrossRef] [PubMed]
44. Kotarska, K.; Wunsch, E.; Kempińska-Podhorodecka, A.; Raszeja-Wyszomirska, J.; Bogdanos, D.P.; Wójcicki, M.; Milkiewicz, P. Factors affecting health-related quality of life and physical activity after liver transplantation for autoimmune and nonautoimmune liver diseases: A prospective, single centre study. *J. Immunol. Res.* **2014**, *2014*, 9. [CrossRef] [PubMed]
45. Janik, M.K.; Wunsch, E.; Raszeja-Wyszomirska, J.; Krawczyk, M.; Milkiewicz, P. Depression: An overlooked villain in autoimmune hepatitis? *Hepatology* **2019**, *70*, 2232–2233. [CrossRef] [PubMed]
46. Milkiewicz, P.; Heathcote, E.J. Fatigue in chronic cholestasis. *Gut* **2004**, *53*, 475–477. [CrossRef]
47. Krawczyk, M.; Koźma, M.; Szymańska, A.; Leszko, K.; Przedniczek, M.; Mucha, K.; Foroncewicz, B.; Pączek, L.; Moszczuk, B.; Milkiewicz, P.; et al. Effects of liver transplantation on health-related quality of life in patients with primary biliary cholangitis. *Clin. Transplant.* **2018**, *32*, e13434. [CrossRef]
48. Raszeja-Wyszomirska, J.; Wunsch, E.; Krawczyk, M.; Rigopoulou, E.I.; Bogdanos, D.; Milkiewicz, P. Prospective evaluation of PBC-specific health-related quality of life questionnaires in patients with primary sclerosing cholangitis. *Liver Int.* **2015**, *35*, 1764–1771. [CrossRef]
49. Raszeja-Wyszomirska, J.; Wunsch, E.; Kempinska-Podhorodecka, A.; Smyk, D.S.; Bogdanos, D.P.; Milkiewicz, M.; Milkiewicz, P. TRAF1-C5 affects quality of life in patients with primary biliary cirrhosis. *Clin. Dev. Immunol.* **2013**, *2013*, 7. [CrossRef]
50. Schramm, C.; Wahl, I.; Weiler-Normann, C.; Voigt, K.; Wiegard, C.; Glaubke, C.; Brähler, E.; Löwe, B.; Lohse, A.W.; Rose, M. Health-related quality of life, depression, and anxiety in patients with autoimmune hepatitis. *J. Hepatol.* **2014**, *60*, 618–624. [CrossRef]

14

Association between Dietary Calcium Intake and Adiposity in Male Adolescents

Jaak Jürimäe [1,*], Evelin Mäestu [1], Eva Mengel [2], Liina Remmel [1], Priit Purge [1] and Vallo Tillmann [2,3]

1 Institute of Sport Sciences and Physiotherapy, University of Tartu, 51007 Tartu, Estonia
2 Children's Clinic of Tartu University Hospital, 50406 Tartu, Estonia
3 Institute of Clinical Medicine, University of Tartu, 50406 Tartu, Estonia
* Correspondence: jaak.jurimae@ut.ee

Abstract: The aim was to investigate the possible association of dietary calcium intake with adiposity, insulin resistance, and adipocytokine values in adolescent boys. In this cross-sectional study, participants were 123 adolescent boys aged 13–15 years, who were divided into tertiles according to their dietary calcium intake. Dietary calcium intake was assessed using three 24 h dietary recalls. In addition, energy intake, body composition, physical activity (PA), and blood biochemical values were also measured. Mean body fat%, fat mass (FM), trunk FM, trunk fat%, and leptin differed between high and low tertiles of calcium intake after adjustment for age, pubertal stage, and PA. For the entire cohort, mean calcium intake was 786 ± 380 mg/day and was related to body mass index (BMI), FM, and trunk fat% but not to insulin resistance or adipocytokine values after adjusting for possible confounders. In addition, only 15.4% of the participants obtained or exceeded their mean dietary calcium intake requirements. These subjects who met their dietary calcium intake had significantly lower body fat% in comparison with subjects not meeting their dietary calcium intake. Odds ratio of being in the highest tertile of FM, trunk FM, and trunk fat% was 3.2–4.4 (95% confidence interval 1.19–12.47; $p < 0.05$) times higher for boys in low calcium intake tertile, compared to those boys in high calcium intake tertile. In conclusion, dietary calcium intake is inversely associated with total body and abdominal adiposity values in a specific group of healthy male adolescents with different body mass values.

Keywords: dietary calcium intake; adolescent boys; adiposity; percentage of body fat; insulin resistance; adipocytokines

---

1. Introduction

Obesity during childhood has become a major health issue that can lead to several chronic diseases and health problems later in life [1]. While some plateauing or decline in the prevalence of obesity has been observed in younger children [2], it is not the case in adolescents [1]. Childhood obesity appears to be the most common cause of insulin resistance in children and adolescents [3], and has been associated with type 2 diabetes mellitus, dyslipidemia, atherosclerosis, and coronary artery diseases [4] as well as with increased morbidity and mortality in later adulthood [5]. Adolescence is recognized as a critical period for the development of obesity [6]. Accordingly, it is important to identify modifiable risk factors during adolescence to prevent lifelong diseases related to obesity.

These modifiable risk factors include dietary habits, as dietary intervention is an important aspect in the treatment of obesity [7]. While it is commonly accepted that various combinations of macronutrients are able to regulate body mass, there is a need to further explore the effects of different micronutrients on body adiposity values [3,7,8]. Among different micronutrients, calcium and vitamin D intake may influence obesity and other health characteristics [9]. Studies with adults have reported inverse associations of calcium intake with body mass index (BMI) [10], body fat% [9], body fat mass (FM) [11], waist circumference [12], insulin resistance [13], and systemic inflammation [14] values. However, only few investigations have examined the association between dietary calcium intake and body adiposity values in children and adolescents with conflicting results [7]. There are studies to suggest that daily calcium intake may play a role in the modulation of body fat during growth and maturation [15,16], while other investigations have not found a relationship between daily calcium intake and body adiposity values in children and adolescents [17,18].

The association between dietary calcium intake with adiposity, insulin resistance, and adipocytokine values during growth and maturation has not yet been clarified. Accordingly, the aim of the present study was to investigate the possible association of daily calcium intake with adiposity, insulin resistance, and adipocytokine values in a specific group of healthy adolescent boys with a wide range of BMI values. It was hypothesized that adolescent boys with higher calcium intake would have lower body fat, insulin resistance, and adipocytokine values compared with adolescent boys with lower calcium intake values.

2. Material and Methods

2.1. Participants

The participants of the study were 123 pubertal boys aged between 13 and 15 years from different schools in Tartu, Estonia. The inclusion criteria for current study were that a boy had to be healthy and took part in obligatory physical education lessons at school. Participants were recruited as a part of larger longitudinal study. Boys using calcium supplementation were not included, nor were those taking any medications or having a clinical history of endocrine or metabolic problems, or cardiovascular, respiratory, or musculoskeletal diseases. All participants had their ordinary everyday diet. All procedures were approved by the Medical Ethics Committee of the University of Tartu, Estonia (Consent No 179/T-4, issue date 16.02.2009), and were explained to the boys and their parents who signed a consent form. Boys were divided in tertiles (low, medium, high) according to energy-adjusted calcium intake [16]. According to the previous study [19], where participants in the low calcium intake group ($n = 26$) compared with those in the high calcium intake group ($n = 31$) exhibited significantly higher values for BMI after adjustments for confounders, we should have had 50 participants per group to have a 0.80 chance (80% power) to detect the difference at 0.05 level of significance between the groups. In our study with 41 boys per group, we had 72% power to detect the difference of similar significance between the low calcium intake goup and high calcium intake group.

2.2. Maturity Assessment

Pubertal development was assessed by self-report using an illustrated questionnaire on pubertal stages according to Tanner [20]. Each boy was given line drawings, pictures, and descriptions representing genitalia and pubic hair development stages. The pubertal stage assessment according to the Tanner method, which uses the self-assessment of genitalia and pubic hair stage, has been previously validated [21] and used in our laboratory with previous studies with boys [22–25].

2.3. Anthropometry and Body Composition

Body mass and height were measured using calibrated medical digital scales (A&D Instruments, Abington, UK) and portable stadiometer (GMP anthropological instruments, Zurich, Switzerland) to the nearest 0.05 kg and 0.1 cm, respectively, with the participant wearing light clothing without shoes. Body mass index (BMI; kg/m^2) was calculated as body mass in kg divided by squared height in meters. Whole body fat percentage, fat mass (FM), fat free mass (FFM), trunk FM, and trunk fat percentage were measured by dual-energy X-ray absorptiometry (DXA) using the DPX-IQ densitometer (Lunar Corporation, Madison, WI, USA) equipped with proprietary software, version 3.6. During DXA measurements, subjects were scanned in a light clothing while lying flat on their backs with arms on their sides. The medium scan mode and the standard subject positioning was used for whole body measurements, which were analyzed using the extended analysis option. The DXA measurements and results were evaluated by the same examiner. The precision of measurement expressed as coefficient of variation (CV) was less than 2% for all measurements [25].

2.4. Dietary Intake

Dietary intake was assessed using the average of three 24-h dietary recalls, including two weekdays (i.e., Thursday and Friday) and one weekend day (Saturday). Participants were asked to record everything they ate and drank for these days, and cup and bowl sizes were provided to help estimate portion sizes. The same dietitian interviewed all participants face-to-face and asked probing questions about their diet recalls. The nutrition data were entered into Nutridata System for Research (National Institute for Health Development, Tallinn, Estonia) and were analyzed for total daily energy (kcal/day), calcium (mg/day), and vitamin D (μg/day) intakes [22]. To estimate the prevalence of nutrient intake below or above the recommendations, the intakes of calcium and vitamin D were compared with their estimated average requirement (EAR), which are 1100 mg/day and 10 μg/day, respectively, according to the Institute of Medicine [26]. Finally, to control for confounding and mitigate for extraneous variation, calcium intake was adjusted for energy intake and expressed as mg per 1000 kcal consumed (i.e., energy-adjusted calcium intake) as suggested previously [27].

2.5. Physical Activity

The Actigraph uniaxial physical activity monitor (model GT1M; ActiGraph, Pensacola, CA), USA) was used to measure physical activity (PA) level and pattern for seven consecutive days. Epoch length was set at 15 s, and data were expressed as counts per min [23,28]. All participants were asked to wear accelerometer on the right hip, allowing removal for sleeping, bathing, and swimming. Physical activity was included for further analyses, if the participant had accumulated a minimum of 10 h of activity data for at least two weekdays and one weekend day [23,28].

2.6. Blood Analysis

After an overnight fast, between 08:00 and 09:00, a 10 mL blood sample was collected from the antecubital vein with the participant in an upright position. Blood serum was separated and then frozen at −80 °C for further analysis. Leptin was determined by radioimmunoassay (RIA) (Mediagnost Reutlingen, Germany) with intra- and inter-assay CVs <5%, and the least detection limit was 0.01 ng/mL. Adiponectin was also determined with a commercially available RIA kit (Linco Research, St. Charles, MO; USA). The intra- and inter-assay CVs were <7%, and the least detection limit was 1 μg/mL. Insulin was analyzed using Immulite 2000 (DPC, Los Angeles, USA). The intra- and inter-assay CVs for insulin were 4.5% and 12.2% at an insulin concentration of 6.6 μIU/mL, respectively. Glucose was measured with a commercial kit (Boehringer, Mannheim, Germany). Insulin resistance index was calculated using homeostasis model assessment (HOMA-IR): Fasting insulin (μIU/mL) × fasting glucose (mmol/L)/22.5 [29].

2.7. Statistical Analysis

Data analysis was performed using SPSS 25.0 for Windows (Chicago, IL, USA). Descriptive data are presented as means and standard deviations (SD). Boys were divided in tertiles according to energy-adjusted calcium intake [16]. Differences between tertiles (Low, Medium, High) groups were assessed by ANOVA using Bonferroni method. In addition, differences between tertiles were assessed after adjustment for age, pubertal stage, and total PA using univariate analysis of covariance (ANCOVA). Spearman correlation and partial correlation (controlling for age, pubertal stage, and total PA) coefficients were conducted to describe relationships of energy-adjusted calcium intake with body composition, insulin resistance, and adipocytokine values. Differences between EAR of calcium and vitamin D intake were assessed by ANOVA. Regression analyses were used to examine the relationships between energy-adjusted calcium intake and body fatness components through two separate models, where body fatness components were inserted as dependent variables and energy-adjusted calcium intake as independent variable. Model 1 was unadjusted model, while Model 2 was adjusted for age, pubertal stage, and total PA to determine the independent association with energy-adjusted calcium intake. Logistic regression analysis was also used to describe the odds ratio (OR) (95% confidence interval (CI)) of being at the highest tertile of each body fatness components according to the energy-adjusted calcium intake tertiles. Significance was set at $p < 0.05$.

3. Results

The study population included 123 adolescent boys, including 4 boys at pubertal stage 2, 30 boys at pubertal stage 3, 55 boys at pubertal stage 4, and 34 boys at pubertal stage 5, with the mean age of 13.9 ± 0.6 years. The mean BMI was 21.6 ± 5.4 kg/m^2, with a range from 13.8 to 45.5 kg/m^2 including 71% normal weight and 29% overweight/obese boys. Participants presented mean energy intake of 1798 ± 535 kcal/day, and the range was 622 to 3300 kcal/day. The mean calcium intake for all adolescent boys ($n = 123$) was 786 ± 380 mg/day, with a large range from 123 to 2460 mg/day. Data indicated that only 15.4% ($n = 19$) of the participants obtained or exceeded their calcium intake EAR [26]. The mean vitamin D intake was 3.2 ± 4.3 µg/day and only 8.1% ($n = 10$) of the participants met the recommended vitamin D intake EAR [26]. Boys who met their calcium intake EAR ($n = 19$) had a mean vitamin D intake of 5.1 µg/day, energy intake was 2330 kcal/day, and body fat% was 18.1 ± 9.1%, while boys who did not meet their calcium intake EAR ($n = 104$) had a mean vitamin D intake of 2.8 µg/day, their energy intake was 1700 kcal/day, and body fat% was 24.0 ± 12.%. These values were significantly different ($p < 0.05$) from the corresponding values in those boys who met their calcium intake EAR.

Body composition, PA, dietary intake, and blood biochemical characteristics of the study population are presented in Table 1. When the study participants were grouped by energy-adjusted calcium intake tertiles, body mass, and body adiposity values were lower with increasing tertile of calcium intake. The participants in the high calcium intake tertile had significantly lower body mass, BMI, body fat%, FM, FFM, trunk FM, and trunk fat% than those in the low calcium intake group. In addition, body fat%, FM, FFM, trunk FM, and trunk fat% remained significantly different between the high and low calcium intake tertiles after adjustment for age, pubertal stage, and total PA. No significant differences between different calcium tertiles were seen in blood biochemical characteristics. However, after controlling for confounding factors, participants in the high calcium intake tertile had significantly lower leptin levels when compared with the boys at the low calcium intake tertile. In addition, no significant differences between the three studied groups were seen in energy intake and vitamin D intake values (Table 1).

Bivariate correlation analysis revealed that calcium intake was inversely related to BMI, FM, trunk FM, and trunk fat% values (Table 2). The correlations between calcium intake and BMI, FM, and trunk fat% remained significant after adjusting for age, pubertal stage, and total PA values. In addition, calcium intake was correlated with body mass and FFM values after controlling for these confounding factors. In contrast, calcium intake was not associated with leptin, adiponectin, or insulin resistance (glucose, insulin, HOMA-IR) values (Table 2). Linear regression analysis showed that in unadjusted model (Model 1), the energy-adjusted calcium intake was negatively associated with trunk FM ($\beta = -0.183$; $p = 0.043$) (Table 3). After adjustment for age, pubertal stage and total PA (Model 2), the association slightly increased ($\beta = -0.185$; $p = 0.042$). There were no associations between calcium intake and other body fatness parameters in Model 1 as well as in Model 2 ($p > 0.05$) (Table 3). In addition, the OR of being in the highest tertile of FM was 4.4 (95% CI 1.55–12.47; $p = 0.005$) times higher for participants with low calcium intake tertile compared to those with high calcium intake tertile (Table 4). Similarly, the OR of being highest tertile of trunk FM and trunk fat% was 3.2 (95% CI 1.19–8.35; $p = 0.021$) and 3.3 (95% CI 1.19–9.05; $p = 0.021$) times higher, respectively, in the participants with low calcium intake tertile, compared to those with high calcium intake tertile (Table 4).

Table 1. Mean (± SD) descriptive characteristics of the studied sample according to tertiles of energy-adjusted calcium intake.

Variable	Total ($n = 123$)	Low Ca Intake Tertile ($n = 41$)	Medium Ca Intake Tertile ($n = 41$)	High Ca Intake Tertile ($n = 41$)
Age (yrs)	13.9 ± 0.6	13.9 ± 0.6	13.8 ± 0.6	14.1 ± 0.6 #
Height (cm)	169.0 ± 8.6	170.7 ± 8.7	167.5 ± 8.4	168.9 ± 8.7
Body mass (kg)	62.5 ± 19.4	70.5 ± 24.1	58.7 ± 15.2 *	58.2 ± 15.4 *
BMI (kg/m^2)	21.6 ± 5.4	23.8 ± 6.5	20.7 ± 4.3 *	20.3 ± 4.4 *
Overweight/obese (n/%)	36/29.3	16/39.0	12/29.3	8/19.5
Body fat%	23.1 ± 11.7	26.6 ± 12.1	22.3 ± 11.4 †	20.3 ± 11.0 *†
FM (kg)	15.2 ± 12.3	19.8 ± 15.4	13.6 ± 9.4 *†	12.2 ± 10.0 *†
FFM (kg)	46.5 ± 10.0	49.8 ± 11.4	44.4 ± 8.6 *	45.3 ± 9.3 *†
Trunk FM (kg)	6.3 ± 5.6	8.5 ± 7.2	5.6 ± 4.3 *†	4.7 ± 4.4 *†
Trunk fat%	21.4 ± 12.1	25.3 ± 12.7	20.7 ± 11.7 †	18.1 ± 11.0 *†
Total PA (counts/min)	398 ± 161	397 ± 165	403 ± 145	393 ± 174
Energy intake (kcal/day)	1798 ± 535	1785 ± 543	1769 ± 561	1839 ± 512
Calcium intake (mg/day)	786 ± 380	515 ± 189	738 ± 240 *	1104 ± 408 *#
Calcium intake (mg/1000 kcal)	434 ± 146	287 ± 60	418 ± 40 *	597 ± 98 *#
Vitamin D intake (μg/day)	3.2 ± 4.3	2.7 ± 3.0	3.5 ± 5.4	3.5 ± 4.1
Leptin (ng/mL)	6.1 ± 8.6	8.1 ± 11.2	5.6 ± 7.5	4.6 ± 6.2 †
Adiponectin (μg/mL)	8.0 ± 4.4	7.5 ± 4.1	8.3 ± 4.3	8.3 ± 4.9
Glucose (mmol/L)	5.1 ± 0.4	5.1 ± 0.4	5.0 ± 0.4	5.1 ± 0.4
Insulin (μIU/mL)	14.2 ± 7.7	15.8 ± 8.5	12.7 ± 6.4	14.2 ± 7.9
HOMA-IR	3.2 ± 1.8	3.6 ± 1.9	2.9 ± 1.5	3.3 ± 1.9

* Significantly different from Low Ca intake tertile; $p < 0.05$; # Significantly different from Medium Ca intake tertile; $p < 0.05$; † Significantly different from Low Ca intake tertile after adjustment for age, pubertal stage, and total PA; $p < 0.05$.

Table 2. Correlation coefficients of energy-adjusted calcium intake with body composition and blood biochemical variables.

Variables	Bivariate Correlation	Partial Correlation Adjusted for Age, Pubertal Stage, and Total Physical Activity
Body mass (kg)	−0.157	−0.211 *
BMI (kg/m^2)	−0.192 *	−0.205 *
Body fat%	−0.167	−0.132
FM (kg)	−0.195 *	−0.190 *
FFM (kg)	−0.104	−0.194 *
Trunk FM (kg)	−0.188 *	−0.150
Trunk fat%	−0.189 *	−0.199 *
Leptin (ng/mL)	−0.111	−0.103
Adiponectin (μg/mL)	0.072	0.130
Glucose (mmol/L)	0.022	0.033
Insulin (μIU	−0.061	−0.059
HOMA-IR	−0.064	−0.053

* Statistically significant; $p < 0.05$.

Table 3. Linear regression coefficients examining the associations of energy-adjusted calcium intake with body fatness components.

	Calcium Intake				
	B ± SE	95% CI	R^2	β	*p* value
Model 1					
Body fat%	−0.01 ± 0.01	−0.03; 0.01	0.13	−0.128	0.157
FM	−14.60 ± 7.58	−29.61; 0.41	0.03	−0.172	0.056
Trunk FM	−7.10 ± 3.47	−13.97; −0.23	0.03	−0.183	0.043
Trunk fat%	−0.01 ± 0.01	−0.03; 0.003	0.02	−0.147	0.104
Model 2					
Body fat%	−0.01 ± 0.01	−0.03; 0.001	0.06	−0.125	0.168
FM	−14.70 ± 7.65	−29.84; 0.45	0.05	−0.174	0.057
Trunk FM	−7.20 ± 3.50	−14.13; −0.26	0.05	−0.185	0.042
Trunk fat%	−0.01 ± 0.01	−0.03; 0.003	0.05	−0.146	0.108

Model 1: Unadjusted model. Model 2: Adjusted for age, pubertal stage, and total PA. B—unstandardized coefficient. SE—standard error. CI—confidence interval. β—standardized coefficient.

Table 4. Odds ratios of highest tertile of body fat components versus other tertiles (medium+lower) of body fat components.

	Body Fat%			FM			Trunk FM			Trunk Fat%		
Ca tertiles	OR	95%CI	*p* value	OR	95%CI	*p* value	OR	95%CI	*p* value	OR	95%CI	*p* value
High	Ref			Ref			Ref			Ref		
Medium	0.92	0.36; 2.35	0.867	1.56	0.62; 3.93	0.342	1.97	0.78; 4.97	0.154	1.24	0.49; 3.12	1.24
Low	2.79	0.99; 7.83	0.051	4.39	1.55; 12.47	0.005	3.15	1.19; 8.35	0.021	3.29	1.19; 9.05	0.021

All models were adjusted for age, pubertal stage, and total PA.

4. Discussion

This study was aimed to investigate the possible associations between calcium intake with adiposity, insulin resistance, and adipocytokine values in a heterogeneous group of 123 male adolescents with different adiposity values. An independent inverse association of calcium intake with different adiposity, but not with insulin resistance and adipocytokine values was observed in adolescent boys. Individuals with higher calcium intake had lower body adiposity values. Furthermore, those boys who met their calcium intake EAR had lower body fat% in comparison with those who did not met their daily calcium intake EAR. Accordingly, it could be suggested that adequate calcium intake is needed to maintain lower body fat values in adolescent boys during pubertal growth and maturation.

Our results demonstrated that lower calcium intake was associated with higher total body adiposity values in adolescent boys in this important developmental age, which is a critical period for the development of obesity [6]. These results are in accordance with a recent study in a large European cohort of children and adolescents [16]. In that study, an inverse correlation of total calcium intake with different adiposity indices was consistently observed in boys but not in girls, and the prevalence of obesity decreased significantly across tertiles of calcium intake [16]. While relatively few investigations have studied the role of calcium intake in modulating adiposity in children and adolescents [16], most of them have supported a significant association between calcium intake and adiposity measures [3,15,16,30], similarly to our results. In contrast, other studies have not found this relationship in children and adolescents [17,18,31]. The relationship between calcium intake and body adiposity has also been evaluated longitudinally demonstrating that lower calcium intake at baseline was associated with an increase in adiposity indices over a six-year period in boys with a wide range of BMI values but not in girls [16]. Similarly, calcium intake was not related to two-year change in body fat in lean peripubertal girls [17]. In addition to possible gender differences, it has been suggested that a certain threshold for calcium intake and/or BMI may be needed to observe the relationship between calcium intake and total body adiposity values [13]. It has also been argued that the effects of calcium intake on body adiposity depend on higher percentage of body fat in children [7].

In accordance with this, the OR being in the highest tertile of FM in our study was more than four times higher for participants with low calcium intake compared to those with high calcium intake and more than three times higher being in the highest tertile of trunk FM or trunk fat%.

Inverse association of calcium intake with abdominal adiposity was also identified in the current investigation, which is in accordance with the results of other studies carried out with 8–9-year-old [32], 9–12-year-old [17], and 12–19-year-old [3] children with various BMI values as well as 7–18-year-old children and adolescents with obesity [33]. Interestingly, Barr [17] demonstrated that calcium intake below the median was independently associated with higher trunk fat% in 9–12-year-old girls. Similarly, calcium intake was negatively correlated with trunk fat% after controlling for potentially confounding variables in our study. It has been suggested that trunk fat may be preferentially affected by calcium intake [17,34], and abdominal adiposity is closely related to metabolic syndrome, type 2 diabetes mellitus, and cardiovascular diseases [3,4].

Another important finding of the present study was the inadequate calcium intake in majority of studied adolescents. It appeared that only 15.4% (n = 19) met their daily calcium intake EAR, similarly to the results of other studies in children and adolescents [3,32,35]. In fact, most studies have observed that more than 90% of studied children and adolescents do not meet the required daily calcium intake [3,32,35]. Therefore, calcium appears to be one of the micronutrients with the highest rate of inadequate consumption worldwide [36]. In our study, adolescent boys with adequate calcium intake had significantly lower body fat% in comparison with adolescents with inadequate daily calcium intake.The importance of adequate calcium intake in adolescent boys should be emphasized because about 45% of bone mineral accrual occurs during early adolescence [37]. This age and maturation period provides a limited window of opportunity for maximizing peak bone mass [38], which is a major determinant of fractures, a major public health problem in adults [6].

Different mechanisms have been proposed to explain the association between calcium intake and body adiposity. For example, it has been suggested that adequate calcium intake increases the oxidative capacity of adipose tissue [32]. Higher calcium intake is associated with reduced 1,25-vitamin D levels, which in turn induce intracellular calcium content to decrease in adipose tissue, stimulating lipolysis, and inhibiting lipogenesis in the adipocyte [39]. In contrast, low calcium intake is associated with high intracellular calcium concentrations, which may then increase the rate of lipogenesis and inhibit lipolysis, resulting in increased adiposity [39]. Furthermore, dietary calcium intake may influence fat metabolism by increased faecal fat excretion [40] and decreased hunger or increased satiety [41]. Anti-obesity mechanisms of vitamin D have also been suggested [16], with vitamin D interacting in a complex system of absorptive and endocrine functions [10]. However, it has to be considered that all these suggested mechanisms still lack confirmation in human longitudinal studies [16].

There was no association between daily calcium intake and measured adipocytokine values in adolescent boys with various adiposity values. Therefore, leptin is synthesized by adipocytes and is directly related to the amount of body fat [42]. While calcium intake was related to body FM in current study, it would have expected to also observe an association between calcium intake and leptin values, similarly to a study with premenopausal women [13]. The differences between the results of our study and that of da Silva Ferreira et al. [13] could be explained by different leptin levels in these studies, premenopausal women having considerably higher leptin and adiposity values compared to adolescent boys in the present study. However, leptin concentration was significantly lower in high calcium intake tertile compared with leptin value in low calcium intake tertile after controlling for energy intake, PA and maturation values in adolescent boys, which was also observed in premenopausal women [13]. Further studies are needed before any conclusion about possible association of daily calcium intake with leptin can be drawn.

The possible relationship of calcium intake and insulin resistance has not yet been fully clarified. Unlike previously reported investigations in adults [13,43,44] and adolescents [28], no association between calcium intake and HOMA-IR as an index of insulin resistance was seen in our specific group of adolescent boys with different adiposity values. While dos Santos et al. [30] found a significant inverse association between calcium intake and HOMA-IR among obese but not normal weight adolescents. In accordance with our results, a recent study reported no relationship between calcium intake and HOMA-IR in adult males, while calcium intake was related to HOMA-IR in adult females [43]. Accordingly, the reported association between calcium intake and insulin resistance that has been found in adults [13,43,44], should be further investigated in adolescents using a direct measure of insulin resistance.

There are some limitations in our study that should be considered. Firstly, this is a cross-sectional study, which limits our ability to make causal inferences. In addition, although the same dietitian interviewed all participants and reviewed their diet recalls with each participant, self-reported dietary intakes are subject to error as it depends on the memory of adolescents, and is susceptible to under- and over-reporting. Another potential limitation is that some significant associations would have not been detected due to slightly underpowered study, although the number of participants was similar to previous cross-sectional studies in this area [3,9,13,19]. The specific information about socioeconomic status and/or maternal/paternal overweight/obesity was also not collected. Finally, our findings are limited to a specific group of Caucasian male adolescents with specific age and maturation range, and wide range of total body adiposity values.

This study has also some strengths. Firstly, objective assessment of PA by accelerometry and body composition by DXA were used in this study. In addition, the present study is one of the few studies that has evaluated possible associations of calcium intake with adiposity, insulin resistance, and adipocytokines taking into account several confounders including pubertal maturation, energy intake, and PA. These findings help to understand the possible associations between calcium intake levels and adiposity values during growth and maturation.

5. Conclusions

Dietary calcium intake is inversely associated with total body and abdominal adiposity values in a specific group of healthy male adolescents with different body mass values. In contrast, no relationships of calcium intake with adipocytokine and insulin resistance values were observed. In addition, adolescents with adequate calcium intake had significantly lower body fat% in comparison with those adolescents with inadequate daily calcium intake. Odds ratio of being in the highest tertile of FM, trunk FM, or trunk fat% was more than three times higher for participants in low calcium intake tertile compared to those with high calcium intake tertile.

Author Contributions: Conceptualization, J.J., E.M. (Evelin Mäestu), E.M. (Eva Mengel), and V.T.; methodology, J.J. and V.T.; formal analysis, J.J. and E.M. (Evelin Mäestu); investigation E.M. (Evelin Mäestu), L.R., and P.P.; data curation, E.M. (Evelin Mäestu); writing—original draft preparation, J.J.; writing—review and editing, E.M. (Evelin Mäestu), E.M. (Eva Mengel), L.R., P.P., and V.T.; project administration, J.J.; funding acquisition, J.J. and V.T.

Abbreviations

BMI, body mass index; EAR, estimated average requirement; DXA, dual- energy X-ray absorptiometry; FM, fat mass; FFM, fat free mass; HOMA-IR, homeostasis model assessment of insulin resistance; OR, odds ratio; PA, physical activity.

References

1. Olds, T.; Maher, C.; Zumin, S.; Peneau, S.; Lioret, S.; Castetbon, K.; Bellisle, K.; de Wilde, J.; Hohepa, M.; Maddison, R.; et al. Evidence that the prevalence of childhood overweight is plateauing: Data from nine countries. *Int. J. Pediatr. Obes.* **2011**, *6*, 342–360. [CrossRef]
2. Chung, A.; Backholer, K.; Wong, E.; Palermo, C.; Keating, C.; Peeters, A. Trends in child and adolescent obesity prevalence in economically advanced countries according to socioeconomic position: A systematic review. *Obes. Rev.* **2016**, *17*, 276–295. [CrossRef] [PubMed]
3. Castro Burbano, J.; Fajardo Venegas, P.; Robles Rodriguez, J.; Pazmino Estevez, K. Relationship between dietary calcium intake and adiposity in female adolescents. *Endocrinol. Nutr.* **2016**, *63*, 58–63. [CrossRef] [PubMed]
4. Gupta, N.; Goel, K.; Shah, P.; Misra, A. Childhood obesity in developing countries: Epidemiology, determinants, and prevention. *Endocr. Rev.* **2012**, *33*, 48–70. [CrossRef] [PubMed]
5. Reilly, J.J.; Kelly, J. Long-term impact of overweight and obesity in childhood and adolescence on morbidity and premature mortality in adulthood: Systematic review. *Int. J. Obes.* **2011**, *35*, 891–898. [CrossRef] [PubMed]
6. Lappe, J.M.; McMahon, D.J.; Laughlin, A.; Hanson, C.; Desmangles, J.C.; Begley, M.; Schwartz, M. The effect of increasing dairy calcium intake of adolescent girls on changes in body fat and weight. *Am. J. Clin. Nutr.* **2017**, *105*, 1046–1053. [CrossRef]
7. da Cunha, K.A.; da Silva Magalhaes, E.I.; Rodrigues Loreiro, L.M.; da Rocha Sant'Ana, L.F.; Queiroz Ribeiro, A.; de Novaes, J.F. Calcium intake, serum vitamin D and obesity in children: Is there an association? *Rev. Paul. Pediatr.* **2015**, *33*, 222–229. [CrossRef]
8. Skrypnik, K.; Suliburska, J. Association between the gut microbiota and mineral metabolism. *J. Sci. Food Agric.* **2018**, *98*, 2449–2460. [CrossRef]
9. Tidwell, D.K.; Valliant, M.W. Higher amounts of body fat are associated with inadequate intakes of calcium and vitamin D in African American women. *Nutr. Res.* **2011**, *31*, 527–536. [CrossRef]
10. Eilat-Adar, S.; Xu, J.; Loria, C.; Mattil, C.; Goldbourt, U.; Howard, B.V.; Resnick, H.E. Dietary calcium is associated with body mass index and body fat in American Indians. *J. Nutr.* **2007**, *137*, 1955–1960. [CrossRef]
11. Jacqmain, M.; Doucet, E.; Despres, J.P.; Bouchard, C.; Tremblay, A. Calcium intake, body composition, and lipoprotein-lipid concentrations in adults. *Am. J. Clin. Nutr.* **2003**, *77*, 1448–1452. [CrossRef] [PubMed]
12. Sadeghi, O.; Keshteli, A.H.; Doostan, F.; Esmaillzadeh, A.; Adibi, P. Association between dairy consumption, dietary calcium intake and general and abdominal obesity among Iranian adults. *Diabetes Metab. Syndr. Clin. Res. Rev.* **2018**, *12*, 769–775. [CrossRef] [PubMed]
13. da Silva Ferreira, T.; Goncalves Torres, M.R.S.; Sanjuliani, A.F. Dietary calcium intake is associated with adiposity, metabolic profile, inflammatory state and blood pressure, but not with erythrocyte intracellular calcium and endothelial function in healthy pre-menopausal women. *Br. J. Nutr.* **2013**, *110*, 1079–1088. [CrossRef] [PubMed]
14. Zemel, M.B.; Sun, X. Dietary calcium and dairy products modulate oxidative and inflammatory stress in mice and humans. *J. Nutr.* **2008**, *138*, 1047–1052. [CrossRef] [PubMed]
15. Keast, D.R.; Hill Gallant, K.M.; Albertson, A.M.; Gugger, C.K.; Holschuh, N.M. Associations between yogurt, dairy, calcium, and vitamin D intake and obesity among U.S. children aged 8–18 years: NHANES, 2005–2008. *Nutrients* **2015**, *7*, 1577–1593. [CrossRef] [PubMed]
16. Nappo, A.; Sparano, S.; Intermann, T.; Kourides, Y.A.; Lissner, L.; Molnar, D.; Moreno, L.A.; Pala, V.; Sioen, I.; Veidebaum, T.; et al. Dietary calcium intake and adiposity in children and adolescents: Cross-sectional and longitudinal results from IDEFICS/I.Family cohort. *Nutr. Metab. Cardivasc. Dis.* **2019**, *29*, 440–449. [CrossRef] [PubMed]
17. Barr, S.I. Calcium and body fat in peripubertal girls: Cross-sectional and longitudinal observations. *Obesity* **2007**, *15*, 1302–1310. [CrossRef]
18. Phillips, S.M.; Bandini, L.G.; Cyr, H.; Colclough-Douglas, S.; Naumova, E.; Must, A. Dairy food consumption and body weight and fatness studied longitudinally over the adolescent period. *Int. J. Obes. Relat. Metab. Disord.* **2003**, *27*, 1106–1113. [CrossRef]

19. Torres, M.R.S.G.; da Silva Ferreira, T.; Carvalho, D.C.; Sanjuliani, A.F. Dietary calcium intake and its relationship with adiposity and metabolic profile in hypertensive patients. *Nutrition* **2011**, *27*, 666–671. [CrossRef]
20. Tanner, J.M. *Growth at Adolescence*, 2nd ed.; Blackwell Scientific Publications: Oxford, UK, 1962.
21. Leone, M.; Comtois, A.S. Validity and reliability of self-assessment of sexual maturity in elite adolescent athletes. *J. Sports Med. Phys. Fit.* **2007**, *47*, 361–365.
22. Jürimäe, J.; Lätt, E.; Mäestu, J.; Saar, M.; Purge, P.; Maasalu, K.; Jürimäe, T. Osteocalcin is inversely associated with adiposity and leptin in adolescent boys. *J. Pediatr. Endocr. Metab.* **2015**, *28*, 571–577. [CrossRef] [PubMed]
23. Lätt, E.; Mäestu, J.; Ortega, F.B.; Rääsk, T.; Jürimäe, T.; Jürimäe, J. Vigorous physical activity rather than sedentary behaviour predicts overweight and obesity in pubertal boys: A 2-year follow-up study. *Scand. J. Public Health* **2015**, *43*, 276–282. [CrossRef] [PubMed]
24. Utsal, L.; Tillmann, V.; Zilmer, M.; Mäestu, J.; Purge, P.; Jürimäe, J.; Saar, M.; Lätt, E.; Maasalu, K.; Jürimäe, T. Elevated serum IL-6, IL-8, MCP-1, CRP, and IFN-γ levels in 10- to 11-year-old boys with increased BMI. *Horm. Res. Pediatr.* **2012**, *78*, 31–39. [CrossRef] [PubMed]
25. Vaitkeviciute, D.; Lätt, E.; Mäestu, J.; Jürimäe, T.; Saar, M.; Purge, P.; Maasalu, K.; Jürimäe, J. Physical activity and bone mineral accrual in boys with different body composition parameters during puberty: A longitudinal study. *PLoS ONE* **2014**, *9*, e107759. [CrossRef] [PubMed]
26. Institute of Medicine. *Dietary Reference Intakes for Calcium and Vitamin D*; The National Academies Press: Washington, WA, USA, 2011.
27. Willett, W.C.; Howe, G.R.; Kushi, L.H. Adjustment for total energy intake in epidemiologic studies. *Am. J. Clin. Nutr.* **1997**, *65*, 1220S–1228S. [CrossRef] [PubMed]
28. Ivuškāns, A.; Mäestu, J.; Jürimäe, T.; Lätt, E.; Purge, P.; Saar, M.; Maasalu, K.; Jürimäe, J. Sedentary time has a negative influence on bone mineral parameters in peripubertal boys: A 1-year prospective study. *J. Bone Miner. Metab.* **2015**, *33*, 85–92. [CrossRef] [PubMed]
29. Wallace, T.M.; Levy, J.C.; Matthews, D.R. Use and abuse of HOMA modelling. *Diabetes Care* **2004**, *27*, 1487–1495. [CrossRef] [PubMed]
30. dos Santos, L.C.; de Padua Cintra, I.; Fisberg, M.; Martini, L.A. Calcium intake and its relationship with adiposity and insulin resistance in post-pubertal adolescents. *J. Hum. Nutr. Diet.* **2008**, *21*, 109–116. [CrossRef] [PubMed]
31. Wiley, A.S. Dairy and milk consumption and child growth: Is BMI involved? An analysis of NHANES 1999–2004. *Am. J. Hum. Biol.* **2010**, *22*, 517–525. [CrossRef]
32. Gomes Suhett, L.; Souza Silveira, K.; De Santis Filgueiras, M.; do Carmo Gouveia Peluzio, M.; Hermsdorff, H.H.M.; Farias de Novaes, J. Inverse association of calcium intake with abdominal adiposity and C-reactive protein in Brazilian children. *Public Health Nutr.* **2018**, *21*, 1912–1920. [CrossRef]
33. Czerwonogradzka, A.; Pyzak, B.; Majcher, A.; Rumińska, M.; Rymkiewicz-Kluczyńska, B.; Jeznach-Steinhagen, A. Assessment of dietary calcium intake on metabolic syndrome frequency in obese children and adolescents. *Pediatr. Endocrinol. Diabetes Metab.* **2008**, *14*, 231–235.
34. Zemel, M.B.; Richards, J.; Mathis, S.; Milstead, A.; Gebhardt, L.; Silva, E. Dairy augmentation of total and central fat loss in obese subjects. *Int. J. Obes.* **2005**, *29*, 391–397. [CrossRef] [PubMed]
35. Magalhaes, E.I.; Pessoa, M.C.; Franceschini, S.D.; Novaes, J.F. Dietary calcium intake is inversely associated with blood pressure in Brazilian children. *Int. J. Food Sci. Nutr.* **2017**, *68*, 331–338. [CrossRef] [PubMed]
36. Beal, T.; Massiot, E.; Arsenault, J.E.; Smith, M.R.; Hijmans, R.J. Global trends in dietary micronutrient supplies and estimated prevalence of inadequate intakes. *PLoS ONE* **2017**, *12*, e0175554. [CrossRef] [PubMed]
37. Bailey, D.A.; Martin, A.; McKay, H.; Whiting, S.; Mirwald, R. Calcium accretion in girls and boys during puberty: A longitudinal analysis. *J. Bone Miner. Res.* **2000**, *15*, 2245–2250. [CrossRef] [PubMed]
38. Jürimäe, J.; Gruodyte-Raciene, R.; Baxter-Jones, A.D.G. Effects of gymnastics activities on bone accrual during growth: A systematic review. *J. Sports Sci. Med.* **2018**, *17*, 245–258.
39. Zemel, M.B.; Miller, S.L. Dietary calcium and dairy modulation of adiposity and obesity risk. *Nutr. Rev.* **2004**, *62*, 125–131. [CrossRef]
40. Bendsen, N.T.; Hother, A.L.; Jensen, S.K.; Lorenzen, J.K.; Astrup, A. Effect of dairy calcium on fecal fat excretion: A randomized crossover trial. *Int. J. Obes.* **2008**, *32*, 1816–1824. [CrossRef]

41. Gilbert, J.A.; Joanisse, D.R.; Chaput, J.P.; Miegueu, P.; Cianflone, K.; Almeras, N.; Tremblay, A. Milk supplementation facilitates appetite control in obese women during weight loss: A randomised, single-blind, placebo-controlled trial. *Br. J. Nutr.* **2011**, *105*, 133–143. [CrossRef]
42. Jürimäe, J. Adipocytokine and ghrelin responses to acute exercise and sport training in children during growth and maturation. *Pediatr. Exerc. Sci.* **2014**, *26*, 392–403. [CrossRef]
43. Kim, J.H.; Lee, S.H.; Park, S.J.; Yeum, K.J.; Choi, B.; Joo, N.S. Dietary calcium intake may contribute to the HOMA-IR score in Korean females with vitamin D deficiency (2008–2012 Korea National Health and Nutrition Examination Survey). *J. Obes. Metab. Syndr.* **2017**, *26*, 274–280. [CrossRef] [PubMed]
44. Tremblay, A.; Gilbert, J. Milk products, insulin resistance syndrome and type 2 diabetes. *J. Am. Coll. Nutr.* **2009**, *28*, 91S–102S. [CrossRef] [PubMed]

Permissions

All chapters in this book were first published by MDPI; hereby published with permission under the Creative Commons Attribution License or equivalent. Every chapter published in this book has been scrutinized by our experts. Their significance has been extensively debated. The topics covered herein carry significant findings which will fuel the growth of the discipline. They may even be implemented as practical applications or may be referred to as a beginning point for another development.

The contributors of this book come from diverse backgrounds, making this book a truly international effort. This book will bring forth new frontiers with its revolutionizing research information and detailed analysis of the nascent developments around the world.

We would like to thank all the contributing authors for lending their expertise to make the book truly unique. They have played a crucial role in the development of this book. Without their invaluable contributions this book wouldn't have been possible. They have made vital efforts to compile up to date information on the varied aspects of this subject to make this book a valuable addition to the collection of many professionals and students.

This book was conceptualized with the vision of imparting up-to-date information and advanced data in this field. To ensure the same, a matchless editorial board was set up. Every individual on the board went through rigorous rounds of assessment to prove their worth. After which they invested a large part of their time researching and compiling the most relevant data for our readers.

The editorial board has been involved in producing this book since its inception. They have spent rigorous hours researching and exploring the diverse topics which have resulted in the successful publishing of this book. They have passed on their knowledge of decades through this book. To expedite this challenging task, the publisher supported the team at every step. A small team of assistant editors was also appointed to further simplify the editing procedure and attain best results for the readers.

Apart from the editorial board, the designing team has also invested a significant amount of their time in understanding the subject and creating the most relevant covers. They scrutinized every image to scout for the most suitable representation of the subject and create an appropriate cover for the book.

The publishing team has been an ardent support to the editorial, designing and production team. Their endless efforts to recruit the best for this project, has resulted in the accomplishment of this book. They are a veteran in the field of academics and their pool of knowledge is as vast as their experience in printing. Their expertise and guidance has proved useful at every step. Their uncompromising quality standards have made this book an exceptional effort. Their encouragement from time to time has been an inspiration for everyone.

The publisher and the editorial board hope that this book will prove to be a valuable piece of knowledge for researchers, students, practitioners and scholars across the globe.

List of Contributors

Patricio Solis-Urra
PROFITH "PROmoting FITness and Health through Physical Activity" Research Group, Department of Physical Education and Sport, Faculty of Sport Sciences, University of Granada, 18071 Granada, Spain
IRyS Research Group, School of Physical Education, Pontificia Universidad Católica de Valparaíso, Valparaiso 2374631, Chile

Carlos Cristi-Montero
IRyS Research Group, School of Physical Education, Pontificia Universidad Católica de Valparaíso, Valparaiso 2374631, Chile

Javier Romero-Parra
Departamento de Ciencias Farmacéuticas, Facultad de Ciencias, Universidad Católica del Norte, Avda. Angamos 0610, Antofagasta 1270709, Chile

Juan Pablo Zavala-Crichton
Faculty of Education and Social Sciences, Universidad Andrés Bello, Viña del Mar 2531015, Chile

Maria Jose Saez-Lara
Department of Biochemistry and Molecular Biology I, School of Sciences, University of Granada, 18071 Granada
Institute of Nutrition and Food Technology "José Mataix", Center of Biomedical Research, University of Granada, Avda. del Conocimiento s/n. Armilla, 18016 Granada, Spain

Julio Plaza-Diaz
Institute of Nutrition and Food Technology "José Mataix", Center of Biomedical Research, University of Granada, Avda. del Conocimiento s/n. Armilla, 18016 Granada, Spain
Department of Biochemistry and Molecular Biology II, School of Pharmacy, University of Granada, 18071 Granada, Spain
Instituto de Investigación Biosanitaria IBS.GRANADA, Complejo Hospitalario Universitario de Granada, 18014 Granada, Spain

Agnieszka Jankowska and Agnieszka Szlagatys-Sidorkiewicz
Department of Paediatrics, Gastroenterology, Allergology and Paediatric Nutrition, Medical University of Gdańsk, 80-803 Gdańsk, Poland

Magdalena Słomińska-Frączek
Department of Paediatrics, Copernicus Medical Center, 80-462 Gdańsk, Poland

Michał Brzeziński
Department of Paediatrics, Gastroenterology, Allergology and Paediatric Nutrition, Medical University of Gdańsk, 80-803 Gdańsk, Poland
Department of Public Health and Social Medicine, Medical University of Gdansk, 80-210 Gdańsk, Poland

Paulina Metelska
Department of Public Health and Social Medicine, Medical University of Gdansk, 80-210 Gdańsk, Poland
"6-10-14 for Health"-University Clinical Center, 80-952 Gdańsk, Poland

Piotr Wiśniewski
Department of Endocrinology and Internal Medicine, Medical University of Gdansk, 80-952 Gdańsk, Poland

Piotr Socha
Department of Gastroenterology, Hepatology and Feeding Disorders, The Children's Memorial Health Institute, 04-730 Warszawa, Poland

Tae-Kang Kim, Zorica Janjetovic and Hui Xu
Department of Dermatology, University of Alabama at Birmingham, Birmingham, AL 35294, USA

Andrzej T. Slominski
Department of Dermatology, University of Alabama at Birmingham, Birmingham, AL 35294, USA
Comprehensive Cancer Center, Cancer Chemoprevention Program, University of Alabama at Birmingham, Birmingham, AL 35294, USA
Veteran Administration Medical Center, Birmingham, AL 35294, USA

Anna A. Brożyna
Department of Medical Biology, Faculty of Biology and Environment Protection, Nicolaus Copernicus University, 87-100 Toruń, Poland
Department of Tumor Pathology and Pathomorphology, Oncology Centre-Prof. Franciszek Łukaszczyk Memorial Hospital, 85-796 Bydgoszcz, Poland

Michal A. Żmijewski
Department of Histology, Medical University of Gdańsk, 80-211 Gdańsk, Poland

Thomas R. Sutter
Feinstone Center for Genomic Research, University of Memphis, Memphis, TN 38152, USA

Robert C. Tuckey
School of Molecular Sciences, The University of Western Australia, Perth, WA 6009, Australia

Anton M. Jetten
Immunity, Inflammation and Disease Laboratory/Cell Biology Group, National Institute of Environmental Health Sciences, NIH, Research Triangle Park, NC 27709, USA

David K. Crossman
Howell and Elizabeth Heflin Center for Human Genetics, Genomic Core Facility, University of Alabama at Birmingham, Birmingham, AL 35294, USA

Mirela Ibrahimovic and Alison M. Mondul
The Rogel Cancer Center, University of Michigan, Ann Arbor, MI 48109, USA
Department of Epidemiology, School of Public Health, University of Michigan, Ann Arbor, MI 48109, USA

Elizabeth Franzmann
Sylvester Comprehensive Cancer Center, University of Miami School of Medicine, Miami, FL 33136, USA
Department of Otolaryngology, University of Miami School of Medicine, Miami, FL 33136, USA

Laura A. Kresty, Katherine M. Weh and Connor Howard
The Rogel Cancer Center, University of Michigan, Ann Arbor, MI 48109, USA
Department of Surgery, Thoracic Surgery Section, University of Michigan, Ann Arbor, MI 48109, USA

Jennifer J. Hu and W. Jarrard Goodwin
Sylvester Comprehensive Cancer Center, University of Miami School of Medicine, Miami, FL 33136, USA
Department of Public Health Sciences, University of Miami School of Medicine, Miami, FL 33136, USA

Vito Francic, Verena Theiler-Schwetz, Christian Trummer, Marlene Pandis, Valentin Borzan, Martin R. Grübler, Stefan Pilz and Barbara Obermayer-Pietsch
Division of Endocrinology and Diabetology, Endocrinology Lab Platform, Department of Internal Medicine, Medical University of Graz, 8036 Graz, Austria

Stan R. Ursem, Niek F. Dirks and Annemieke C. Heijboer
Department of Clinical Chemistry, Endocrine Laboratory, Amsterdam Gastroenterology & Metabolism, Vrije Universiteit Amsterdam and University of Amsterdam, Amsterdam UMC, 1105 Amsterdam, The Netherlands

Martin H. Keppel
Department of Laboratory Medicine, Paracelsus Medical University Salzburg, 5020 Salzburg, Austria

Nicolas D. Verheyen
Division of Cardiology, Department of Internal Medicine, Medical University of Graz, 8036 Graz, Austria

Winfried März
Synlab Academy, Synlab Holding Germany GmbH, 68163 Mannheim, Germany

Andreas Tomaschitz
Health Center Trofaiach-Gössgrabenstrasse, 8739 Trofaiach, Austria

Jae Hoon Jung and Sook Hyun Park
Department of Pediatrics, School of Medicine, Kyunpook National University, Daegu 41404, Korea
Division of Neonatology, Kyunpook National University Chilgok Hospital, Daegu 41404, Korea

Soriah M. Harvey, Vanessa E. Murphy and Megan E. Jensen
Priority Research Centre Grow Up Well, Hunter Medical Research Institute, School of Medicine and Public Health, University of Newcastle, Callaghan, NSW 2305, Australia

Peter G. Gibson
Priority Research Centre for Healthy Lungs, University of Newcastle and Hunter Medical Research Institute, Callaghan, NSW 2305, Australia
Department of Respiratory and Sleep Medicine, John Hunter Hospital, New Lambton Heights, NSW 2305, Australia

Michael Clarke
Metabolomics Australia, Centre for Microscopy, Characterisation and Analysis, The University of Western Australia, Perth, WA 6000, Australia
School of Molecular Sciences, The University of Western Australia, Perth, WA 6000, Australia

Rita Moretti, Maria Elisa Morelli and Paola Caruso
Neurology Clinic, Department of Medical, Surgical and Health Sciences, University of Trieste, Strada di Fiume, 447, 34149 Trieste, Italy

Rose Marino and Madhusmita Misra
Pediatric Endocrine Unit, Massachusetts General Hospital and Harvard Medical School, Boston, MA 02114, USA

Alejandro De-la-O, Lucas Jurado-Fasoli, Manuel J. Castillo and Ángel Gutierrez
EFFECTS 262 Research Group, Department of Physiology, Faculty of Medicine, University of Granada, 18071 Granada, Spain

Luis Gracia-Marco
PROFITH "PROmoting FITness and Health Through Physical Activity" Research Group, Sport and Health University Research Institute (iMUDS), Department of Physical Education and Sports, Faculty of Sport Sciences, University of Granada, 18071 Granada, Spain

Francisco J. Amaro-Gahete
EFFECTS 262 Research Group, Department of Physiology, Faculty of Medicine, University of Granada, 18071 Granada, Spain
PROFITH "PROmoting FITness and Health Through Physical Activity" Research Group, Sport and Health University Research Institute (iMUDS), Department of Physical Education and Sports, Faculty of Sport Sciences, University of Granada, 18071 Granada, Spain

Nurul Nadiah Shahudin
Faculty of Sports Sciences & Recreation, Universiti Teknologi MARA (UiTM) Cawangan Pahang (Kampus Jengka), Pahang 26400, Malaysia
Centre for Community Health Studies (ReaCH), Faculty of Health Sciences, Universiti Kebangsaan Malaysia, Kuala Lumpur 50300, Malaysia

Mohd Jamil Sameeha and Nor Aini Jamil
Centre for Community Health Studies (ReaCH), Faculty of Health Sciences, Universiti Kebangsaan Malaysia, Kuala Lumpur 50300, Malaysia

Arimi Fitri Mat Ludin and Zahara Abdul Manaf
Centre for Healthy Ageing andWellness (H-CARE), Faculty of Health Sciences, Universiti Kebangsaan Malaysia, Kuala Lumpur 50300, Malaysia

Kok-Yong Chin
Department of Pharmacology, Faculty of Medicine, Universiti Kebangsaan Malaysia, Cheras 56000, Malaysia

Ewa Podgorska, Agnieszka Drzal, Martyna Elas and Krystyna Urbanska
Faculty of Biochemistry, Biophysics and Biotechnology, Jagiellonian University, Gronostajowa 7 Street, Krakow 30-387, Poland

Zenon Matuszak
Department of Medical Physics and Biophysics, Faculty of Physics and Applied Computer Science, AGH University of Science and Technology, al. A. Mickiewicza 30, Krakow 30-059, Poland

Jan Swakon
Polish Academy of Sciences, Institute of Nuclear Physics, Krakow 31-342, Poland

Andrzej Slominski
Department of Dermatology, Comprehensive Cancer Center Cancer Chemoprevention Program, University of Alabama at Birmingham, Birmingham, AL 35294, USA

Agnieszka Kempinska-Podhorodecka, Monika Adamowicz, Mateusz Chmielarz and Malgorzata Milkiewicz
Department of Medical Biology, Pomeranian Medical University, 70-111 Szczecin, Poland

Maciej K. Janik
Liver and Internal Medicine Unit, Medical University of Warsaw, 02-097 Warsaw, Poland

Piotr Milkiewicz
Liver and Internal Medicine Unit, Medical University of Warsaw, 02-097 Warsaw, Poland
Translational Medicine Group, Pomeranian Medical University, 70-111 Szczecin, Poland

Jaak Jürimäe, Evelin Mäestu, Liina Remmel and Priit Purge
Institute of Sport Sciences and Physiotherapy, University of Tartu, 51007 Tartu, Estonia

Eva Mengel
Children's Clinic of Tartu University Hospital, 50406 Tartu, Estonia

Vallo Tillmann
Children's Clinic of Tartu University Hospital, 50406 Tartu, Estonia
Institute of Clinical Medicine, University of Tartu, 50406 Tartu, Estonia

Index

www.ingramcontent.com/pod-product-compliance
Lightning Source LLC
LaVergne TN
LVHW060544210926
848485LV00005B/1259
9781639275649